'Fox has achieved something rema[...]
her as one does for a friend, but the[...]
touch of the Mitfords in her funny,[...]
I loved it'
Sarah Perry

'Generous, engaging and laugh-out-loud funny, Fox's
memoir is a reminder that the willingness to share experience, good, bad and sometimes bloody terrifying, is one of
the best parts of what makes us human'
Julie Myerson

'Part journal, part pitch-black comedy, this extraordinary
account of childhood abandonment and life-threatening
illness is also a painfully intelligent meditation on
vulnerability'
Rachel Cusk

'Life-enhancing... Original and wonderful'
Sunday Telegraph

'Fox is a brilliant storyteller and a beautiful writer'
Evening Standard

'Delightful and moving... Fox's writing brims with
joie de vivre'
Spectator

'An exceptionally involving memoir'
Observer

'[...] savage and
[...]liance'

5430000098588 6

GENEVIEVE FOX

Born in New York, Genevieve Fox lives in London where she works as a journalist and editor. *Milkshakes and Morphine* is her first book.

GENEVIEVE FOX

Milkshakes and Morphine

A Memoir of Love and Life

VINTAGE

For Richard, Reuben and Sebastian

1 3 5 7 9 10 8 6 4 2

Vintage
20 Vauxhall Bridge Road,
London SW1V 2SA

Vintage is part of the Penguin Random House group of
companies whose addresses can be found
at global.penguinrandomhouse.com

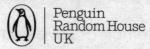

Copyright © Genevieve Fox 2018

Genevieve Fox has asserted her right to be identified as
the author of this Work in accordance with the Copyright,
Designs and Patents Act 1988

First published in Vintage in 2019
First published in hardback by Square Peg in 2018

penguin.co.uk/vintage

A CIP catalogue record for this book is available from the British Library

ISBN 9781784706692

Printed and bound in Great Britain by Clays Ltd, Elcograf S.p.A.

Penguin Random House is committed to a sustainable future
for our business, our readers and our planet. This book is made
from Forest Stewardship Council® certified paper.

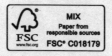

'So the darkness shall be the light, and the stillness the dancing'

from 'East Coker', *Four Quartets*,
T. S. Eliot

CONTENTS

1

THE INTERLOPER

It doesn't hurt, but I know it is there and I know it shouldn't be. Interloper. I have touched it a couple of times already, clocking the chutzpah of it: how, silently and without any warning, it has taken up residence, uninvited. Nasty.

It's nothing, I tell myself, getting ready for bed some ordinary November night. My hands, which are undoing my jeans, want to be up there, where the thing is. One hand breaks away, flies up to my face. The index finger zeroes in on my chin and traces a line across my neck from one side to the other, as if in mock execution. Halfway along, it meets the camber of the lump and stops, follows it over the top and down the other side. Whatever this is that has moved in is bigger than a pea, smaller than a Malteser, and as firm. Odd, I think, my mind having now caught up with my hand.

Richard is in bed, reading. I hurry over to him, tripping over two rolls of Christmas wrapping paper right in front of me. I am not usually nervy. Nerves have made me clumsy.

'Feel this.'

'What?'

I take his hand and place it on my neck, just to the right of my throat.

'Can't feel anything,' he says, his eyes still on his page.

He is doing that blokeish thing with his fingers, keeping them together like a paw. He pats half-heartedly. 'Nope.'

'Here.'

He pats some more. 'No. Probably your glands.'

I do occasionally get swollen glands; they have come and gone since I was a teenager. The medical term is lymphadenopathy, and it's the lymph nodes to the right of my trachea that have been the ones to play up. Spooky, I think later, maybe they were a sign of things to come. Until very recently, I did not know the word lymphadenopathy and I have not used the word trachea since school. I've never needed medical terms and always tried to ignore bodily functions. I am Gwyneth Paltrow's worst nightmare. I have never *listened* to my body, pampered it, fuelled it with moon food and unprocessed bounty. I don't wear Lycra in public, drink liquidised kale or shy away from sugar as from something diabolic. I do my thing; my body does its thing. A temple it has never been.

My science teacher at school, Barney, was one of my favourite teachers. I especially loved him for letting me and a friend blindfold him on a lab stool and spin him ferociously, just for the fun of it, but I could never stomach physiology. Even now, just thinking about blood vessels and arteries and metres of colonic tubing makes me queasy. House renovations have a similar effect; when an old building is being gutted, the beams and plumbing and wiring horribly exposed, I see entrails. And so, I've treated my body with the same disregard I do our old boiler: I've simply ignored any niggling malfunctions and pressed on.

Unusual, then, that my body is the first thing I think about the following morning. What is it doing, housing this furtive, insensate lump? Although I try to put it out of my mind, by the third morning I feel the calling of that merciless oracle, Google. If I check out my symptoms online, I will be able to put my mind at rest. Then again, doing so could have the opposite effect, and so I spend the rest of the day resisting its siren call. By nightfall, I capitulate. I take my laptop to bed, shutting the door before keying in 'lump in neck'. Down comes an avalanche of possibilities. Swollen glands. Cyst. Skin tag. A goitre. Salivary calculus. Tuberculosis. Thyroid cancer. With a tap of the 'Next' tab more and more unseemly possibilities descend. Snow-blind, I decide to pull out while I still can: I delete my search history, slam the laptop shut on my anxiety.

On the fourth morning, I decide Richard is right. The lump is a case of swollen glands, probably stress-related.

The trouble is, I am not stressed, unless one counts fretting over a house move and its renovation and having a puppy who uses the freshly laid oak floor as a litter tray. We did leave leafy Primrose Hill for urban Tufnell Park, so the move was traumatic, for sure. But I've got over it. More than got over it. In fact, I am a bit *Eat, Pray, Love*, which is my personal shorthand for a novel feeling of being tethered, spiritually. As opposed to physically, as if I were a goat, say. The eating and the love were already sorted. I love to eat, really love it. And, to misquote the poet Geoffrey Hill, I love my husband and my children … I celebrate the love-choir. It's the spiritual equanimity that's taken me by surprise; years of intermittent searching and questioning and very occasional prayer would appear to have amounted to something. Also, for a while now, I have wanted to delve inwards, to take the leap into silence and see what I can find there. Three months from now I'll be marooned inside my own head, unable to concentrate enough to read, write or even watch movies. Silence will feel like torture, and solitude – something else I often crave – its antechamber.

Five days since sensing the lump, I wake up to find it has had a growth spurt.

Richard is snoozing.

'Feel this.'

Once again, I place his fingertips on my neck.

'I can't feel anything.'

I take two of his fingers and place them on the little ball. It rolls beneath my skin. Take it out and you could play table football with it.

'Oh, yeah. It's just your glands. Don't worry.'

'Hmm.'

'Go and see the doctor, if you're worried.'

The first available appointment is ten days away, which is fine. I am in no hurry. If the ball has bounced elsewhere by then, I have the spots of dry skin on my face that I can mention instead. I have been meaning to have these sun-damage blemishes checked out for a while. I become a cyberchondriac in the meantime. I go back to Google and key in 'lump in neck' again. Various benign conditions come up, but I skirt over these; it's the killer diseases I am after and so, alone in cyberspace, I catastrophise myself to death. The cyst, the stone in the salivary gland and the random benign lump all get short shrift as I move inexorably to an oropharyngeal tumour, a tumour somewhere in my head and neck, non-Hodgkin lymphoma, Hodgkin lymphoma, thyroid cancer (again), salivary gland cancer, nasopharyngeal cancer, cancer of the larynx, throat cancer. The possibilities multiply and as they do so, one thing, at least, becomes clear: if the lump doesn't hurt, isn't tender, moves about and is getting bigger, then it needs to be looked at. If it has been there for more than four weeks, the GP should refer me immediately to a hospital specialist.

Three days after I make the GP appointment, I wake to find the lump sticking out under my chin like a bulge in a silk pocket. The skin around it is hot and red. I show Richard. No tapping or patting this time.

'Go to the doctor. Today. Get an emergency appointment.'

It is Wednesday, 27 November 2013.

'Hello, sur-ger-ee.' The receptionist's voice is part of motherhood for me; I have been taking my children to this practice since they were babies. Her defensive, disembodied voice has just enough lilt in it to make it human.

'I'd like to see a doctor today, please.'

'Sorry, we're fully booked.'

'Please.' My own brisk voice is gone. Something weepy and weak has taken its place.

'Is it an emergency?'

Thank goodness. She is not inured to a plaintive tone.

'Yes.'

'What's the problem?'

'I've got a lump in my neck and it's bright red and it's suddenly got huge.'

'Ten-thirty with Dr Whitley.'

'Thank you.'

An hour later I sit in the surgery and rehearse the symptoms in my mind as I wait for my name to flash up on the LED announcement strip above the reception desk. I've got a lump, it is growing, it doesn't hurt, it's firm to the touch and it moves around. It has been there four weeks, maybe more. Don't chicken out. Don't underplay the symptoms. Remember the statistics: 46 per cent of cancer patients are diagnosed late, reducing the chances of successful treatment. I think of my fellow journalist and late friend Ruth Picardie, who told a girlfriend and me about a lump in her breast during one of our late night powwows at Soho House and how she hadn't done anything about it. We made her promise to go to a doctor that week. She did, had a fine-needle biopsy and an ultrasound scan soon after, only to be advised by a breast surgeon that the lump was benign and did not need to be removed. After giving birth to twins, the lump came back, as big as a golf ball this time. An aggressive cancer was diagnosed and she died within a year, aged thirty-three, just shy of her twins' second birthday. I think of another colleague, the *Telegraph* journalist Cassandra Jardine, who kept coughing a few desks away from me, was persuaded to squeeze in a visit to the doctor between interviews and was given antibiotics for a persistent dry cough. It turned out to be adenocarcinoma, a cancer of the lining of the lungs. She died twenty-two months later, aged fifty-seven, leaving behind her five children, aged between thirteen and twenty-two, and her husband. Tell people you've got cancer, and many will list tales of survival. I know there are plenty out there; right now, I can't think of a single one.

My name comes up on the digital ticker tape. Genevieve Fox to Room 2. My usual GP is away. The man behind the desk looks about twenty-one. Does young mean he will be a box-ticking penny-pincher reluctant to refer patients to hospital specialists unless absolutely necessary? Or does it mean he is keen and conscientious? I take no chances. When he asks how long the lump has been there, I up the count to six weeks, no question. I explain its rate of growth, the fact that it doesn't hurt, the works. I get the urgent referral. I will be seen in two weeks, the legal limit. I've got this nailed, I think, as I walk out into the winter sun and get on my bike. *And all shall be well, and all shall be well. And all manner of thing shall be well.* Hang on a minute. What's St Julian of Norwich doing inside my head? I'm singing next, quietly at first, then so loudly the pigeons on Chalk Farm bridge take flight as I pelt out a medley of survival disco anthems. 'The only way is up'; 'All Right Now'; 'I've got all my life to live, I've got all my love to give, And I'll survive'. Steady, I think, all you've done is go to the doctor. I switch to 'It's Raining Men' instead. As portents go, there's none cheerier.

2

THE GIRL IN THE PHOTOGRAPH

Three shiny kids dressed in matching university sweatshirts stand in front of a pleated photographic studio curtain and smile at the camera. Their arms are hanging down by their sides. The boy, who is a head taller than the two girls, has black hair cut around his ears, strong cheekbones and straight, gleaming teeth. His smile is effortless. The bigger of the two girls, who is standing to his left, has personalised her outfit: she wears striped trousers, a pair of clip-on plastic earrings that hang off her little lobes, and there's a sheen of lipstick on her mouth. She is trying to look grown-up but the fullness of her smile gives her away. The smaller girl, whose fringe is cut sharp across her forehead, is clutching her plain trousers with one hand and grinning. Any second now the giggles she is holding back are going to burst right out of her.

The giggler is me, aged three. The clean-cut, chiselled boy is my older brother, eight, the girl with the earrings and the lipstick my five-year-old big sister. Our American father was a professor of law in New Jersey when this picture was taken, which explains the sweatshirts.

From time to time I put this real picture up on an imaginary moodboard alongside various snapshots from my early childhood in America, some real, most taken from memory since I only possess a handful of photographs from this period. I take a look, and consider whether I like what I see. If I don't, I swap the images around, or wait until I come up with some fresh ones – composite memories created out of snatched details I pick up here and there about my first years spent in New York, New Jersey and Connecticut back when we were a family.

I like my American moodboard. It is pretty upbeat. Ideal family. Two parents, three kids, a car, a cat. I don't have an actual photograph of the five of us together, but I can imagine the scene, and I do. I have got pictures of my parents, though, and they often look fancy, like they are about to go somewhere swanky. The woman, who either does an easy smile to camera or a self-conscious, cheeks-sucked-in pout, is sometimes wearing a long dress. At other times she is in a cocktail frock or a casual day dress with nipped-in waist. In one black and white photograph, which now sits in a frame on a shelf in my kitchen, she is in a train carriage, a fox stole around the neck of her dress coat, looking sultry. In another, she is sitting on a sofa, wearing a dark, ruched silk dress with a fresh rose on her lapel, the satin hem peeking out, and, beneath it, a hint of frilly petticoat is just visible. She's adorned herself in another fur stole and there's a funny white scalloped hat splodged on her head, which she is resting nonchalantly on one hand. She looks straight at the camera and pulls the same sultry face. When I look closely I can feel how soft her pale skin is and the cold of her wedding ring. The man matches her looks, dressing up in full white tie or a seersucker jacket and cotton trousers. At other times he wears jaunty short-sleeved shirts with bold graphic prints. His head is always slightly to one side and his lips are slightly parted, as though he has cracked a joke just before the camera shutter closed. The kids are similarly well turned out. The girls wear matching outfits for important occasions. In summer, they wear Peter Pan collar dresses emblazoned with hand-stitched tulips. On Easter Day they wear lemon coats and white gloves.

Two years after that university photograph was taken, we moved to England. There's a new moodboard to go with this life, my new UK life, though I don't like it half as much as I like my American moodboard. The snapshots on the UK moodboard are memories and a few real photographs from the first three years of our new life, the best photograph the only one of Mother with my sister and me. The picture was taken for the passport my sister and I travelled on when we flew to England, Mother all bouffant hair and a tidal wave of a white fur collar, and the two of us in matching, Blackwatch jackets. There is less glamour on this moodboard, and no group shots. The man – our father – is nowhere to be seen, the boy, eleven now, is rarely around. The woman – our mother – has swapped organza gowns for bright Seventies kaftans for the cocktail hour and slacks and polo necks for daywear. The girls still wear matching outfits, but only now and then. The look is different, though the colours are bright and hopeful. After that, there are memories, lots of them, and plenty of photographs of me growing up from the age of nine onwards. But they do not gel, at least not into something I want to pin up on the walls of my mind. They are better off stashed away in imaginary drawers, under beds, in old boxes.

The American moodboard continues to offer plenty to work with. I like everything on it, even the mundane stuff, the weird stuff, the stuff that suggests complications, the stuff where memories show up their true, mutable nature, changing what was into something different altogether. Here's a photograph of my sister standing up in her cot in our apartment in New York, holding on to the railing and crying, I think in protest at me, the intruder, her baby sister, born in Manhattan fourteen months after she was born in Hartford, Connecticut. Then there's a memory of me in a velvet dress, sitting on my father's lap as he does up the straps of my patent Mary Jane party shoes; another of Father standing over a frying pan as he makes toffee for breakfast. Toffee, for breakfast? It can't be true, but it's what I remember. I also remember walking to kindergarten, located on a different floor of our apartment block, and realising, halfway down the hall, that I have forgotten to put on any pants. Then, by way of reparation, I buy a packet of Rolos, or whatever the American equivalent is, from a vending machine and I find a boy at kindergarten to hide with me in a cupboard. We don't come out until we've worked our way through the whole tube. I remember, or think I remember, being remonstrated with, but gently so. The world was safe then. It had known parameters.

Before the kindergarten class went out to play we had to stand in a line. The teacher would tell us to zip up our lips and we would, pinching our index finger and thumb together and running them across our mouths. Once we were outside in the playground, we did the same thing in reverse, and all those words we had been holding in for ever were set free. One sunny day, I played on the swings. It must have been a weekend, or after kindergarten was over. My English aunt was watching over me. When my toes touched the skyline, high up where she could not get me, I sounded out the letters I had heard others say. F-U-C-K. My aunt, who had olive skin, black horse's hair and a potato nose covered in tiny holes, shouted up and told me to stop swearing. I swung my legs harder. She was my mother's fraternal twin – not identical, I was always quick to point out later, given her appearance, and more besides – but I wanted to get away from her, even then. There was something sticky about her. She had latched on to our family like a barnacle. Instinct told me to shake her off. Three decades later, I would still be trying to do so.

Mother brought us to England in 1969. Father did not come with us because he was dead. One minute he was with us, one of us, then he was gone and we were off on an aeroplane to England, where my maternal grandparents lived. Our Siamese cat, Cleopatra Boadicea, came with us. We moved into Marine Gate, a white art deco apartment complex that sat like a luxury cruise liner on the cliffs overlooking Brighton beach, and Mother enrolled my sister and me in a Catholic convent school. My UK moodboard starts here, with a photograph of my sister posing with her head to one side, her little white teeth glinting, one hand under her chin. I am next to her, the pair of us in our navy school blazers with black and white braided trimming, white shirts and black and white ties. In the first week a nun slapped me across the cheek for saying potato chips. I should have said crisps. Don't be impudent, she said. I was six years old and I didn't know what impudent meant but the slap knocked my American accent out of me soon enough. The nuns were easily offended. One nun made me stand in between the legs of the blackboard easel after my alarm clock, which had been lying in wait in my pencil case, went off in class. It made a nice change to stand in there, hidden between the slabs of black. But then the gusset of my favourite tights – black diamonds on a white background – started slipping down. The nun spotted me hitching it up. Unladylike, she snapped, ordering me to come out. Stand with your face against the wall. With pleasure. It was better than washing my mouth out with soap and water, which was what we had to do after we had said something bad.

I loved those nuns. Some of them were warm women beneath their icy blue wimples. Others gave their order, the Sisters of Charity, a bad name. Rumours abounded in the playground that one of the older nuns had thrown salt into the eyes of a boarder, aged five, who was crying because she was homesick. They did like things just so. We had to genuflect when we passed the grotto where the Virgin Mary stood, come rain or shine, on the way to chapel, and wear our skirts with modesty. The main nun, the Mother Superior, checked the gap between hem and kneecap with a tape measure. Two inches was the maximum allowed. The nuns ran a shop off a side room in the chapel. The bestseller was holy water, sold in small plastic bottles; the water had come all the way from Lourdes. One afternoon, when Mother came to collect me, I clung on to the waist of my favourite nun, protesting that I didn't want to go home. I didn't know it then, but I only had two years left of Mother. When I rewind to that scene, as I often do, even now, I see her getting out of her car and watch myself running to the nun instead of to her. I feel the squidginess of the nun's waist and my hands sinking into the small of her back. I cannot feel my mother, any part of her, nor can I see how I could have chosen the Catholic sister over my mother, even for a second.

The mother who drove us to school in the lemon left-hand drive she had shipped over from America was different to the one who picked us up. Morning Mother was a blur of big, messy hair and sleepiness. Sometimes, when we were running late for school, which felt like all of the time, she pulled up outside a bakery to buy something for our packed lunches. She came back with two white paper bags, one for me, one for my sister, containing a white roll, buttered, a thick layer of ham folded up inside, and a packet of crisps. The boys and girls who had school dinners ate Spam, lumpy mashed potato and salad cream. Another rumour went round that one girl, forced to eat her lunch, threw up over her plate, and was then forced to eat that too. We had milk in first break. Instead of being kept in a refrigerator, the quarter-bottles sat in crates on the edge of the playground. When we helped ourselves, peeling off the aluminium lids and dunking our straws, the milk was warm. It was how the English drank their milk, and it seemed barbarous. My sister and I loved milk so much, by the time we left America we had been nicknamed the Cats. Warm English milk was something we had to get used to, along with bright yellow butter spread thick on crusty white bread and candy sold in big glass jars that sat, out of reach, on shelves behind the shop counter. Before being put in small white paper bags the candy was weighed by ladies in aprons that were more like dresses with the sleeves cut off. Not candy. Sweets. Mother gave us 40p on Fridays to go to the sweetshop near the old gasworks and we would come back with a stash of Black Jacks, Bazookas, Refreshers, Tooty Frooties, Sherbet Dip Dabs, lemon bonbons and Flying Saucers. One day my sister and I took our secret society – code name the Bear Club, members: two (my sister and me) – on a field trip to the store. Armed with a mirror which we held in the palm of our hand at ground level, we looked up the skirts of customers. We did the same with the nuns in the playground.

Afternoon Mother was a Seventies dream in cowl-neck jumper, slacks and slick make-up. 'I have to put my face on,' she would say solemnly, and I would picture her, behind her closed bedroom door, fixing a scalped face on to her own. In between waking from her afternoon nap and picking us up, her overly plucked eyebrows had turned into brown crescent moons, her lipstick was on and her hair was backcombed into something puffy that curved back over itself, rolling away like the South Downs. She didn't wear a wig when she collected us, saving these for the cocktail hour at six. On a hot summer's day, Mother took us to Preston Park instead of going straight home and, if the sprinklers were on, my sister and I would take off our uniforms and dare each other to run under the spray and across the spongy wet grass in our pants. At the weekends I sometimes went off on my red scooter on my own, but usually I played with my sister. One day we rang Mother from a call box and when the pips went, we shoved in the twopence coins and, putting on a fake voice, told her that her daughters had been killed in a car accident. That's the only time I remember her being cross.

Mother displayed her three brown wigs on white polystyrene mannequin heads lined up on her dressing table. Sometimes, when she was out, I pretended to be her. I would put one of the wigs on, matching it with one of her fur coats and a pair of her wide-legged velvet trousers, ignoring the dummies watching me with their hollowed-out eyes. We all liked dressing up and I did so for my wedding to Sydney, my teddy bear, when I was seven. I wore my sister's hand-me-down First Holy Communion dress, the one I had worn for my own First Holy Communion a few months earlier. Grandma had made it out of white lace, and it had a high neck like a priest's collar and sat just above my knees. Sydney, who was the colour of Golden Nuggets and almost as tall as me, wore a pair of my knickers and a bow tie. Everybody came to the wedding except my brother, who had been swallowed up by something called boarding school soon after we came to England and never seemed to be around. Grandma, my aunt, my sister, Elsie our cleaner, Libra our Labrador, and of course the mother-of-the-bride all watched me walk down the aisle, which we had formed by moving around the living-room furniture to make a walkway.

I don't know what music we chose for the occasion, perhaps John Pertwee singing 'A fox went out on a chilly night' from my prize album, *Children's Favourites*, or something from *Fiddler on the Roof* or *Paint Your Wagon*. Mother loved those musicals and she played records all the time. She loved Maria Callas singing Schubert and Kathleen Ferrier singing Mahler, too. It's tragic, she would say, lowering the stylus on to the vinyl, and we knew what she meant. She had told us that this beautiful woman with the wavy hair and wide mouth had died, aged just forty-one. My mother sang at the Wigmore Hall just like Kathleen Ferrier, I would say later, not knowing a single thing about the Wigmore Hall. I was mimicking Grandma: My daughter sang at the

Wigmore Hall, she would say, or, My daughter studied singing at the Guildhall School of Music, to which a grown-up would respond with the *ooh* noises grown-ups make that capture something being both impressive and sad or of no interest at all. They could hardly say, so what? You can't disrespect those who mythologise their precious dead.

A few months after my mock marriage, Mother sent my sister and me to boarding school, too. Moira House School for Young Ladies was a red-brick building on a hill on the outskirts of Eastbourne, a seaside town forty minutes down the coast. Brighton had the Seven Sisters cliffs. Eastbourne had Beachy Head. There was no beach on the headland, just grass, and a long drop; it is a popular suicide spot. I don't know what Mother thought boarding school could offer over a real live mother at home. I was seven and the youngest boarder in the school. Later, I told people that Mother sent us to board because she knew she was dying; I presumed she was weaning us off her, getting us used to her absence. That's what I told people. Three decades later, I discovered she simply thought it was the done thing. Who knows how much else I've got wrong about her.

I went with a new green trunk with brass buckles, a flip lock and studs around the black edges. It was packed with everything on the clothes list: seven pairs of underpants, one pair of waist-high navy gym knickers made of old people's flannel with elasticated leg holes, one black leotard, one ankle-length evening dress (Christmas term only), two nightdresses, one bed jacket, one pair bed socks, one art smock (non-regulation), one pair pleated grey regulation woollen games shorts disguised as a skirt for hockey and netball, grey woollen V-neck sports sweater, two red Aertex shirts (winter term, white for summer), two pairs woollen knee-length grey socks; two pleated, belted navy smocks like the ones the St Trinian's girls wore, and five long-sleeved shirts of choice. Miscellaneous: one laundry bag, one blanket, one woollen scarf, one writing case. Shoes: one pair flat day shoes, brown or black, one pair formal shoes, one pair Dunlop Green Flash trainers, one pair black gym shoes, one pair hockey boots, one pair slippers. One hockey stick (winter term). One black regulation swimsuit.

The biggest item was a grey woollen hooded cape with red lining and straps on the inside that you criss-crossed and pulled around your waist and did up with a button. It must have been designed by a feminist: it had an inside pocket like men's jackets have. I used it for stashing Creme Eggs and slabs of toffee bought when, as one of the school's four Catholics, we made a candy dash after going to Mass in town on Sundays; the poor, arriviste Protestants, or Prodidogs as my Ireland-born Catholic grandmother referred to non left-footers, had to walk in crocodile straight back to school. I pitied them. The fact that they had a groovy vicar who delivered his sermons whilst cycling around on a bicycle only deepened the gulf between us. We had gone up to London on the Brighton Belle and bought the uniform in Harrods. Mother and Grandma sewed on the name tapes. Later, when other people bought me my clothes, I would remember Grandma saying of her daughter: Thelma always bought the best for the girls. All adoring mothers of course say the same thing about their daughters, but for me it was proof that Mother's love for us was particularly special.

I wore one of my new nightdresses on my first night. I had been put in a bedroom with three other girls on Blue Landing, where the youngest slept, and we had been instructed earlier in the day not to leave our 'dorm' to go to the 'loo' after 'Lights Out'. Caught short in the middle of the night, I spotted a bin, hitched up my crisp nightie and peed into it, the urgent liquid sounding out against the enamel. I slid the bin under my high-legged metal hospital bed. Not far enough. When one of the older girls rang the handbell on the landing outside our door at 7 a.m. the following morning, I swung my legs into the darkness and straight into the bin. It emptied across the lino and spread across the floor.

I had been a boarder for nearly a year when a letter arrived from Mother. There was nothing unusual about that. She was a good letter-writer and she wrote frequently, always in blue ink on blue headed paper. Three sentences in, she mentioned that she and Richard – Richard Williams, the man she had met at the golf club and who had sent her a bouquet of red roses the next day and had been visiting us for the last year, who drove a maroon Jaguar with silver spindled wheels, wore double-breasted suits and cravats, put pomade in his hair and bought us candy on Fridays – had got married. At least that's what she told me. 'But you still call Richard Richard,' she wrote and I thought: I get it, you're telling me that Richard is not our father. We are not to call him Father. That was a relief, because I thought then – and the side of me that has never let go of that picture on my American moodboard of us as the golden nuclear family still thinks – that Father could never be replaced, especially not by a man with a moustache.

Richard Williams was a Good Thing, although later, after everything ended, I never once told anybody about him, not even my best friend Louise, my accomplice in the blindfolding of our biology teacher. I struggled even to tell my own Richard, years later.

Richard Williams complicated my orphan narrative, which I would spend careful years reducing to something as brief and palatable as possible. His existence required more explanations and, as time went on, all I ever wanted was to get my orphan status out of the way and move the conversation on, away from what felt more and more like an embarrassing condition. It was easier to leave that whole chapter out. Besides, if people knew Mother had married again they might think that Father had not been perfect, which of course, to my mind, he was. Grandma and my aunt would later say that Mother marrying Richard Williams had been wrong, that he wasn't a patch on Father. Lyttleton Fox, they would tell those who hadn't even known

Father, knew JFK. At my aunt's funeral, her husband said in his eulogy that his dead wife's dead brother-in-law had known JFK. I think Father might have been at the same school as the American president or met him, once, or maybe even he just saw him in a crowd. I don't know and I don't care. It's Wigmore Hall syndrome all over again. Lyttleton was a gentleman, they would proclaim. Richard Williams was a Bad Man, they would mutter, he was a gold-digger. That sounded rather wonderful and like something from a fairy tale. But when they said he drank too much, I thought, that's an odd thing for my aunt to remark upon, considering.

I think I loved Richard Williams. He used to sit me on his knee when he drank his whisky and soda. One day he gave my brother the Japanese Rising Sun flag he had taken in 1945 as an acting captain in the Indian Army during the recapture of Burma in the Second World War. He was promoted to acting major, which didn't stop him acquiring a wooden propeller blade and a brass cylinder, both of which he also gave my brother. He often took us for spins in his Jaguar, which had leather seats and a pull-out drinks cabinet in the walnut dashboard. We drove to pubs in the countryside. Mother and Richard would go inside and my sister and I would sit on the back seat, sipping warm Coca-Cola through straws and eating crisps. Sometimes we all sat together at picnic tables in the pub garden and ate Chicken in a Basket. The novelty basket was made out of wicker and lined with a red napkin that matched the ketchup I oozed all over the chicken, which wasn't a whole chicken nestling in a basket as if to lay eggs, but one of its legs or wings. Chips were piled up on one side. At some point, the spins assumed a different purpose: they became house-hunting trips instead. One old house we saw overlooked a graveyard and Mother looked out of a top window and said, I don't want that view. In the end we moved to a house with a garden on one of those roads that say PRIVATE: RESIDENTS

ONLY, and have gravel lanes with miniature potholes and a golf course nearby. Libra the Labrador fitted right in.

The house, in a village called Ditchling, less than ten miles from Brighton, was the storybook kind. It was a rectangle with a roof like a gym skirt, a front door bang in the middle, lollipop trees either side and a big, round sun high in the sky. That's how it felt, at least. We were only in that house for one summer, maybe a bit longer. It was always hot. Too hot. There were glass doors on to the back garden, which had a bright green lawn that rolled out flat like a sheet of marzipan, and rose bushes either side, which Richard planted for Mother. It was the house of death. If there was a time when Mother was well when we lived in that house with its drive and its tended flower beds, I don't remember it.

That summer term I came back to it at weekends. I was a weekly boarder and Richard or Mother collected us every Friday night and drove us back on the Sunday evening. I would stand at the common room window, holding on to the bars that prevented us from falling out on to the curved drive below, and watch for the Jaguar to pull up. When I spotted the silver spokes, I would grab my white vinyl overnight case containing my teddy bear and knitted woollen rabbit, and run down the back stairs of the Victorian building, out of the side door past the kitchen bins, and down the tradesman's steep steps to the pavement.

One Friday evening I was holding on to the window bars, waiting for Mother or Richard to turn up to collect my sister and me. It was dusk. The day girls were long gone, the other weekly boarders had been collected hours earlier, and the full-time boarders had already gone down to supper. Punctuality wasn't Mother's strong point – I'm my mother's daughter on that front – but tonight felt different. The light was fading and the air was very still. Sometimes, when you are waiting for someone and the appointed hour has passed, you sense that your hope is spent and that the waiting will not end. Something like desolation sets in. It set in then. The housemistress eventually came and told me that Mother was not coming. She was not well and we were to stay at school that weekend. 'I am sorry, darling,' Mother said later, when we spoke on the telephone, not in the dank, graffitied call-box cubicle off Blue Landing where calls to the outside world were usually made, but in the housemistress's living quarters – a special privilege. Mother's voice was soft and sweeter than honey. There was such love in it. I told her it didn't matter, not a bit. But it did matter. I felt stranded, which was a new feeling. So was the realisation that I had the power to make a grown-up feel better by lying.

I was in alien territory from then on. It was as if, with that phone call, a pocket was created within the air that everybody else breathed and my sister and I slipped into it, unbeknownst to others. Mother's dying had begun. Everything shifted to accommodate it.

My sister and I quickly became a two-girl get-well industry. We made elaborate cards and presents. They were gestures of love, not heartfelt admonitions for recovery. Grandfather, our mother's father, had died the year after we moved to England. But it didn't occur to me that Mother would die, not for a single moment. No one told us she had breast cancer, or liver cancer. I've never been sure which she had, but have somehow settled on breast. Or maybe they did tell us. Either way, it would not, could not change things. She was love, and love wraps around you. It holds you as you bend into a harsh wind or stretch towards the sun. It does not disappear. That is not what love does.

Mother was sick and she would get better. She just needed to be looked after. Libra had been hit by a car and gone to animal hospital and recovered. I had lain under the desk, Father's desk that Mother had shipped over from America – I had lain under it with Libra, and made sure that she healed. I would do the same with Mother. Her recovery was just a matter of time.

My best gift was a miniature sickbed, fashioned from a packet of notelets which formed the mattress. Sitting on the living-room floor, the sun streaming in through the French doors, I made the sheet out of a Mansize tissue. I folded it down at the top, just like we were taught to do at school, taking care to do sharp hospital corners. I added a blanket cut from a square of felt and made a small pillow out of more tissue, folded up. We used to make figures out of pipe cleaners and clothes pegs back then. I don't remember squeezing a figure under the sheets. I only hope I didn't.

By this time Mother was upstairs in bed, under her own sheets. I remember the roses on the wallpaper that she said were driving her mad from the counting of them, the shiny chestnut bureau and my grandmother – and my aunt – flapping through the house. Richard Williams was there, too, of course, but it is the women I remember and their well-intentioned whispers. One night Mother walked from the bathroom to her bedroom and I overheard Grandma say to my aunt: 'She shouldn't have such hot baths. They'll kill her.' Oh good, I thought, if it is only a matter of skipping a hot bath, then there can't be that much to worry about.

I was happy for Grandma to be in the house, but I didn't like my aunt being there. She had a habit of swooping in on Mother's life, no matter where we lived, as if her own, liquor-fuelled life weren't enough to keep her in it. Her twin's illness legitimised her parasitical habits. As for her husband, a man who is repeatedly scratched out of any photographs, real or imaginary, he was mercifully absent. Before, back when he was still alive, Father had banned my aunt's husband – we never called him 'uncle' – from our home. I didn't know then what his offences had been, aside from repeatedly borrowing money, but his grey and white greasy hair, side-parted, the strands piled on top of each other, his nylon slacks and his temper alone marked him out as undesirable. Once, during a picnic in

America, he choked on a chicken bone and some Boy Scouts hung him upside down and cleared his airways. It was hard to forgive them for that.

The morning they came to tell us Mother was dead my sister and I were camping in a tent on the marzipan lawn. I knew she was dead when my aunt unzipped the door of the tent: it was an act of intimacy not ordinarily in her remit. Later that morning, she took us for a walk down the private gravel road. She extended her clammy hand and I knew I had to take it. Grandma took the other one. That was my first taste of my new state: being hostage to the whims of adults.

After Father was gone, there had been Mother. It had mattered, not having a father. It was awkward – different – and no child likes to be different, particularly if the nuns have marked your card and there are some boys in the playground who track you down for speaking in a weird way. I missed him, in a not-knowing-what-I-missed way. But my world was essentially still whole. Now Mother was gone too and it had a puncture in it. Out there, in the new world, there was nowhere to take cover. We were animals in flight.

3

D-DAY

The Interloper has a life of its own. It is doing well, for now, enjoying its moment of glory. But soon it will be history. I've had two lumps already, in my breast, and they sent me reeling, too, if only for a short while. The first appeared two months into breastfeeding Reuben. In the four days between finding the lump when we were on holiday in North Wales and seeing a consultant on Harley Street, paid for with an American Express card, I thought Mother's breast cancer had finally come for me. The lump was a milk cyst. So was the next one, which I found just before Bassy's first birthday. Life, birth, tissue mass, milk ducts, benign cysts. What is alarming invariably turns out to be routine cell tissue stuff.

The referral letter arrives. Please come to the UCLH Macmillan Cancer Centre, it says. No thanks. Not necessary. I haven't got cancer.

Macmillan. Coffee mornings. Cake sales. *I am doing a coffee morning for Macmillan because they were so marvellous when my mother was dying.* A friend said that to me only months earlier. I go and see my GP because the Interloper has got bigger and I want to see if she can have the Macmillan appointment brought forward.

Understandable, she says, but you've got nothing to worry about. I had a lump on the side of my face and it turned out to be benign. I want to believe her because I've known her for years and we have mutual friends and she has young children too, all of which makes her real and what she says believable. But I don't believe her. I have such a bad feeling about the Interloper. I ask her why it's the Macmillan *Cancer* Centre. That always worries patients, she says. It doesn't mean you've got cancer. It is just where you go.

Before the appointment, in the first week of December, my old friend Fliff drops round for breakfast. I've known her since I was sixteen, when I switched from my girls' school to Canford, then a boys-only boarding school in Dorset that took girls in the Sixth Form, 44 of them, in a school of 500 boys. When I walked into my first English lesson I saw a copy of Plato's *Republic* sticking out of a tweed jacket pocket belonging to a boy with foppish hair; the first time I walked towards chapel for the morning service a voice bellowed 'Hands!' as in, get them out of your pockets; a term later, three boys from my house turned me upside down and rammed me head first into a laundry basket of worn Y-fronts. The Plato boy – Billy – became my best friend, but the girls lived together, and stuck together. Since then, Fliff and I have talked about everything life can throw at you, from heartbreak and how she'd had the chance to twist Margaret Thatcher's head off when she did her make-up at Downing Street, to the Dutch thinking it's normal to buy sex toys for their teenage daughters. No topic is out of bounds. Until the Interloper. I can't bring myself to mention the fact I am off to the hospital later that morning to get it checked out. Instead we discuss how avocado on sourdough has become the breakfast rage, how Tufnell Park is full of litter, and whether she should ditch ceramics for midwifery. Then, just as she is leaving, I mention the lump. It's nothing, I say, just a stone in my salivary gland. Of course it is, she says, and I watch her eyes widen as she clocks my worry. Call me later, when it's all over, she says, and we'll have a laugh.

I get to the UCLH Macmillan Cancer Centre and wish she had come with me. I am seen by the consultant head and neck and reconstructive surgeon. His jawbone is as fine as her first jock of a boyfriend's, and he has olive skin and dark hair. This is a good omen: handsome and cancer don't go together.

Weeks later, I tell a friend that my Greek oncologist is a dish. Richard, who is with us, grimaces. How could I even notice the consultant's looks at a time like that? No time like the present, I might have said, but don't. The fact is, there is a disconnect between what I say and the tinnitus of fear in my head. I don't know how to explain any of this to him, how to articulate it. When, in the weeks to come, people ask me how I was told I had cancer, I include the initial consultation and throw in the handsome oncologist. They don't expect it and it makes them laugh, which gives all of us a reprieve. It also moves the camera away from me for a moment. I am a shameless extrovert, usually; now I abhor all the attention I am garnering. With cancer, you learn early to be careful what you say to people: you edit your thoughts, mindful that it is selfish to be relentlessly truthful.

Dr Dish looks down my throat.

'Can't see anything,' he says. 'You'll need an ultrasound.'

I could have told him he wouldn't be able to see anything just by looking down my throat. The GP tried that and couldn't get a good enough look either.

'Fine. When?'

'There's nothing til next week.'

'The GP said I would get an ultrasound today,' I whine. 'He said I would get an answer today.'

Maybe the GP didn't say that, but this is what I think he said, this is what I am expecting. Dr Dish says that if I take the form he gives me to the lady in the ultrasound department over in the main hospital, she may be able to fit me in the following day. But I am working at the *Guardian* the next day so ought to take the appointment next week. I stand on the street, undecided, before erring on the safe side. The ultrasound receptionist is friendly and helpful. She explains that the list is full but if I do come back tomorrow at twelve sharp she will bump my appointment request to the top of the radiographer's waiting list and, fingers crossed, if he has time, he will fit me in. She'll put in a word for me, she adds.

The next day I slip off for an early lunch and, breaking the habit of a lifetime, arrive on time. The receptionist remembers me, and as she takes my form, she winks. I take my place on a plastic chair in a grey holding pen off the main reception area. Most of the seats are occupied. Plastic bags and holdalls and handbags squat at people's feet. No one is reading anything. A few people check their phones. Most people just sit. This is all new to me; later, it will become normal, to wait amongst others also waiting, our eyebrows raised in readiness or lowered in denial, none of us reading or doing anything at all, an occasional exchange or announcement of a name breaking the sick, sad quiet. Today, though, I have my newspaper, which I hold up near my face so that no one will try to talk to me or catch my eye. I've been drinking water all morning, says the woman next to me. I'm dying to use the toilet. How revolting, I think, lowering the newspaper and turning to face her. But I can't, she says. I'm not allowed. I hate the word toilet. Mother told us never to use it; use lavatory, she said, or Ladies' Room. I smile at my neighbour and tilt my head to one side and I think, please don't talk to me any more.

An hour and a half later, my name is called. The radiographer is chatty. He asks what I do. I say I am a freelance newspaper journalist. A very good friend of his is an arts journalist, he says as he moves about amidst mystical machinery and unidentifiable objects on a metal trolley. He names the writer. Do I know him?

Yes, I say, I know his work, he's good. The conversation is confusing me. How can it be that this radiographer, who is also, dare I say it, rather dashing, can look and feel like someone I might well be friends with and who knows people like me who work out there in the real world? I have left my known world and dropped into his; I don't want them to be linked. I need there to be a separation; it will help me believe that all this is not real and will soon be over.

He puts gel on my neck and runs a metal gavel under my chin. We both look at the screen and I get a Pavlovian thrill. To me, ultrasounds mean looking at my unborn babies at the twelve-week and twenty-week scans. Then I remember I am not looking for a curled-up woodlouse of a foetus with an alien head and four dinky protrusions, but something small and round and unwanted.

'Aha, there's the culprit – a stone in your salivary gland.'

That's what he should have said. What he actually says is:

'It's not your salivary gland.' He says a few other things, too, but I am no longer listening. Then I hear him say: 'We'll need to do a biopsy.'

Biopsy away, I think. I had those with the breast lumps.

He produces a needle big enough to pierce a donkey's hide. His assistant anaesthetises the Interloper. I shut my eyes. In goes the needle, out it comes. He puts a small Band-Aid on the hole. Leave it on overnight, he says, to avoid infection. I peel it off on my way home. I don't want the boys to see it.

On the following Saturday I take Reuben to Denmark Street to buy him a bass guitar for his fifteenth birthday, which is on Christmas Eve. We drive and on the way I fight back tears. What if this is the last outing I make to buy him a birthday present? 'I won't be able to read them *Pippi Longstocking*,' Ruth Picardie wrote of her infant twins when she was dying from breast cancer, 'or kiss their innocent knees when they fall off their bikes.' I am lucky; I've had years of my boys, but I want more. In the store, Reuben sits on a stool and tries out a few instruments. His fair hair falls over his face. His long, alabaster fingers ply the strings. Normally I would walk around the store and keep out of his way. I keep close, unable to take my eyes off him. I take his picture with my phone. He grunts.

It is a tradition, coming to Denmark Street, just the two of us. We got his first half-size classical guitar here when he was eleven years old and we've bought a full-size guitar, two basses and two amps since. We've been into every store on the street. I stop myself devouring the sight of him as he chats to one of the Hendrix lookalikes and nonchalantly interject at the key moment to negotiate price. I go over my budget, of course I do, and throw in a hard case, too. We get lost getting back to the car and when we find it, we've got a parking ticket. I am only very slightly irked, which I see surprises Reuben, so I rant like I normally would. But my mind is on What If. It is the wire wrapped around the heart, tight, getting tighter, every now and then yanked a little tighter still, the wire cutting a little deeper. What if I only have months to live? Well, there is a last time for everything – a suddenly meaningful cliché. But *when* is the last time, and what is the form for dealing with it – with all the last times? Do we mark off each last, like Robinson Crusoe notching up the days on his wooden cross on his desert island? The last Christmas Eve. The last of my sons' birthdays shared altogether. The last Christmas Day with all of us together. The last stroking of Bassy's eyebrows. The last smell of Reuben's hair. The last love, unspoken, felt, defining, between Richard and myself.

It is diagnosis day: 20 December 2013. We take the tube to Warren Street. It's a five-minute walk to the UCLH Macmillan Cancer Centre. I am wearing one of my favourite dresses as we're entertaining later and I won't have time to change. The wind is messing up my hair, which I've pointedly taken the trouble to blow-dry. The appointment to get the results of the biopsy is at 2 p.m. We have to be out of there and home by 3 p.m., when Richard's mother is arriving from Liverpool. She's staying for Christmas. At 6 p.m. eighteen adults and children are coming over for Secret Santa. It is a tradition we've shared since our children were at nursery, primary and, some of them, even secondary school together. I've tried to make the party a few days earlier without acknowledging to myself why but, forty emails and dozens of texts later, this is the only day we can all make. I decide it is another good omen. The tree is rammed with baubles, and we've got heaps of food and drink and presents. It would be rude for anything to spoil the festivities. And, like I say, I've done my hair.

We have left the boys at home to await their grandmother's arrival and look after our schnauzer puppy. As we approach the Centre, built on the old site of the UCLH maternity hospital where both boys were born, I tell Richard that this is the one and only time we will walk down this street. We will go to the pub afterwards, he says, which is unusual for him, a decorous drinker. One quick drink and then we'll put all this behind us. Every cloud, I think, wondering whether to have a really good single malt whisky or a warming whisky mac.

We take the spiral stairs up to the first floor. When I was here two weeks ago to see Dr Dish (who, technically speaking, is my Mr Dish since he is a surgeon and surgeons do not, for reasons unknown to me, take the title of doctor) I clocked the Macmillan nurses in their navy, white-trimmed uniforms and their soft shoes. I watched one approach a seated couple she clearly knew already and stand in front of them, noted how they both craned their necks towards her as she spoke. One of them obviously had cancer; that's why they had a relationship with a Macmillan nurse.

I tell Richard not to come in with me, to increase my chances of not needing him.

'If anyone comes out to get you,' I say, 'you'll know it's bad news.'

We sit in companionable silence and wait.

'Genevieve Fox.'

My name is a statement; it gives away nothing. There is no lilt in the voice of the man who announces it. He is well trained in neutrality. Standing by the reception desk, he does not smile as his eyes scour the waiting area. I stand up, he nods, I follow him.

It is a short journey – no more than thirty paces – and I am conscious that it could lead me somewhere I have never been. Or spin me right back to where I started. The door to the consulting room, the same room in which I first met with Dr Dish, is open. This time, there are four people in the room. One man sitting, one man standing, one young woman standing by the window, and the Macmillan nurse I had seen talking to the couple minutes earlier. So. I have cancer. There are four people in the room. If I had been spared, only one person would be here to give me the results.

Desire, all I have ever wanted, want, might want, is reduced to a swiftly calculated, single compromise: let me not have only months to live. I accept the cancer, I accept it and will deal with it with as much grace and fortitude as I can muster, but on the condition that you give me at least six months.

Give me more and I will open myself to you. I promise.

Nobody moves. They are actors on a stage just as the curtain is raised. Wanting to turn back, I step inside the room. The tableau stirs; the seated doctor points to the chair opposite him.

'Please,' he says.

I sit down. He pulls his chair towards mine.

'How are you today, Genevieve?' His knees are less than a foot away from mine. He leans in towards me. This is bedside stuff.

'I'm fine.'

He leans in closer.

'How are you in yourself today?'

In myself.

Catatonic with dread. Petrified. Overwhelmed by a longing that I can feel under my ribs and in my stomach and in my legs to be anywhere but here.

'I'm fine, absolutely fine.'

The others have not moved.

'There is only one way to tell you this. The tumour is malignant.'

'Can someone get my husband, please?'

'Of course.'

There is a shuffle and the man who is standing leaves the room.

Into the lonely silence silent tears course, swelling the surprised riverbanks.

My skull is not fit for purpose; it cannot contain my brain and whatever else is in there. It is a seething, steaming, chthonic mass.

Richard walks into the room. His face has turned into silly putty. It is ashen and it droops. He sits on the chair that has been placed by my side and puts his hand on mine. A tear falls, love's messenger. *Head and neck cancer. Tumour. Scans. Tests. Find primary. Surgery. No surgery. Chemotherapy. Radiotherapy. Remove tumour. Shrink tumour. Your Macmillan nurse. Write to you. Wait. Find out. Make decisions. Meetings. Clinics. Christmas. New Year.*

'You seem very calm.'

'Well,' I say, and my voice tails off.

'Any questions?'

Am I going to die? If so, when? 'No. Thank you.'

I nod as the consultant speaks. When I think he has finished I nod some more to indicate that I have understood that we will get the prognosis in the New Year.

I take my hand away from Richard's and draw myself up tall. I am ready.

On leaving the consultant's room, I move planets. I am on Planet Cancer now. We see things differently here. Richard, who lives on Earth, goes up to a bottle of sanitiser affixed to the wall by the stairs and squeezes some disinfectant on to his hands. The sign next to the decontamination liquid reads: CLEAN HANDS SAVE LIVES. I watch, in disbelief, as he rubs them together. So, my husband thinks I am contagious. He is on the side of the well. I marvel at his lack of tact.

But then, out on the street, he takes my hand in his. That's twice in an hour. He only ever holds my hand on high days, holidays or under negotiated circumstances. Out walking the dog, I occasionally take his hand, simultaneously pointing out a tree twenty metres ahead of us. You only have to hold my hand til we get to that tree over there with the big leaves, I say. He fancies himself as an arborealist – we both do, though neither of us can identify even the commonest trees – but sometimes I can trick him when he unfurls his hand and say, oh no, I meant that tree with the jagged leaves, and get an extra metre or two out of him. Today his hand wraps around the whole of me. I make a guttural noise to keep down my river cry. There is no mention of the pub. We stand on Tottenham Court Road and he hails a taxi. It's normally fun to get into a black cab; it's a rescue in a rush, or a treat after a night out. Now, knowing what we know, it's a bullet and it's heading for our children. We've only just hit Hampstead Road when a woman telephones from the hospital. You need to come in on the 23rd of December and then again on the 24th and you must eat and drink or perhaps you must not eat and must not drink and I think, back off, two hours ago I didn't even have cancer and, by the way, the 24th is my son's birthday and I tear into my handbag for a piece of paper and a pen and try to write down something of what I think the firm, friendly stranger at the other end of the phone has been saying to me.

When we get home my mother-in-law's suitcase and a hotchpotch of bags are lined up in our hall. Knitting needles stick out of a tote bag. The gold rim of an Assorted Biscuits tin glints next to gifts wrapped in shiny Christmas paper. In another bag, the tip of her collapsible walking stick peeks out between a jar of Horlicks and a bunch of bananas. We call the boys down, and go into the living room. Margaret is embedded in the corner of the smaller sofa in the bay window, her velvet slippers already on, an empty mug and a plate on the side table. I see the golden crumbs and think: she's got started on her Rich Teas. Dave, the young family friend who has driven her down from Liverpool, perches on the other sofa, as if to say, I'm not stopping. He's neat in blue jeans and tucked-in polo shirt and white trainers bright as albino rabbits. *Hello Gen. Everything all right?* Margaret says as I lean in to kiss her. She kisses me back, lips on cheek. *The journey was fine. How long was it, Dave? Four hours, Margaret. Yes, that's right, four hours. We stopped, of course.* I think about how she used to move her head towards mine and merely kiss the air, and about what we've shared over the years. *We had our sandwiches. Our own, not service station sandwiches. It was quite quiet, really, wasn't it, Dave? It was, Margaret, yes.* The boys come in. I hug them. They hug their grandma. She asks them for their news and I watch them, hawk-mother now. And she turns to Dave. *You'll be wanting to get back, Dave. Dave has to get back. To the girls. And to Jenny. What time will you come for me next Saturday, Dave? We won't stop on the way. I know you'll want to get back. To the girls. And to Jenny. We'll be home by lunchtime. The girls love their dancing, don't they, Dave? They do, Margaret.* Dave says he'll get going and after he has left, Richard makes tea. Margaret wants to know who is coming for Secret Santa. She knows most of the children and their parents, too, and wants to hear how they all are. *Secret Santa, though. What a lot of work for you, Gen. All those people. You're not cooking for sixteen, are you? You do love your parties, Gen.* I slip upstairs and, bedroom door closed, yelp and heave. I grab a pillow and hold it over my face to block out the noises I am making, throw it off and, down in the bathroom, splash cold water on to my face. There must be no pauses. No gaps. No thinking until we've got through Christmas.

The boys carry their grandma's bags up to the spare room and we all go down to the kitchen in the basement. There's a bigger, L-shaped sofa there, and Margaret sets up camp. Her library book, a copy of *The Westmorland Gazette*, her knitting bag, the remote control, the fudge we have just given her and her glasses are laid out on the table beside her. Once she's on that sofa, she stays put. She isn't a mother-in-law who does. She is a mother-in-law who sits, charging the atmosphere with her low-key love. Her small navy handbag, bulging indecorously, sits at her feet like an overfed lapdog. Once, when we went on a day trip to Windsor Castle, she had to empty its contents in front of a security guard. Out it all came on the table: pills, glasses, sewing kit, nail scissors, tissues, wallet, key ring with photos of Richard and his brother Mark when they were little boys, and a super-size Mars Bar. Oh, I wouldn't dream of eating it, she told the guard, the colour rising in her powdered cheeks. It's for emergencies, you know.

I leave Margaret with the boys and go upstairs to clean the fire grate and lay a fire. A few coals remain, shrunken to peach stones, and ashes have fallen through the bars. I crouch down and as I make my first sweep with the dustpan brush the couplet *'Golden lads and girls all must, / As chimney sweepers come to dust'* sounds off in my head. The lines are famous, hackneyed even; as a schoolchild I learned the poem they come from, 'Fear no More' from Shakespeare's *Cymbeline*, off by heart, and we sang this hypnotic dirge in choir, too. Now, sweeping up the ashes, the jaunty couplet that ends the first stanza hurls itself right at me; winded, I drop the brush and sit back on my heels. *Come to dust*, these three words, repeated at the end of the two stanzas that follow, no longer seem to be there to create eerie echoes and emphasis. They mean something, and their meaning is clear: carbon is all I am, a living organism, tomorrow's ash.

The fire is burning its mortal coal as the children and adults form a makeshift circle on the living-room floor for Secret Santa. Butterflies are on the rampage inside me. Margaret has swapped sofas – she's back on the small sofa behind me in the bay window. Ten-year-old Maya has taken up position by the Christmas tree, her red Santa's hat and black boots lending her an officious air. The packages, kept anonymous in newspaper and tissue paper, are right by her feet – there is no chance of any sneaky prodding or squeezing. She booms out the rules of the game, which we dispute, even though we're playing it together for about the eighth time and know the rules, and we talk over her and then, one by one, we choose our numbers from Santa's hat and adults and children alike cheer or groan, depending on what number we have drawn, the higher the better. Then Maya starts pulling numbers out of the hat. Three! Twelve! Six! Six. No one claims it. Come on six! Your number's up, someone says, and I think, there's an idiom. And on Maya goes, until all the numbers are distributed.

After a Christmas tea, the children and teenagers disperse and we sit down to supper, which is when I do something I would never normally do. I clock our friends' jobs. Of the eight of us, three are medics. One is Caroline, Head of the Palliative Care Team at UCLH, married to Hans, Head of Immunology at the Royal Free and Director of the UCL Institute for Immunity & Transplantation, and the third is Paul, a consultant neurologist. A fourth has recently been seriously ill. I've inadvertently arranged a mini medics' convention. It's only now I find out quite how serious the sick friend's condition was and he tells me how hands-on and supportive Caroline and Hans have been. Supportive in what way? I hear myself asking him. Helpful by doing what? Calling how often? My inquisition is entirely selfish: I want to know what it means for friends to be supportive, what it is one even needs. Turning to Hans, I ask him how the research into immunotherapy is going. It is not unusual for me to ask him about his work – he is the mastermind behind the PEARS building, a brand new £55 million cancer research centre being built next to the Royal Free Hospital in Hampstead – but it is disconcerting to find myself one of his statistics; not that he knows as much. Our news may be hot off the press, but we have no intention of ruining anybody's Christmas by sharing it. It's our secret and we have not yet been alone with it in our house; the longer everyone stays, the longer we won't have to be. I want them to stay all night. I watch them, and listen to the clamour, see how engaged everyone is in conversation, life-lust lighting up the festive table. But they do leave, and we are left, and we fall, headlong, into the expanse of our unspeakable, new now. We don't sleep that night, or any night that follows. We look at each other often, hold each other, divide up last-minute shopping tasks. We don't look forward to anything, not even to Christmas Eve, because it is another day that takes us away from our known reality.

We get to Christmas Eve, and I wake early. I have another scan mid-morning. I dress like a bauble: black and gold sequinned pencil skirt, a silky top, a chainmail gold necklace and chunky black patent heels with a gold buckle.

'You're not going to the hospital like that, are you?' Richard says. 'You'll make the scanner short-circuit.'

Yesterday I had an MRI scan. Today I've got the PET scan the admissions clerk was calling about when we were in the taxi on D-Day. When it's over I'll hurry up to Lemonia, our favourite Greek restaurant in Primrose Hill, for Reuben's birthday lunch. He celebrated BC, or Before Cancer, with his friends, and we gave him the bass, but we give him a couple of extra presents, like we always do on the day itself, and then I say I've got to go out and both boys' foreheads zigzag. Where to? they ask, indignant. We always do family stuff on Christmas Eve. I mutter something about last-minute shopping.

It's not a complete lie. I've realised that if I do kick the bucket in the next six months or a year, I won't have left them a code of conduct or way of being. Having failed to tell them anything of value in this regard, they will need someone else's words to live by, so I'm making a quick dash to the bookshop near the hospital to buy them some poetry. It is a big ask of any poet but, since an emergency audit reveals me to be a mouse amongst men, a necessary one.

4

WORDS TO LIVE BY

The poetry section is upstairs at the back, as always, poetry the disagreeable habit never shared in polite circles. A series of round tables is covered with short stacks of books. I run my fingers over them, not looking at the titles, my head too full of all the life lessons I have not given the boys: how to love, how they must put happiness above money and ambition, how they must be good and kind and always try to put themselves in others' shoes, how they must look out for each other, brothers united. That's it, I think, leaning on a book, they need to stand by each other. I glance down, move my hand. It has been resting on *The Picador Book of Funeral Poems*.

I turn to the individual poets lined up in po-faced A to Z formation on the shelves. There aren't that many of them; if it were adult colouring books (by which I do not mean X-rated but, rather, calming pictures of beaches or flowers) or a manual on how to be happy and sugar-free I was after, I would be spoiled for choice. No matter. My index finger is already teasing out an Auden spine. I can't buy them Auden, though, much as I love him. He is the muzak of poetry nowadays, thanks to that Nineties romcom *Four Weddings and a Funeral*. Imagine if the boys think that's how I discovered the English-American poet. I've had a crush on him since I was fifteen and came upon the lines 'I shall never be/Different. Love me' in 'Anthem for St Cecilia's Day'. A homosexual wordsmith offering himself up as defenceless, vulnerable and in need of love, I couldn't believe it; the fact that I got it all wrong and that the 'I' in question was a personified Music in a poem that uses music as a metaphor to explore the power of God's grace is by the by. We live and learn, and perish the thought that the boys should learn the wrong things about me. This posterity business is trickier than I thought. Perhaps I should have gone down Mother's route, and left nothing.

The reworking of the Ten Commandments in Auden's 'Under Which Lyre', his Phi Beta Kappa poem which he read at Harvard in 1946, are hard to beat though. I'll take 'Thou shalt not live within thy means' and 'Read *The New Yorker*, trust in God;/And take short views' to my grave. If I manage to get the boys to have these on mental speed-dial before I get there, then it's job done, as Graham our builder likes to say. I keep scouring the shelves just in case there is something better, but what is it I am looking for? Poetry that will resonate with two freshly motherless teenage boys and with the motherless adults they may become. Vain, shallow and moved by my own mortality, I decide my choices must also reflect well on me, even if using someone else's legacy for my own is somewhat wanting. As it is, no one measures up, obviously, and I dismiss this chain-store behemoth – and the entire literary canon – as a bit limited.

And then I spot Ezra Pound, lovely, flawed Ezra. He was a defender of Fascism, a shameful anti-Semite, and he did go on. But even as I think this, the precision-perfect lines, 'As if the snow should hesitate/And murmur in the wind/and half turn back' from his poem 'The Return' play in my poetry jukebox of a head, and I think, *half turn back*. The poem is about ancient warrior gods, once 'Wing'd-with-Awe', inviolable', now diminished and reluctant to return to earth. *The snow can't turn back.* What about me? I think. I can't turn back. The poem, suddenly, is all about *me*, my life, my death. At this stage of the cancer game, I could make a barcode speak to me. Oncologists should add another side effect to the list: raging egotism. Or maybe it's just me? Either way, I start blubbing, definitely more for myself than for the boys, and grab a tightly folded tissue from one of those packs grannies and new mothers – and now me – carry around with them and blow my nose with Asperger gusto. Sylvia Plath, nestling close to Pound, gets showered with phlegm. I should buy the book, to save shoppers from my germs, but I won't. She had two children herself and put her head in the oven, which is a bit off-message for my purposes. I think of Elizabeth Jennings, who suffered much mental anguish in her life, and adored her mother. 'O you are/The way a blackbird sings/ And shapes the air' she wrote years after her death. When I first read those lines, in my twenties, I gasped. I interviewed Jennings around that time, in a café next to the bus station in Oxford. She wrote to me beforehand of her nerves before any interview, asking if I would mind meeting her in this particular café because 'my room is a shambles of books and music boxes etc' and it is 'a nice quiet place and I am a regular'. She sat across the Formica table from me, her back as bent as a fishing rod when a huge fish has taken the bait. I wished she wasn't in an old raincoat on this warm day in May and that she didn't have swollen feet and I wanted to say: If you can write like that about your mother, words so tender, are they not enough to heal you?

They're not, are they? I am beginning to see that now. Words are not enough.

On my way out of the poetry section, I spot Walter de la Mare. I remember him being good on children, or childhood, and being a Catholic, like Elizabeth Jennings. And big on fairies, too, and moonlight and animals and then I think of Bassy and how, when he is tucked up in bed, he is my elfin creature covered in moss and that when he sleeps I run my fingers over his eyebrows and I heart-soar at the magic of him. So the pair might be a good fit. I buy it, along with the Auden, and hurry off to the hospital, clutching the books to my chest like liquor in a brown paper bag.

Christmas has emptied the hospital. It's like *The Day of the Triffids*. The main concourse is empty, all the drooping heads and shuffling legs and vacant eyes gone elsewhere for the festive break. I take the elevator downstairs and find the imaging department. I've got the pick of chairs, but there is no wait. My name is called and a woman tells me to go to the loo and take off all my clothes except my knickers and put on a baboon gown. She says gown. I add 'baboon'. You expose your bottom if you forget to do up the ties lower down.

'Have you come for a PET scan?' she asks when I find my way back to her.

No, I've come for a gin and tonic.

Given that there are no other patients here, that it is Christmas Eve and that she has a clipboard in her hand, she must know why I am here.

I am not cancer-nice, not yet. I am still an island, craggy, access limited. I do my toothless, puffed cheeks polite smile instead of replying.

She puts her head to one side.

'Come this way. We'll get you ready for your scan.'

We. She thinks nothing of her use of the inclusive, filial pronoun. To her, it is a habit of speech, but it settles me, makes me feel as if an entire team of medical staff is gunning for me. I follow her into a shiny side room, its shades of grey and blue and flashes of metal so unfamiliar two weeks ago but now just part of the landscape here on my new planet. I sit on a bed, or whatever you call a narrow stretcher on wheels with adjustable railings, and my legs dangle over the edge like a child's. I don't swing them. I'm not in the mood, and I'm not a child either, though I'm certainly getting an insight into why not knowing what's going to happen next vexes nervier children. A rectangular white metal bin stands alongside a blue one. 'USE YOUR FEET, NOT YOUR HANDS', says the sign on the white one. The sticker on the blue bin reads: 'HOSPITAL PRODUCTS ONLY'. That's me, I think, a hospital product. Richard once had a friend whose job was to dispose of hospital waste. I picture myself inside a giant metal bin full of squishy human organs, my hands pressed palms upwards, trying to push my way out.

'Have you eaten or had anything to drink?'

'No, just a cup of tea.'

'With sugar?'

'Yes.'

She shakes her head and tuts like a disapproving aunt. She's joined the Sugar Police.

'I only have four granules. Less than a quarter of a teaspoon.'

'You're not supposed to eat or drink for 24 hours before your PET scan. Didn't you read the letter?'

Actually, I don't know what a PET scan is and I certainly did not read the letter which presumably outlined what I should expect and how I should prepare. Who would read such a letter? Besides, I need a cup of tea in the morning. I've come close to violence without one, once raising a bread knife to a university flatmate who tried to engage me in conversation and get me to try her porridge before my morning fix.

'We'll do a test anyway. See how much sugar is in your system. Just the one cup, was it?'

There's a needle, a pinprick and bits of plastic and cellophane and cotton and she leaves the room. Ten minutes later she is back. Everything is fine, she says, we can do the scan. We'll give you an injection and you won't feel anything, maybe just a bit cold for a second or two and you will be radioactive. Just for a few hours.

Shut up, nice nurse, keep the radioactive stuff to yourself. It is Christmas Eve, for heaven's sake, it is my son's birthday, I shouldn't even be here. From this moment, I am a Damien Hirst shark, suspended in an alien environment until normality resumes and I am where I should be: in the Greek restaurant, celebrating Reuben's birthday. We will be sitting in a booth, like we always do, and we will order our usuals: halloumi, houmous, spanakopita, calamari and louvia for us all to share as starters and then fish kebabs for Richard and me and chicken kebabs for Margaret and the boys. Warm pita bread will be served in a basket, along with olives and short sticks of vinegary raw carrot we won't eat. The restaurant will be bustling, the waiters in their black trousers and white shirts friendly and frantic. *And all shall be well.* The nurse injects the radioactive liquid, called a radiotracer, into my right arm. Later, I read on the NHS website that the radiotracer is a form of radioactive glucose and that cancer cells take up sugar more vociferously than other cells which explains why, in the weeks to come, people will tell me not to eat sugar and I will think they are being faddish when in fact they are being rather sensible. In my case, more of the radioactive glucose will accumulate in the tumour in my neck and, hopefully, in the primary tumour. These will show up as red on the scan.

Lie down, says the nurse, for an hour. A whole hour! I do so, like an obedient dog. It's novel, lying down when you're not tired, sick or hungover. I don't see why I can't sit up and read a book. I eye up the carrier bag with the Auden and Walter de la Mare in it and think about getting off the couch and sneaking one of them over. But, unusually, I do what I am told and stay put.

Hospital time is mercurial. An hour, in which you do nothing, not even think, can last a matter of minutes, or it can stretch out as long as your lifetime. I doze off, and I am running under that sprinkler in the park near school. Mother is watching – she is with someone, Grandma maybe – as I cavort in my pants with my sister, our summer uniforms and our sandals discarded on the spongy lawn. We vanish and then Richard, Reuben and Bassy appear, looking like they did when I left them this morning, except that they are older. They *look* the same, but I know they are older and that they have lives I don't know about and then they've gone. I am Tiresias, blind, between two lives, seeing more than I bargained for.

All the while, time, which is also weightless, bears down on me, has me bending like a weeping willow until the tips of my leaves touch the tips of the blades of grass beneath me, which they shouldn't. That's not what willows do; they bend, but only so far. There should be a gap between the tip of the blade of grass and the tips of the narrow leaves. The gap is life; it is being alive; it is the breath and the pause that open up fresh understanding, a new knowing. It is why the American poet Emily Dickinson punctuates every line of her poems with one, two, sometimes even three dashes. You hear life in the gaps she creates, and the questioning. The gap must not be closed.

Eventually, the nurse rouses me and takes me into the scanning room. I lie on a plastic table with a giant donut of a scanner at the other end. Six or seven times the table seems to move in and out of the circular scanner and I wonder what the person who lay here before me is doing now. Having a cup of tea, I hope, or wrapping the final Christmas presents and readying the stockings. I shimmer off in my bauble skirt the moment the scan is finished and, the first to arrive at the restaurant, flick through the Walter de la Mare I've bought for Bassy. Pausing at random, I read: 'Ahoy, and ahoy!'/ 'Twixt mocking and merry –/'Ahoy and ahoy, there,/Young man of the ferry!' It's drivel. What did I buy this for? I wish I had bought some Pound instead; it would give me an excuse to tell the boys my story about revising the American poet for my Finals. Stir-crazy, I stole into my flatmate Donald's tiny bedroom – so tantalisingly tidy and free of the discarded clothes and the yellow Post-It notes nailed to my own floor with drawing pins. The impaled bits of paper represented the ants Pound watched in his outdoor steel cage as a prisoner-of-war in an American military camp in Pisa in 1945. I arranged myself at Donald's desk and got stuck into my revision. Soon bored, I opened his underwear drawer, in my defence, already slightly open. Seeing the neat stacks of boxer shorts, I pulled out a pair – nice, bright ones covered with Egyptian pyramids – and put them on my head. Then I got back to work.

I am picturing Donald's face as he walked in to find me there with his knickers on my head when Reuben and Bassy arrive with their grandmother. I was just thinking about a poet I liked at St Andrews, I say. I chortle. They groan. I give Reuben the Auden. Another birthday present, I say, feeling beneficent. Yeah, thanks, he says, not looking at it. I come over all Tiresias again and see into the future: it is a world where words don't matter and people do not seek answers in literature. Which is excellent. I no longer need to compile a legacy of words to live by for the boys, since they wouldn't read it if I did, and cross it off my To Do list.

After lunch we pitch up at our old next-door neighbours' for their annual Christmas Eve drinks party. Martin, the host, hands me a glass of Bolly and I think, thank God someone serves proper champagne. Better still, the table against the wall is lined with it, so there's no danger of Prosecco as a backup, an all too common ruse in these straitened times. Jo, Martin's wife, is talking to JC, irrepressible owner of L'Absinthe, the neighbourhood French restaurant. His *potatoes dauphinoise* and *tarte tatin* are two of the seven wonders of the edible world.

'Sorry to interrupt, but could you do the catering at my wake, JC?'

This is the question I want to ask. But what's the etiquette? Should I ask him now? He might give me, or rather Richard, a *bon prix*, put on the spot like this by a customer-cum-corpse. I decide against it, but make a mental note to tell Richard I don't want a buffet. *Buffet.* The very word is dispiriting.

The local carol service, to which most of the drinks party traditionally debunks, is quite the opposite. It is uplifting and melancholy at the same time, as Christmas carol services are. Richard often gives it a miss. This time he comes, voluntarily. Toddlers act out the Nativity. Joseph is smaller than Mary this year and the stars are wandering all over the apse. I get through most of the carols, admittedly bleating not bellowing as I usually do, until 'Away in a Manger'. I make the mistake of looking at Richard. His eyes are rivers trying to provide enough surface to stop the whole world from flooding. I have to open my own wide. We get to the bit about blessing all the children in thy tender care and my voice warbles. My own tears betray me, living feeling so urgent suddenly, so necessary and wonderful; if this were a movie I would hug my husband and the stranger next to me, hug anyone within reach, and I would tell them how much I love this world, say thank you, tell them how good life has been to me. You don't need to be scared witless that your time might be up in order for Christmas to make you feel happy and morose and finished all at the same time. But it helps.

We skip another annual festive drinks with old Primrose Hill friends and head home, every minute accountable, time something to wade through, and something to cherish. As soon as we're home, we pile into the upstairs living room to lay out the stockings and read 'The Night Before Christmas'. Richard is Camcorder Man, as always. More posterity in the making. He zooms in on the Christmas tree, pans across to the empty stockings I've laid out on the hearth, the glass of milk and cookies for Santa and the single carrot for the reindeer. Why do we always leave just one carrot, I think. There are at least six reindeer. Pepper the puppy bounds through the living-room door. Richard turns the camcorder on her, then follows her as she makes for Santa's cookies. Bassy scoops up the plate just in time. I keep my eyes on Richard and the camcorder. I want to be ready when he turns it on me. He pans to Margaret, back in her spot on the sofa in the bay window. She smiles for him. I'm standing next to her in front of the mantelpiece, so he should film me next. I get my smile ready. Instead, he twists forward in his armchair so that he can get a better angle on Reuben, who is lolling on the big sofa to his right. What about me? I'm not a ghost. Not yet. Film me.

Get on with it, says one of the boys. Start reading.

All right, I say, holding up the print-out of the poem I've been holding in my hand. We do have a hardback, illustrated edition of it somewhere, which would better suit the enormity of the occasion, but I can't find it. Richard points the camcorder at me. Finally. I look into the lens and smile, then I start reading, my voice an am-dram whisper.

"Twas the night before Christmas, when all through the house . . .'

I've read 'The Night Before Christmas' on Christmas Eve since Reuben was two. I first heard it at the new house we went to stay in the Christmas after Mother died and I know to start quietly, building up to full voice when the reindeer are charging across the rooftops and about to drop the kids' presents down the chimneys.

'Not a creature was stirring, not even a mouse;
The stockings were hung by the chimney with care . . .'

But it shouldn't be me reading the poem, not this year when the world is spinning on its axis and my voice could give me away at any minute. I get twenty lines in. St Nick whistles and calls out to his reindeer:

'Now, Dasher! Now . . .'

'Vixen' gets lost in the back of my throat.

'What's the matter?' the boys ask.

Stupid bloody idiot.

'Gen, what is it?' asks Margaret.

Ping-ping. Richard turns off the camcorder. The cancer is our secret; our sorrow will not go on record.

'What? Oh, nothing. It's the poem. It gets me every time.'

It never has before. I usually relish the sound of my own voice. I can feel everybody's eyes on me. I avoid Richard's, take a deep breath, and launch back in. The presents are delivered, the reindeer head home and Santa signs off in customary fashion:

'And away they all flew like the down of a thistle.
But I heard him exclaim, ere he drove out of sight—
"Happy Christmas to all, and to all a good night!"'

Our own night is one of wakefulness and fears we do not share with each other. I curl into Richard and want, very badly, to grow old with him. I hadn't realised how I take our dotage for granted. It is a given, like his love, not something I have to ask for, yearn for, negotiate. He always jokes that he won't look after me when I am old because I will be a cantankerous ingrate and I've said that's fine by me, I won't look after him either. He doesn't want me to. I am not a body wipes and spoon-feeding sort of spouse. We'll be the Twits, he laughs. But he also says, we'll have a fine old age, rent out the house half the year and live somewhere hot, go to galleries, take the grandchildren out, read all day. When he plans out loud like that I know I am his heartbeat, and he is mine, my heart's hearth. This could be my last Christmas with Richard, not only the last with the boys; the fact hasn't registered with me until now. I reach my arm over his chest. At least he'll have the bed all to himself and there'll be no fights about when to put the lights out, but it's a bit bloody previous, I think, and then, whoosh, something grabs me, catapults me into a pitch-dark terror. My closed eyes are open now and alert. I am standing on a road in the dead of a Stephen King night, waiting for a truck to thunder round the bend and run me over. I can't make myself move out of the way.

Christmas Day is usually being woken early by Bassy after Richard and I have stayed up to wrap presents til two in the morning, fumbling for my first cup of tea, chasing it with a champagne sharpener and opening our stockings. It's presents and paper everywhere and everyone forgetting to eat the smoked salmon and eggs we've got for breakfast and me dragging the boys off to church and them alternately scowling and laughing the whole way through the service. It is changing into the new outfit I have kept for Christmas Day and cooking and eating and drinking, it's pulling crackers and taking it in turn to read out the jokes and me saying we should watch the Queen's speech and being overruled and eating Milk Tray and Bendicks Bittermints and, in the early evening, looking at my own presents Richard always showers me with and reading my new books and feeling content. This year the traditions are observed, but there's a numbness in the air and a sadness in the heft of Richard. How far can he bend without touching the tips of those blades of grass himself?

I resolve to shore him up with love.

That night is another without sleeping. All the slow, post-Christmas days follow. The cheeses and Christmas cake don't get eaten, more bottles are left unopened. We see friends. When one says their close relative, two years younger than me, has just died of cancer I get up abruptly and leave the room. I forgot, I say, I have an appointment, so sorry, and I head out. I get in the car, our secret so heavy now and cold, the world outside frozen. We need to cross the ice to get to the places we usually go and we can't; we can't negotiate the ice.

A couple of days later I go for another scan and then New Year's Eve looms. Friends, eating, drinking, late-night karaoke, that's the usual formula. But I can't face another performance and neither can Richard. I ask Bassy's godmother, Vicky, one of the other Boxer Shorts university flatmates, if we can come and stay with her and her husband, Martin, in their house in the countryside just outside Bath. I've already told her what's going on and she knows we are waiting for a prognosis. We drive down the day before New Year's Eve and get lost coming out of Bath, as usual, but don't argue about it, which is unusual, and then get lost again on the country roads. The fields are endless, the trees smug, knowing as they do that they will be around for ever. Another new year is nothing to them.

Finally the tyres are crunching the potholed gravel track leading to The Ranch, our nickname for Vicky's house, which sits in a dip, overlooking a valley. The boys and puppy pile out of the car; Richard and I take our time. Vicky is outside, waiting for us, smiling her expansive smile that animates her whole body and I think, oh no, this is a mistake, I can't do this. It's the first time we've been with someone who knows. A hugger, she hugs me even harder than usual. Avoiding eye contact, I will her to let me go.

There is tea, the obligatory asking after Chilli and Basil, Vicky's aged, ailing cats who have taken over an entire suite downstairs: the study and the adjoining utility room. There is a walk, some sitting about on sofas, reading, then drinks in the living room while Martin and the boys repair to the kitchen to make a Chinese banquet from scratch. Pepper scratches at the door of the study. She can smell the cats.

'I've saved some salmon for Chilli,' Vicky says, as she hands me a plate of salmon blinis.

'Ah,' I say, when I should say more, but I don't, because I am a bad person-with-cancer rather than the soft-touch type.

Most cats die at fifteen. Vicky's cats are twenty-two and unspeakable. They have been ever since she adopted them as scrawny, abandoned kittens in Hong Kong in 1989. Myself and the fourth Boxer Shorts university flatmate, Nell, flew out to stay with Vicky shortly after their arrival. Each night Nell and I bedded down on the sofas in the living room and, before the sun had even risen over Discovery Bay, they would be up, skitting across from dining table to shelf to chair like crazed, caged leaping monkeys. They used our faces as springboards. We cursed them and swatted them away. When she moved back to the UK in 2003, Vicky brought them with her. In 2006, Martin and Vicky decided to marry. I took Martin to one side. There'll be four of you in the marriage, I wanted to say. Instead I asked: How do you feel about the cats? He raised his eyebrows in reply, too loyal to say more. They won't last for ever, I said. But they are still here, eight years later, one blind and incontinent, the other arthritic and immobile.

Vicky runs through the plans for New Year's Eve. A walk, a pub lunch and in the evening a country and western night – burgers, poker, a double-denim dress code, and as much Dolly Parton as we like. We can go to the local church too, she suggests, and bang out the old year. We always do it, don't we, Martin, and the pair of them recount how, in Asia, where they have each lived in the past, it's a tradition to bang out the old year in order to make way for the new one. You grab woks and saucepans and wooden spoons and any instruments you can lay your hands on, they say, and everyone makes as much noise as they can. I want to put my hands over my ears at the very thought. I don't want to bang out this year. I want it to last for ever so that next year does not happen. Sounds fun, I say.

The next day we stop off at the local church after the pub, but there's no banging. There isn't a saucepan to be seen. They must have forgotten. I am so relieved. On the way home Pepper starts limping. She's cut her paw, or got a thorn in it. Vicky takes a look at it as soon as we get back, and digs out the number for the vet, just in case. She's so caring, and she hasn't even got cancer. Then again, Pepper is eminently likeable. The evening unravels, as planned: burgers, poker, country music. We don't make it to midnight. Otherwise, we have kept up appearances. We go to bed. We don't sleep.

My defences come down on New Year's Day. Martin takes Richard and the boys off for a walk so Vicky and I can have some time together. We slope off to Babington House, a Soho House outpost I've always wanted to go to. I love a bit of bucolic chic, usually. We sit next to the open fire in the library and I don't even look around the room. I am cold. I move out of my armchair and sit on the fender, and then I continue the trading with Death that I began in the consultant's room twelve days earlier.

'I will settle for two more years, just not six months,' I inform Vicky. I speak matter-of-factly, as if she will be passing on what I say to someone else, and my authoritative tone will affect the decisions taken. 'I can't do six months.'

'I know.'

'I am not afraid of being ill. I am not afraid of dying.' I am not sure if this is true. 'I just don't want the boys not to have a mother.' I am clear on this one.

'I know.' And she does know. Her own mother, Jeannie, was orphaned as a child and she has told Vicky, and me, about what it was to grow up without parents. Jeannie is the only other orphan I know. I've met plenty of half-orphans but, without meaning to sound competitive, they don't count. The first time I stayed with Jeannie when we were down from St Andrews, she astonished me by talking about being an orphan, openly, as if it were a fact and no reflection on her, and about the loneliness and the unloving aunt who brought her up.

'It is my worst fear,' I tell Vicky, 'but I never thought it would actually happen.'

'Of course you didn't,' she replies. Wisely, she does not say that it might not happen.

'I want the full deal,' I sob, 'motherhood until the boys are at university.' And then I make myself shut up, but really, I want to say that I want more. Much more. I want to live to see my sons grow into middle-aged men with nostril hair. I want to drink champagne at their weddings – or Conscious Couplings or whatever the marital fashion will be by then. If they have children, I want to live to see them, too, and I don't want a walk-on part in their histories of love. I do not want to be a faded picture on their moodboards.

Vicky is looking at me, waiting for me to say something else. I shut my eyes and ask for grace, but it is just a word. I do not know what I am asking for. I look at her instead, she holds my hand, my shoulders heave, and with my eyes I tell her. I tell her of the heart's hollow that being motherless creates, how the grief lodges beneath your skin, how the loneliness and the longing are the air that you breathe and that sometimes, when the longing is so intense that you want to say, *please, no, I've had enough, just bring her back*, you feel as though you are suffocating. And no one has any idea how you are struggling to inhabit your new, motherless self and to find your way in a world in which you are no longer safe. If the boys become motherless, how will anyone know that they, too, are no longer whole? How will they know that the boys feel as though something is missing?

I want. I want. I want as though the verb had been invented for me. My desire alone defines it. It is as though I have never wanted anything before. I have not: not like this. From the deep, down where the root-hairs reach, down where the cancer cells are multiplying, the cry rises: LET ME LIVE.

Finally, I say: 'We'd better get back to the boys.'

Vicky hugs me, and this time I succumb and let the tears out. Then I go to the bathroom and splash my face with cold water. It is raining hard when we get outside. I turn my face into it. I turn my face. *Seek my face.*

Later that morning, in the car on the way home, Bassy says: 'Why did we have such a quiet New Year?'

'Yeah,' says Reuben, 'why didn't we have a party at home?'

I look at Richard, and then I say:

'We just felt like doing something different.'

5

BREAKING BAD

Each time I imagine myself telling the boys I have cancer, Mother photobombs the scene. I picture them sitting either side of me on the big sofa in the kitchen and there she is, sitting at the far end, looking just like she did the last time I saw her alive. Her brown hair is schoolgirl long and scratchy as a daddy-long-legs, some of it pulled back over her head and tied at the back with a ribbon. Her crisp kindling wrists are poking out of the sleeves of her floral cotton nightie, a plastic wristband on one of them. The only difference between now and the last time I saw her, in the nursing home in Brighton, is that back then she was propped up on pillows as puffy as her stomach, which bulged through the sheets, fat with victorious cancer cells. Now she's perching on the arm of the sofa, unsupported but still in her nightie, waiting for me to speak.

I can't speak. I don't want to frighten the boys, and how can they not be frightened? Once I've told them, there will be no going back to a time when the world was steady. Once I've told them, they will think I am going to die. Mother was ill and she told me she was going to get better – and then she died just the same. Too bad. It is time to do our duty as parents and shatter their world. Also, if I do tell them sooner rather than later, I can say I am going to be all right which, though technically untrue in the absence of a prognosis, isn't a blatant lie. After the prognosis, whenever that may be, I don't want to lie to them. There's a practical consideration, too. In four days' time I am having exploratory surgery in my neck to enable the oncology team to check for cancer cells in my lymph nodes and decide on a treatment plan. The procedure will entail a day and a night in hospital, with the possibility of full-on surgery the following week. I can't spring that shock on them. Besides, the strain of withholding the truth is making my skull ache. It is getting hard to talk to the boys about anything, knowing what I am holding back.

In the end, though, Richard and I can't tell them, can't agree on what is best, decide to put it off a bit longer. Three more days pass and it gets to Friday, the day before the surgery and the overnight hospital stay, and we still don't tell them. Instead I nonchalantly mention that I am going out with Julia, another university friend and Reuben's godmother, who is over from Madrid, and that I will be staying the night with her down in Brixton. Why do you have to stay over, Bassy asks. It's a fair point. We're going dancing, I say, we're hitting the town. *Hitting the town.* This isn't a phrase I ever use; I sound like a suburban Fifties housewife let out for the night.

Richard isn't taking me to UCLH, nor will he visit in the evening. We've agreed that it is better if he stays with the boys, carrying on as normal. Julia will meet me at the hospital, then come back during evening visiting hours and again the following morning, when Laurence, an old school friend and Bassy's godfather, will collect me. My overnight bag is packed with entertainment. There's the *Vanity Fair* I got in my stocking, Rilke's *Selected Poems* (I've never read him, so 24 hours to myself seems like a good opportunity) and *The Goldfinch* (another Christmas present; everyone's talking about Donna Tartt's novel and I like being in the loop), my laptop, make-up and my new pink cashmere slippers.

Julia is waiting for me in the hospital foyer. Up we go to some mystery reception area and she stays with me until it's time to put on another baboon gown, then it's down to 'theatre' soon afterwards. I'm a prop, stretched out on a mobile hospital couch. My friend's got a famous dog, the anaesthetist volunteers. My friend is Millie. Or maybe she says Milla. You know, from *Made in Chelsea*. I don't know; my cocktail party conversation skills suddenly elude me. She describes what Millie/Milla's dog – Herman, or Herbert, maybe it's Sherbert – can do and all I can manage is: I've got a dog. Then I can't compete because Pepper, I suddenly realise, has no extracurricular interests or party tricks. The needle for the general anaesthetic spares me further humiliation; in it goes and when I come round I am entombed in starched sheets. I sniff the pastel air and through the big windows to my right I can only see sky. I remember now. I am in the Tower, home to all the wards. I am up on the ninth floor. A lilac antimicrobial privacy curtain forms a dividing wall to my left; a noise like a spluttering train is coming from the other side of it. The other half of the curtain is stacked back on the overhead rail, leaving me on display like a performance artist. The patient directly opposite is looking straight at me, waiting for me to do something, to make a noise myself, perhaps, or to say something now that I am awake. Who knows how long she has been waiting for me to come round. I cut her with my razor eyes. Better she knows immediately that the fact of our hospitalisation engenders no sense of kinship in me. She is old and haggard and looks like she's got no puff left in her. Do not talk to me. I get out of bed, look through the window, see the cars down on Euston Road, note the BT Tower, all so familiar and unfamiliar, turn around to take in the ward. Five beds altogether, three on my side, two opposite me, only two with their privacy curtains drawn closed. On the bed diagonally opposite mine a body is curled in the foetal position, the crown of the head just visible at the top of the bed covers. From it a round of raging words fires into the wall. I pull the curtain across the front of my bay and climb back on to the bed.

I should have brought earplugs, I think, as I lay out my magazine, book and laptop on my table, a brilliant, swivelling thing that can go across the bed or sit perpendicular to it. I call Richard and tell him all is well, then I sit and stare, sit and doze. Julia turns up with sushi for supper, which I don't feel like eating, and we chat, and then visiting hours are over and she leaves. I am shocked to find myself here, alone, in a hospital bed. Doubtless one always is. During the night the spluttering train keeps spluttering, and in the morning I go to the bathroom and glance at where the noise came from and see a lady patient in the bed next to mine with a hole in her throat. Julia returns at eight o'clock with an almond croissant, which I wolf down. When the consultant comes to do the ward round he is impressed; most throats wouldn't tolerate a croissant following the surgery, he says, and I purr. Instinctively, I want to be a good patient and do well at the small things, in the subconscious belief that it will bode well for the final outcome.

Some time between the consultant's visit and being discharged a Catholic priest floats past the beds. He is in costume – black suit, surplice, dog collar. I sit up, to show how alive I am.

'Morning, Father.'

He can keep his last rites to himself.

'Oh. Morning.'

Father Whoever-he-is sounds caught out, as if he wasn't expecting to find himself here. I know how he feels.

He is hovering by the window, his expression neither smiling nor grievous – a study in openness. Julia, who stood up when he arrived, remains standing. We watch as he reaches for the hand sanitiser on the wall and rubs his hands together. Priests do that these days, before Communion, but I don't think he should do it now, in front of the living and the perhaps-dying.

'Lovely view,' I say. 'The BT Tower and everything.'

'Yes.'

'Hello. I'm Julia.' She steps towards him and offers her hand. The handshake, she tells me later, is limp, which does not surprise me. His entire physique is concave and apologetic. Julia launches into sherry-before-Sunday-lunch mode, telling him how she is over from Madrid, that she is a teacher, that's she's home for Christmas and how the break has, fortuitously, coincided with her university friend's hospital admission. Here she gestures towards me. I pick up the baton. I am in for a minor, exploratory procedure, I say, keen that the Disciple of Death should know I am on the side of the living, at least for now. It is not as if he has asked.

'Oh,' he says. 'Ah, yes. Right.' Then he wishes me well and, after another squeeze of the sanitiser and rubbing of hands that marks the well from the unwell, he is off. Julia looks at me. I look at her.

'That was a bit rubbish,' she says.

'Not even a prayer.'

'Shall I get him back?'

'If he'll come back.'

The woman I thought had given up on God in her early twenties because the Anglican Church had an exclusion policy on gay love is running down the ward, calling out: 'Father! Father! Excuse me, Father!'

She comes back seconds later with the man-in-black in tow.

'I don't like to impose,' he says. 'Usually the patient or their relative will give me clues. They'll say which church they go to. That sort of thing. You said you were over from Madrid,' he continues, turning to Julia. 'I didn't want to impose on your friendship and your time together.'

What he does not say is that, as with the travelling salesman of old, strangers are wont to shut the door in his face or, worse, lynch him, reporting him to the authorities for spiritual interference. Either that or, as Julia later says, he is so careful not to offend that he has lost sight of the priest's brief to reach out. I explain about the boys, how they don't know I am in hospital because we can't bring ourselves to break the bad news.

'Honesty,' he says, no trace of hesitancy in his soft voice now, 'go for honesty. It is essential. Honesty. In everything. Especially with children.'

If I tell them I am ill, the past might repeat itself, I say, and I give him a snapshot of my childhood. I explain that I don't even know how long I have to live. My eyes well up, which infuriates me. I am a grown-up; I am over my own childhood losses. Slowly, he draws out key facts, first establishing that I have a fully extant husband.

'And he is . . .?' He lets his voice trail off.

'Oh, he's a great father,' I say, realising that he does not assume that the existence of a husband means he is a good thing. 'He's very loving.'

He nods, and then he asks about the boys, how old they are, what their personalities are like, how I think they might respond to being told I am ill. I dodge the last question: I don't know the answer.

'Better to tell them. They sound like they will be able to cope. They will mature as a result, rise to the occasion. It won't be easy for them, but it is better for them to know. They must be in on it from the very beginning,' he continues, his voice insistent now, 'and might feel betrayed if you conceal everything from them, even for a few more weeks.'

He asks about my treatments next. With chemotherapy and radiotherapy on the cards, he says, hiding such an obvious illness from them would be impossible, and too stressful for me. Then, with great wisdom, he suggests that it is vital that the whole family be with me on what he calls my journey, at every stage.

'You are in it together,' he says, 'and it might bring you closer together. You will need their help.'

There's a thought. The idea that the boys might help me is anathema; I protect them, I help them. I have never seen mothering as a two-way process. Over the years, and to this day, I mention my own mother and father just enough to stop them from asking questions or to make either parent remarkable by my own omissions. Bassy was eight when I first mentioned that my mother had died 'when I was very young,' and I've never told them exactly how old I was when each parent died or how I fared after that. Why would I?

Laurence picks me up and I am home by Saturday lunchtime. As soon as we have time together, I tell Richard what the priest said. OK, soon, he says, we'll tell them soon. In the meantime, we decide to enlist Caroline, the palliative care friend who was at the Secret Santa dinner; part of her job is to help parents break the news of terminal illness to their child or, when parents find that impossible, to tell the child herself. Richard doesn't want to use the word cancer. I do. For both of us it is still the C word; I feel sure Caroline can advise us and act as mediator. I can't face calling her straight out to tell her what's going on, so I send her a casual text. *Call when you've got a mo*, or something equally carefree. And of course she doesn't, not straight away. Need is so hard to spell out.

Meanwhile, I reassure myself that the boys are part of a generation that will view cancer for what it often is nowadays: a curable illness, a chronic disease. They won't choke on the word, like Richard and I do, and see tombstones and hearses flashing before them at its very mention. One in every two people living in the UK is expected to develop cancer at some stage in their life, but many will be habituated to its prevalence and, seeing how people survive it, won't be terrified of it. Half of those now diagnosed with cancer are predicted to survive for at least ten years. The disease, and living as a survivor of it, will be normalised.

Hans alone has got over 200 scientists and clinicians studying the immune system and developing new biological treatments, far less punitive ones. The future of cancer therapy is to move away from chemotherapy and radiation therapy in favour of exploiting the precision of the immune system, enabling it to selectively attack cancer cells and leave normal tissue intact. Plus there's the fact that over half of deaths from cancer occur in people aged seventy-five or older. At worst, Reuben and Bassy's generation can reasonably hope to live long enough to be grandparents, all else being well. That's if air pollution doesn't kill them, they don't get run over by a bus or fatally bitten by a deadly spider, which happened to the most handsome boy at my school, in his back garden in north London.

Not knowing how long I've got myself, I do an audit of The Few Important Things I Have Shared That Might Influence The Boys in a Positive Way.

1. I stopped eating meat when I was nineteen because of the cruel husbandry of mass-produced meat and battery eggs then in common practice.
2. The East End gangster Reggie Kray, who had a photograph of me in a strapless fuchsia silk ball dress on his cell wall, once requested that I visit him in Parkhurst prison. He used to write to me following the research I did for his book *Slang*, which the writer Francis Wyndham – a close friend of my half-brother, who had got me the research job – helped him produce. The Home Office vetted me in the comfort of my Little Venice home and gave me the green light but – at the last minute – I didn't go, mindful that Reggie had nailed Jack 'the Hat' McVitie to the floor through his throat and that it didn't do to humour

murderers, especially ones that might be released and come round for a chat.

3. When the boys were seven and five, I ripped out pictures of Margaret Thatcher from a colour supplement and together we burned them on an open fire in a rental cottage in Walberswick in Suffolk. They already knew the 'Maggie Thatcher, Milk Snatcher' chant, so we recited it together.

4. A few years later, I sorely wanted to pour my can of Coke over the former premier when she stood behind my chair during her tour of the *Daily Telegraph* offices. I stopped myself.

5. I don't shop at Primark.

6. I bang on about how the drugs trade is immoral and exploitative.

But what will the boys remember about me? Probably just me shouting. Or how I made them make their first Holy Communions. They think, erroneously, that I believe in God, hands down, no questions asked, and are embarrassed when I wear my All Saints black leather belt studded with 'Jesus Rocks' because they do not think it is to any degree ironic. They know, I think, that I avoid squashing spiders, even though I am scared of them, and ants too. So I put this on the list.

7. It is wrong to squash spiders and ants.

And that's about the best of it. Given this paltry offering, why do I worry that the boys won't be able to navigate the world without me?

The priest said the boys will be able to cope, with the news of my illness at least, that they will mature, implying a capacity for resilience I have not factored in. I hate the thought of them learning resilience they way I've learned it. I've kept my childhood from them precisely because I don't want to spook them into thinking that parents don't last, that one day they might come back from school and I will be gone, or wake up in the morning and not be able to find me.

Before the boys were born, I feared getting breast cancer, and wanted to live to at least the same age as Mother had: forty-two. When I hit forty-two I cheered, only to realise that Reuben had only had eight years of me, Sebastian six, and I wanted both of them to have me for at least as long as I had Mother: nine years. I had Reuben when I was 34, so I needed to get to 43. But Bassy was also entitled to nine years of me, and that took me to the age of 45. When I dropped them off somewhere, or said goodbye to them, I very often thought: I hope I see you again later today. Kiss kiss. I love you. You never know what tomorrow brings.

I often shared my fearful calculations with Richard, talked about the legacy of loss and the filial dramas that played out in its wake, and always he said: I love you, you've got me now, we've got our own family.

One day, walking across Chalcot Square in Primrose Hill, I realised that our co-parenting could not continue to be played out in the shadow of my own losses and I resolved to let go of my fears. I put them in a box, along with memories I did not care for, sealed it up. I did not want to curse the boys, then aged ten and eight. Five years later, I got the cancer diagnosis.

Orphans have always augured ill; like their fictional counterparts, they are outsiders, free agents, agents of destruction. Free, they lose their way, as poor Jude does in Thomas Hardy's *Jude the Obscure*, or, like Superman and Batman and Robin, are superheroes whose rescue missions are made possible by their freedom, as are the antics of orphan poster boy and wizard Harry Potter. What a contrast he is to the often dour, archetypal offerings of nineteenth- and early twentieth-century fiction: *The Secret Garden, Huckleberry Finn, Oliver Twist, Anne of Green Gables, Jane Eyre*. I devoured each hero's adventures, and internalised their journeys. But by the time I came across Jane Fairfax in

Jane Austen's *Emma* or the orphaned siblings in Henry James's *The Turn of the Screw* as a young adult, I was alert to the use of the orphan as a literary device, and I minded it. It's not that a mirror was being held up to my own life, but rather that to see the orphan's prescribed trajectory – abandonment, dependence, seeking connection whilst finding your own way – writ large was humiliating, and depressing.

Having neither ties nor redress, orphans work perfectly as agents of change, as well as of redemption; weak, they are the touchstone that reveals the weakness and failings in others. For that reason, and others besides, they are dangerous, unknown things and not always to be trusted. To his uncle and aunt, Harry Potter isn't so much dangerous as a nuisance and a punchbag, as is Roald Dahl's James, who escapes his sadistic aunts for adventures inside a giant peach. Both are part of a generation of literary orphans that have fun. The dangerous orphans are the ones who rebel and try to escape their lot; they are proud and they hate their dependence on others. Think of Caliban or Jane Eyre. Wretched, brutish Caliban is not only a hybrid creature whose mother was a witch. He is also an orphan. He is dependent on the tyrannical Prospero whom he once loved and who has enslaved him. Caliban rebels; his rejection of fine language in favour of foul is part of that rebellion. His monstrous form further separates him from the civilised world and the moral order Prospero is hell-bent on creating on his island. Caliban's otherness defines him. He is without connection, and, as with all orphans, whether fictive or real, that makes him both vulnerable and potentially fearless. Jane Eyre, whom I have always loved, is of course the most fearless orphan of all, but she pays a price for it. Her loneliness is acute and she is, at a profound level, ashamed of her orphan state. She embodies freedom, but she is not free: the desire to belong burns inside her, a fact seemingly contradicted by her fierce independence.

If the orphan state defies the rules of nature, it's not surprising the natural world is full of stories about them. In his book *Pathlands*, about walking in rural England, the nature writer, pilgrim and occasional shepherd Peter Owen Jones recalls encountering an orphan sheep on a Sussex farm. He knew she was an orphan and hand-reared because, he writes, 'she didn't mind being stroked'. And he goes on, 'Hand-reared sheep never really fit in with the flock, they never quite lose the imprint of their human foster parents, it leaves them not belonging to either . . . I see the orphans thrown together in a pen not knowing where they are, but the most important thing of all is that they have no mothers. When a lamb has no mother it has no map; when the bond is broken between the lamb and their mother they become a lost sheep.'

He continues: 'I was once on a farm in Devon and was told about a hand-reared ewe called Judas. She lived in a slaughterhouse and when the lorries arrived crammed with nine-month-old lambs Judas would be placed at the bottom of the lorry ramp: her job was to lead the lambs into the slaughterhouse holding pen and she did this many hundreds of times throughout her life.'

I try to get hold of Caroline again. She doesn't pick up. I send another text, another misleading one in which I make it sound as if I just want a catch-up. Then we get to Sunday lunchtime and, panicked by the impasse Richard and I have now reached, I send the text I should have sent first time round. *Caroline, I need to talk to you urgently.* She calls straight back.

'Sorry I missed your calls,' she says. 'We've been at a wedding. What's up?'

'Well . . .' And then, after much circumlocution, I spit out the C word. We arrange to meet in our local pub later that afternoon.

It's a big pub, and it's practically empty. Richard and I wait for Caroline. I reach across the table for Richard's hand. We talk for a bit, then our words fizzle out in another failed raid on the inarticulate; T. S. Eliot on the anguish of what cannot be said has often come in handy over the years, but never like he does now. Caroline arrives in a whirlwind of love and concern and, expertly, swiftly, she brings us to a place where we can both see that we must tell the boys forthwith. We agree on later this evening. Then she asks how we think we might tell them and I whisper the words I've been practising in my head.

'Boys, we've got some bad news . . .' Caroline leans in. I try to speak a little louder. Richard looks down at his hands. 'You see here, this lump in my neck.' I point to the Interloper. 'I've been to see the doctor and it turns out it is malignant but I am going to be all right.'

Richard's eyes well up. I keep going. Malignant. Will they understand that? Should I leave it out? I realise I left out the word cancer, too, and tumour. I used the word 'but', which was a mistake. 'But' is always ominous. I try again.

'Boys, we've got some news, some bad news – about me. I don't know if you've noticed that I've got this lump in my neck. I've been to the doctor and it turns out it is a tumour. I've got cancer, but it's treatable, and I'm going to be OK.'

'That's good,' Caroline says. I hear the 'but' and make another mental note to leave it out. I am a young tree, freshly planted. My budded branches reach out to my sons. The roots feel the effort and themselves reach deeper into the unknown earth.

I try again. 'I've got cancer *and* it's treatable. I'm going to be OK.'

We walk home, dragging our feet, pushing against the blizzard of dread and sorrow, blinded. What good are statistics? The fact is, the boys will only have a mastery of them when they are older. Cancer is not a good word; to suggest that it is, is to obfuscate, it is to play with semantics until you tease the word into something that does not catch at the back of your throat. I don't think I can say it, and why must I on this dark Sunday night made for shutting out the world and curling up together in front of the fire and watching a family movie? Once inside our house, we circle the silence, putting off the moment that will last for ever, heart-heavy. Eventually, I call the boys down to the kitchen. Pepper is curled up on the floor. I wait for them on the sofa and when they trundle down the stairs, I pat the cushions either side of me, holding out my arms that should be protective wings, holding out my arms and opening my heart and knowing, as I do so, that my outstretched arms say what I cannot say:

Please, not me, not yet.
I hold out my arms. I open my heart. Protect me.

The boys sit either side of me. I close my outstretched arms around them. I never want to let them go.

Richard is sitting on the arm of the sofa, in Mother's spot. She, mercifully, is nowhere to be seen.

Willing my voice to stay strong, I begin:

'Boys, I don't know if you've noticed, but I've got this lump . . .' I touch my neck. And then I'm off, I don't know what I am saying, the words are a dead man drumming. Then I've said it. Cancer. I've got cancer. Instantly, Reuben folds into me, his lithe body covering half of me. He sobs, heaves. Bassy gets up, comes round to his brother's side. 'RooRoo,' he whispers, using the nickname he had for his big brother when he was a toddler. It is a magic spell now; he is using it to get back to somewhere safe. He wraps himself over his big brother, so that, piled up, we look like we are playing sardines. Bassy does not cry. He is very still.

'It's all right,' I say. 'I'm going to be all right.'

Richard starts talking, very loudly and very fast. I hear words like hospital and chemotherapy and radiotherapy. I turn to him sharply, willing him to stop spouting these treacherous words.

'Don't glare at me like that,' he says.

My God, I think, we are going to argue. He is telling them too much, propelling them into a future that is medicalised and scary, so I say, louder than him, I am going to be fine, over and over. We are like characters in a play, not hearing each other, trying to change the way things are with words. But words are shifting shadows of reality. Facts are fixed.

'Can we watch TV now?' asks Bassy, getting up. Reuben's sobbing is steady now. I draw him closer, my exposed heart open to the elements.

6

FROM THE OUTSIDE IN

Nine months before she died, Mother wrote her will, making her stepson our guardian. You'd think she would have chosen her twin sister – married, with no children of her own. But she believed in her stepson, our father's son from his first marriage, in a way she did not believe in her twin. She thought the world of him. They had been in close contact since our arrival from America. So she asked him to be our guardian, even though he was a twenty-seven-year-old travelling journalist, not long back from reporting the Vietnam War, and with a small son and family difficulties of his own. I have often wondered how she expected him to cope with such a monumental responsibility. I suspect she felt it was her duty both to keep us from her twin's clutches and to keep us on the privileged trajectory she and Father had set us on. And why did he accept? He liked our mother very much, he wrote to me many years later. He felt it was a courageous decision on her part and he also accepted for Father's sake, he said, and because he felt it was his duty.

My maternal grandmother might have been another option, but she was seventy-one, so there wasn't much mileage in her. I always assumed that was why we did not live with her. What she did offer was very good pastry, which she used to make blackberry and apple pie, and a natty dress sense. She was still wearing denim skirts and bold blouses and, wherever possible, a hat or big sunglasses, sometimes both, and gold chains with lockets at the end. She used to be a milliner and though she measured in at five foot, tops, she wore her big hats over hair that was more golden than grey. She wore a dark blue felt fedora in winter and, in summer, a straw hat. Her lipstick ignored the seasons. It was always candy pink. She smoked long, thin cigarettes in brown paper called More, and her fingernails flashed with daubs of red varnish. Each nail must at some stage have been fully covered with varnish, but I only remember them in their chipped glory reaching for her ration of Green Shield stamps from a shopkeeper or for her bottle of snuff from her handbag. She brewed tea in novelty teapots – thatched cottages, Winston Churchill driving a tank, his helmeted head the lid – and served it in white china cups with gold edging. The tea often came with a thick slice of fresh white bread and butter, the butter pasted over and on top of itself like oils on canvas. After drinking tea, I think eating was what she loved best. She was always popping Liquorice Allsorts into her mouth or tucking into ice cream and wafer sandwiches.

When we first came over from America she lived in a bungalow with a husband – our grandfather – but no fridge. She would buy a block of vanilla ice cream from her local parade of shops and bring it home wrapped in newspaper, carrying it in a net bag that drooped from the weight like one of her pear drops. She'd cut the buttercup brick, placing a slice between rectangular wafers, and then suck it, as if she had no teeth. The end of the wafer would turn soggy and change colour and taper into a bird's beak. I spent days of my childhood sitting opposite her, watching her eat her ice-cream sandwiches, the black mole on her upper lip occasionally disappearing beneath a blob of vanilla, and trying to work out the nature of her breasts, which were in the wrong place, low down near her waist. Everything shook when she snored. The mole, her tiny torso, Winston Churchill in his china tank. Her pink lips puffed up and down and made a putting sound that quickly built up to a helicopter with hiccups.

Grandfather grew blackberry bushes under netting and beans on poles in the back garden. Once we let off a firework and it chased him along the path that went down by the side of the house and made his knobbly knees go up and down like a piston. He was Scottish, though nothing about him indicated what this might mean, and he had been a language teacher. He had a list of things to teach me, which he kept in his head. By the fireplace in the front room he taught me how to play chess, tell the time and swear in German. *Dummkopf!* he would say and my own head would burst from giggling. Out on our walks on the South Downs he taught me how to identify the butterflies that somehow knew when he was coming and flew about us or alighted on gorse bushes just so we could look at them. He showed me how to peel an apple in one continuous strip that, once it fell, kept on curling, as if searching for the fruit it had just been protecting.

When we walked, his tread was firm and purposeful. He was a tall man and in the bungalow he was bent. Out on the Downs he unfurled, charging down the path behind the church with its diamond tower and up Nore Hill and on to the flat so that you had to run every now and then to catch up. I used to have to do that with Father, too. Grandfather made you notice things you never otherwise saw, not just the butterflies but birds he knew by name, and the bursts of purple flowers, each a mass of fingers curled in on themselves as if holding something precious. As he strode, he sang, usually 'I'll take the high road and you'll take the low road.' His voice was deep and he sang out. I joined him and together we worked the rhythm of the song with the rhythm of his stride and each time we got to the chorus and the climactic 'On the bonnie, bonnie banks of Loch Lomond' we were booming. But because Grandfather had magical ears, he heard the birds' songs, even so. Hear that? See that? And I had to stop to hear and turn to see the skylark already on its way and the Red Admiral now a black line in the cornflower sky. Mother used to drop us off to stay with Grandma and Grandfather and on the morning she came to get us, Grandma would put our hair in curlers and take us out on the bus with them still in so the curls had time to set. Sure enough, when Mother arrived we looked our best.

Mother had died in August, which was handy as far as term times went. There were only a few weeks to go before we had to be back at school in early September. Plans were being made for us to move to London with my half-brother, into the house he had already bought months before Mother's death in anticipation of looking after us. In the interim we stayed with his mother, Father's first wife, in her big house in a village in the Sussex countryside, and it was there we went for our first exeat weekend and half-term post-Mother. Father's first wife had married an Englishman three years after her divorce. At the time, I had no idea how extraordinary it was for her to have her ex-husband's children to deal with, or how it felt to her husband, once an army major. They had two children, both of whom felt like adults to me, confident and gregarious. When their son took my sister and me up to London Zoo and carried me on his shoulders, I thought he was a gentle giant, and an old one at that. It turns out that when we appeared from nowhere he was only sixteen or seventeen, and his sophisticated big sister was only eighteen or nineteen. Our arrival must have been pretty odd for them, and for my half-brother and half-sister, too. The whole thing was what grown-ups would call unsatisfactory, a muddle, a case of making-do when really nothing satisfactory could be done. One day I put on my best dress, the wine-coloured polyester one I wore for Mother's funeral. Richard Williams was coming to take my sister and me out for lunch. I waited by the front door of the Regency house for the sound of his wheels on the gravel. The appointed hour came and went. I walked down the drive to the gate, in case he hadn't wanted to come up to the house and was waiting in the country lane. But he never showed up, and he didn't call either, and I went back inside.

The Sussex house was an old vicarage and it hummed with its own rhythms and routines and ways of doing things. If you went into the drawing room, as the living room was known, before the house had yawned itself awake, the embers of the previous night's fire would be gone and a new one would have been laid while the house was sleeping. Logs stretched across the grate, sitting on twists of newspaper, waiting for a match. Then the house would stir and breakfast would be prepared, served in the dining room. Scrambled eggs and tiny sausages waited in silver containers on the sideboard. You put whatever you wanted on your plate, which in my case was as little as possible to cut short the ordeal of being in the dining room at all, and then went and sat down at the shiny wooden table. Cold toast waited in triangles in a silver rack. The butter was pounded into a ramekin and had ridges across it like a ploughed field. If you got down to breakfast too late, the food would have vanished.

The house had a main staircase just right for swanning down if you had changed for dinner like the grown-ups did and a narrow back staircase for charging up and down and accessing the other end of the house. The nursery was at this end, and so was the annexe where Ana, the cook, and Lucio, her husband, lived with their young daughter who had short curly hair and never came into the house. Now and again my sister and I were taken into their flat, accessed by the door that we would otherwise never open, to say hello and the little girl would be there. Ana and Lucio were from Portugal and one day they were going to return and build themselves a mansion.

Lucio was short and dapper and rather glamorous. He had dark hair with shorter, tighter curls than his daughter and always wore a white jacket and black trousers with polished black shoes. His wife had big hips and, aside from those rare moments spent with her in her flat, I only ever saw her in the functional kitchen that was three times the size of the one at Marine Gate. I had a child's palate, and an American one at that. The only vegetable I liked was cucumber, sliced, with the seeds cut out of the middle. Ana's cooking, with its creams and purées and chicken bereft of bright orange breadcrumbs filled me with dread. Mother had told us to eat what we could, and since we knew what we were eating, our plates usually ended up clean enough. And if they weren't one could ask for clemency, knowing it would be granted. But now we often ate in the house of strangers and uneaten food caused offence; I knew I had to force everything down. I heaved a lot. Not on Christmas Day, though, when Ana cooked a mighty turkey. She got up in the dark to put the dog-sized bird in the oven. It emerged hours later, succulent and delicious. We had seven Christmases in that house and it always buzzed with talk of Ana, what a feat the cooking of the turkey was, how amazing she was. But I hardly ever saw her; I rarely even went into the kitchen.

At lunch and supper, or what in our new world we called dinner, we sat down and waited for Lucio to serve us. The first time he stood on my left-hand side and offered me a bowl of vegetables I turned my upper body towards him and reached out for the serving spoon and fork as I had seen everybody else do. I had been watching to see how it was done. The adults kept talking as they scooped up whatever was in the bowl, a momentary glance all they needed to locate the spoon and fork, then there was a quick nod at Lucio, a nod back. They made it look easy. But when it came to my turn I was nervous. I needed to get this right, I needed to get everything right now.

Our survival depended on it. Lucio held the dish out for me. I reached out, immediately fumbled. The serving fork was on the left and the spoon was on the right. Left-handed, I had to get the spoon into my left hand. Everybody's eyes were on me – the inconvenience, the bother who did not belong here. I felt self-conscious all over, in my toes, my stomach bog pit, my pink-flare face. When you stick your fleshy tongue out to receive Communion and there is the panic that the priest might put the wafer too far back and you'll have to rasp your throat and roll your tongue back on itself to shift it somewhere so you don't choke, that's how it felt. Only worse. Lucio remained quite still and gave no indication of either impatience or disdain. After a moment, he picked up the spoon and moved it to the left of the fork.

Cutlery remained a stumbling block. Mother had always told us we had good manners, but now it seemed she had been wrong. I knew about putting my knife and fork together when I had finished eating, but that was about it. I didn't know that if you wanted more you turned your fork upside down, that it was alright to flatten a cluster of peas with the prongs and then bring the victims up to your mouth, and I was very slow on the uptake when it came to knowing which knife, fork or spoon to use. They were laid out in columns on either side of the plate. The adults never dithered. They grabbed their cutlery and launched in. I dithered, waiting to see whether they would use the big knife or the small knife, the spoon on the right or the spoon that sat above the plate, handle facing left. Then, one glorious, sun-filled, life-changing day, a lunch guest saw me hesitating and she whispered: 'You know, there's a trick to this. It's terribly simple. You work from the outside in.'

I left the Sussex house with a passion for croquet and a sense that things were about to change all over again. There had

been talk about us moving to London and now here we
were, my brother, sister and I, filing into a tall Georgian
terraced house in Islington. It was joined to the identical
houses either side of it with invisible seams, little to tell them
apart save for the colour of the front doors and the lives
within. The long windows had panes divided into squares
and got shorter the closer to the sky you got. Some of the
gateways had swirls of wrought iron overhead and they all
had spiky black railings to stop you from tumbling into the
basements. There were huge trees, lamp posts shaped like
Narnia lanterns and, at one end of the vast square, a
playground and tennis courts.

The tall house had a staircase that kept going up. I followed
it right to the top, where the ceilings were lower and the windows
were set back like sunken eyes. This was to be our own floor,
and we were sharing it with the nanny, who hardly spoke. As
we walked in and out of the empty bedrooms, we were told we
could choose our own wallpaper, which was intended as a treat
but felt like another opportunity to do the wrong thing. I suspect
we seemed ungrateful, think we sulked and skulked, definitely
tried everybody's patience. Downstairs was for the grown-ups.
It was the early Seventies: black, glittery, feathery Biba had
opened on Kensington High Street and the Rolling Stones were
all lips and riffs. That's how Downstairs felt to me: funky and
fearless and out of bounds. Downstairs, no one did the humming
bits in Lee Marvin's husky 'Wand'rin' Star' or got excited about
Shirley Bassey and Harry Secombe on TV. Cocktail hour with
Mother in her wig, plucked eyebrows and swirly-print maxi
dresses and us staying up in our nighties was history. Now it
was David Bowie questioning life on Mars and Mick Jagger
singing the sadness in Angie's eyes in long, twisted vocals that
made Mother's favourite song, John Denver doing 'Leaving on
a Jet Plane,' sound like choirboy antics. There was wood on
the floor now and the doors were made of it too, grainy wood

that looked like shaved tree trunks with bits in. Floppy cushions with miniature mirrors sewn into the fabric lay about on low, languorous sofas and people with curly hair and long limbs came in and out, forever puffing all manner of smoke into the singular air.

This new existence was short-lived and we were back at the Sussex house within a matter of months. It felt like we were creating fissures in other people's lives, lives which already had fissures running through them, as adult lives do, of course. I didn't know that then and presumed that, until we came along, the landscape was intact and that it was the three of us who sent fault lines zigzagging across it.

Determined as my half-brother had been to look after us, it was too much and my father's first wife sought an alternative solution: someone else to look after us, long-term. But who? On 8 November 1973, three months after Mother died, a carefully worded advertisement was placed in *The Lady*, the weekly women's magazine that has been running classified advertisements for butlers and housekeepers, nannies and gardeners since 1885. Two decades later, my half-brother, who had kept both the advertisement and the fifty or so replies, asked me if I wanted to have them.

THREE RECENTLY ORPHANED CHILDREN

need kind, loving, cheerful and intelligent lady (can be single, divorced or widowed) or married couple in 30–50 age group to make a home for them.

All three bright and very rewarding. Boy (15), shy, articulate, bookish; girls (10 and 9), musical, interested in horses, gardening, sophisticated for age. All at Sussex boarding schools.

Accommodation in East Sussex (possibly in wing of country house near guardian's parents) provided.

Guardian and his parents wish to stay in close but non-interfering contact.

A wage is to be paid but essential requirement for successful applicant is ability to create happy family atmosphere for children to return from school.

Box 7893.

'Perhaps you could let me know wages,' writes a butler's wife from Banffshire, Scotland. If the price is right, she is prepared to make the move down south. 'It is not easy to know how to respond to the advertisement,' writes a mother of three who, unaccustomed to life in service, is less pragmatic. She has a big house filled 'with a great deal of noise and activity', she is 'VERY bookish!', '2nd son – musical, and hopefully going to choir school. 3rd son – artistic and takes ballet lessons – hopefully a budding Nureyev!' The first child doesn't get a mention, so presumably has no accomplishments.

'Have you found someone to love the three children yet?' writes another. 'I can't get them out of my mind.' She and her husband 'do not drink or smoke, we have a healthy respect for all religions, and a deep & personal belief in God. We are vegetarians and love animals – our daughter lives at Windsor Castle, and looks after the Queen's horses . . . My husband was with an advertising agency. Then he ran the Human Rights Society . . . You may have seen me as Mrs Brown in the French film *Anne & Muriel*, directed by François Truffaut?'

I haven't, but suddenly I am fantasising about *la vie de bohème* we might have had with these humanitarian vegetarian *intellectuels*, François dropping round of an evening, all of us in black polo necks, sipping red wine from tumblers in a fog of existential smoke rings. But then I read on. 'We have many interests and I have had experience with old ladies, mental patients, cripples, the blind, & prisoners.' Orphans would have rounded off her list quite nicely. 'Life,' she adds, 'is full and rewarding.' In the fifty-plus letters of application, experience of the disabled, a love of animals and a compulsion to do good are common threads. As a charity proposition, we offer a bonus ball – we pay. The position is one of upmarket fostering. One couple has a son of their own and two girls they adopted after the mother died and the father left them in an orphanage and went off to Australia. Why would they take us on? What sort of people are they? Big-hearted, evidently, and I still scorn them.

Rather them than the couple from Bristol 'of good education & smart appearance & approach'.

'We hold a joint position at a large Public School for boarders in charge of the dining halls & welfare of the pupils age [*sic*] from 11 to 18 years. Previous positions held are:
– Housekeeper & Steward to the Vice Chancellor of the [*sic*] Bristol University.
– Housekeeper & Butler to the British Ambassador & family in the Middle East
– Housekeeper & Butler to Henry Ford II & family.'

From an ambassador and a car magnate to lowly orphans – could they endure the comedown? They might wreak their resentment on us; it would be like being thrown to Aunt Sponge and Aunt Spiker.

Autonomy is what appeals to Frustrated from Twickenham, working at the time of application in 'such a post' as the one advertised 'in the house of an MP'. There are three children in her charge; she names each of them, and their schools, in the case of the boy, a famous one. 'I understand all their needs & ailments and give them a happy home & atmosphere to live in. When I am in full charge, we are one happy family.' The

emphasis falls on the 'when' like a claw on the shoulder. 'The
Parents,' she continues with viperous capitalisation, 'have been
away twice – on 4-monthly world tours & many shorter periods.
My problems start when Mummy & Daddie [*sic*] return, spoiling
the children in every way, undoing all my hard work. The
children at once start playing everyone up. It's most frustrating
for me & so bad for the children. I feel I am patient & happy
& want to stay so. However, I feel this cannot continue . . .
I would rather leave before trouble begins.'

I fear it already has.

Alan Bennett would hang moving monologues off these
applications. I, defensive, see only dimwits and losers. 'My
furniture is in storage in Ventnor,' proffers a widow with an
eleven-year-old daughter, working as a secretary on the Isle
of Wight. Perhaps Ventnor is an upmarket storage facility,
and she mentions it in the hope it will reflect well on her.
A housekeeper working on the Arundel estate writes that
her gardener husband 'takes sandwiches and can't face the
cotton-wool bread' and so 'I decided to make my own.' She
owns a knitting machine. 'We had a Wool-shop once,' she
notes in brackets. A fifty-year-old from Dorset is 'very lonely
and want[s] more than anything to be needed.' She can
back off. A divorcee reduced to working in a boarding school
and with no home for her children wonders if it might be
possible to 'merge my needs with the obvious great need of
the three children?' No. It might not. Needs. Need. I don't
want these briers sticking to me. A 'school from school', she
says, 'is no alternative to the happy home atmosphere one
seeks to give any child who spends eight months of the year
in school'.

The next applicant is straight out of a Victorian novel. She
outlines her marriage in order to explain her suitability, and
availability. 'I married the man I loved on his conditions.'
What a dread juxtaposition: love and conditions. Those

conditions were that they would not have children since the husband already had a son by his former wife. Nine godchildren, their siblings and being 'lent' friends' children have served as surrogates. 'I seem to be Auntie to everyone!' Meanwhile, the man she loved has had a change of heart. 'Seven months ago, my husband quite suddenly decided he was a loner & didn't want to be married any more. I am recovering from the shock & trauma & understand that so many men of his age feel like this . . .' They still live together, unable to afford to live separately. 'Apart from the loss of my husband, I think my greatest grief is that I shall have no one of my own to look after.' Well, you're not having us. Only someone who needs to love would take on someone else's children, obviously. I do not want to be the stuffing that fills the gaps in a stranger's heart.

'My dear young people,' begins a former occupational therapist in the final letter, 'I wonder whether your guardian showed you the very well worded advertisement in *The Lady* which told a little about you all, and the very sad reason why you need someone to help make a home for you.

'After looking at the ad I wondered a great many things about you all – what you were really like (the inside person I mean, that has the feelings, not just the polite outside one shows to strangers).' How distasteful. 'What are the things you really want in the person who will try to see you through the rest of your growing-up years?' Then, just in case addressing the three of us directly isn't cringeworthy enough, she decides to tell us 'something about myself, and why I am writing this letter, so that you and your guardian can think about whether I might be the sort of person you are looking for'. Three typed pages later she's detailed her marriage to a Canadian, their divorce, the death of her sister-in-law and taking on the care of the brain-damaged baby nephew, bringing him and her daughter to England, the daughter's 'ghastly' grammar school and how the nephew 'looks on me as his real mother now'. The brother, meanwhile, has fallen in love and wants his son back. 'I shall soon be a "spare" Mum looking for a family.' Have us, then: any 'mum' will do. She lists her uninteresting interests, which include going to places 'where history is made' (has she actually noted our ages?) and recommends a 'Family Council (the only way to run a household of any kind is on democratic lines). Trying to make a household run smoothly so that everyone puts in some work, and gets some of their own needs met is a real challenge.' Indeed. Then she moves on to 'the growing-up process'. 'The oldest of you is already into adolescence, and you two girls will be starting in a few years . . . Some people find it a lot more painful than others.' That's enough of that, thank you.

While my half-brother sifted the applications, he was also pursuing the possibility, mentioned in the advertisement, of us moving into the wing of a country house. The country pile was a wonderful thing with at least six roofs and endless windows. I'd have to draw the Ditchling house over and over to make it compete for size. There were sheep in the garden that was more like a park and the grass kept going until it met the South Downs, which rose up around it like a fur collar. The house, called Firle Place, was in the same village as the Sussex house and, as well as visiting over Christmas, we sometimes went for tea, or to spend the day. The lady who lived there was called Diana and she had something about her: not just warmth, a good line in cardigans and the title of viscountess, but an air of freedom and fun that whistled through the stone house and made it feel soft. She devoted hours to teaching my sister and me Racing Demon, the favourite of all her card games. No one cleared a croupette faster and she taught us a fast hand. I remember the thwack of the cards hitting the green baize and the excitement of shouting 'Out!' at the top of our voices.

Diana had offered us an apartment in a wing of the house. She and her husband the viscount didn't want rent, suggesting only that we might pay for the architect and alterations my half-brother had already identified. My half-brother was pleased, noting that we would live in considerable style. But the legalities of the arrangement turned out to be complex, and included issues of tax and questions of remuneration for capital improvements. My half-brother was also concerned by the fact that the tenure would be unsecured. The estate's lawyers had advised that 'the Fox children and their governess could with safety only be that of guests for an extended period'. In the event of the viscount dying, we would most likely be given six months' notice. The lawyers also noted that an approved governess must be in place by the time we took up residence. My brother duly explored an alternative in which his 'very charming orphaned dependants', as he described us, rented or bought a property on the nearby Glyndebourne estate, home to the bucolic opera house; its owners were close friends of my half-brother's family.

We had already spent time there, and would do so over the next few years. I met my first pug at a Glyndebourne Christmas tea party. It rescued me from Denis Healey and I've had a soft spot for these snuffling, much-maligned mutts ever since. The tea party was in the seventeeth-century manor house and I found myself struggling to make conversation with a big, baggy man sitting next to me, his eyebrows bushier than Basil Brush's tail, only pitch black and frazzled, as if he had just had a fright. Struck dumb by his appearance and my shyness, I saw no escape, until one of the family pugs came along. It stood in front of the Shadow Chancellor, glanced up at him and then reached out a paw and tapped his shiny black shoe as if it was telling him off for something. He guffawed, I giggled and we both relaxed into conversation.

My brother fared less well when, the three of us standing on the touchline before the beginning of the traditional Boxing Day football match, one of the players came up to him and put a whistle in his hand. Males of various ages ran about kicking the ball to each other, in teams of course, heading for their respective goals. I may not have been sporty, but I knew the basic rules. One team goes one way, the other goes another. The rules seemed to be lost on my brother, who blew the whistle at random. In the end, the players, a friendly lot, couldn't stand the chaos and he was stood down. My sister and I squirmed. It didn't do our image any good at all. Nor did mezzo-soprano Janet Baker when she paused, mid aria, during a rehearsal to ask if those in the stalls could please shut up. All eyes were on my sister and me. How, she asked, could she be expected to continue with the racket we were making? We often sat in on those rehearsals. It was a novel way to spend our time and meant that live opera was never anything to be frightened of, providing there wasn't a diva in the house.

The other novelty about the Glyndebourne visits was Nanny Parkin, who had also been nanny to Father's first wife's children by her second marriage and now looked after the Glyndebourne children. The children called her Nanny Parkin, and so did the adults. I thought that was very odd and somehow infantilising, for her and the other adults. Nanny Parkin had various children in her charge but she took us under her wing as if we were just three more additions and no bother at all. We were often at the top of the house or down in the nursery, as kitchens often seemed to be called, having tea, which meant supper, with her looking after us all. One of the children was the same age as me, or a bit younger, and she was very friendly and open and quite happy to let me join in with whatever she was doing, which often included riding her enormous horse. Once she even let me take the chunky carthorse out on my own. I could barely get it to move, and on my return pretended that we had charged up the bridle path and out into the open countryside when in fact we had only got as far as the gate leading to the bridle path at a plod. The gate was closed. Opening it required me to get the horse to walk into it, lunge at the catch and, pulling the gate open, simultaneously get the horse to reverse. I could not do this. Defeated, I turned around. Back in the stable, I made like a Pony Club girl and removed the tack and brushed the horse down. Within seconds I became sandwiched between its mighty belly and the stable wall. I thought I was going to be flattened to death. When I eventually freed myself, I walked back across the field, the manicured lawns of Glyndebourne's back garden ahead a comforting sight. But I couldn't reach the house. A ditch deep enough to swallow two dozen divas cut me off, and I had to find a different route back. One of the grown-ups later told me that the invisible trench was called a ha-ha. It was just about the best word I had ever heard.

While a place for us to live was explored further, polite rejections were written to most of the *Lady* applicants. One or two were subjected to an initial telephone interview with my half-brother – who somehow managed to attend to such matters in between reporting from war zones, interviewing rock stars and attending to his own family – and were duly rejected. 'A person has to be chosen with great care,' he wrote to the Glyndebourne family when sounding out the housing possibilities there. In fact, he did have one person in mind. But where we lived remained a work-in-progress. A cottage on the Glyndebourne estate was not an option and the Firle Place trustees eventually declared us unsuitable tenants. The generous offer was reluctantly withdrawn and in the interim we stayed on in the guest bedroom at the Sussex house with my half-brother's mother.

I sensed there was something exceptional about her, and that confused me because my grandmother and aunt cast her as a wicked witch, their words against her slowly-poured poison in my ear. She was a Bad Woman; that's what our aunt said, over and over. She offered no specifics and her language was sloppy; it got sloppier, and toxic, after a few whiskies, so I never knew what made Father's first wife bad. I adopted a policy of mistrust, to keep myself covered. In her dealings with us, Father's first wife was kind, and driven, I think, by a mother's instinct to help her son to manage his own life less encumbered. In the Christmas holiday she took us up to London to stay in her Chelsea apartment near Sloane Square. We went to the movies and for shopping excursions. My half-sister – Father's eldest child – sometimes met up with us for tea at Peter Jones. There are several pictures of her on my UK moodboard, each quite different from the others, so that sometimes it's hard to think of her as the same person. In one, a black and white photograph taken by Lord Snowdon, which hung at Marine Gate, the Brighton apartment block we lived in with Mother, she is a quietly smiling, beautiful teenager in a rugged polo neck sweater, artfully examining the cracks on a bare wall with her index finger, the better to show off her fine profile and high cheekbones. In another, she is a striking debutante standing at the foot of a swirling staircase, one hand on the banister. She is wearing the pearl and sapphire choker she would leave to my sister and a white ball gown with short, puffy sleeves, her dark brown hair pulled back over her luminous face, her blue eyes looking out, sparkling into a world in which she is still, for now, engaged. I look at the photograph and, rewinding the clock, I think, which gentleman will be lucky enough to have the first dance?

In the portrait of her she hung above the mini fridge and kettle in her bedroom in the halfway house for sufferers of poor mental health she lived in in Chelsea, she isn't looking out, she isn't looking down, she is just being. She does not see, does not want to be seen; a liminal figure on a Louis XIV chair whose arms do not embrace her or provide comfort, her entwined hands rest on her mustard-coloured skirt. There is no sense of movement, no sense that she has just sat down, or might soon be off somewhere. She cuts the figure of a young woman with no sense of entitlement, no claim on the world. Her schizophrenia robbed her of a full life.

When she boiled the kettle, the steam shot up over the painting. She knew it did, and she didn't mind, as if the damage to the painting by Bloomsbury artist Duncan Grant, a family friend, was of no consequence. She didn't like the painting. 'I look like I am away with the fairies,' she once told me and I didn't know how to reply. It was such a sad thing to say, and I wondered if, and this was an alarming thought, she had a sense of her self before the voices took up residency in her head, before the treatments started, the round of ECT, the first dose of medication that made her jaw lock. As a child, I knew her only as withdrawn and frail and brittle. At the Sussex house she had the same bedroom she had had as a child and she was often alone in it. On occasion I visited her and when I stepped from the hall into her room, it felt lonely and wrong. It felt like a child's room, and she wasn't a child. Sometimes she went away, to a hospital or a clinic, and we went to visit her and she was so skinny it was haunting, her wordlessness also all wrong, and everything about her felt lonelier still.

I enjoyed the trips up to London with my father's first wife. There was a solitaire game on the coffee table in her apartment, its base and the balls made of marble. One morning, kneeling down as I played, loving the softness of the carpet, and the light all around me, I realised that, in this moment, I was happy. This was confusing, and it joined other feelings that kept ambushing me just when I thought I was holding steady. I liked Father's first wife, very much, and I knew that this wasn't right – she was related to us, but only indirectly and for all the wrong reasons, and we were with her for all the wrong reasons.

One day we were introduced to a woman called Tamsin who lived a street or two away from Peter Jones in a narrow house in a narrow street. We had tea with her. She had brown hair, wore pearls and the sort of skirt that the housemistresses at school wore. Her hands were very big, bigger than I knew a woman's hands could be, and she wore a large round watch on her wrist, a man's watch. Her house was too small for her stature, as if she were a giant in a doll's house. There was a desk at one end of her rectangular living room. It had a series of cubbyholes, like a warren, and a letter-holder made out of papier mâché and painted with tiny flowers. At the other end of the room was a fireplace with a tapestry fender and, like everywhere we went now, small tables with objects displayed on them: glass paperweights, silver picture frames, trinket boxes, china dogs in pairs, their bodies facing each other but their heads turned outwards. By the fire was a small chair that sloped on the sides. It didn't have any arms, and the back and sides had dimples in them with buttons on top. Its proportions were right for the room, but not for Tamsin. We did so many visits and met so many new people that it was always a relief to get away. But now we kept being taken back to this particular house, first for tea and then for lunch that was prepared in advance in the tiny basement kitchen.

After dinner on the first Christmas Eve of our new life, everybody gathered in the living room of the Sussex house. My half-siblings' stepfather was installed in an armchair, his dress shoes that looked like slippers firmly on the ground, a book in his hands and the Christmas tree lit with real candles flickering behind him. My sister and I sat on the floor in front of the fire, not knowing what was going to happen next. And then the room fell silent and he began reading 'The Night Before Christmas'. I had never heard the poem before but the deepness of his voice felt just right for it and so did his dark eyebrows and the inky night outside. When, years later, I decided to read the poem to my own children, I noted where I was plucking the tradition from, and felt I was drawing from the wrong well. And then

I thought, it's a poem to be shared, my half-siblings' stepfather was always kind and I have such cheering memories of him reading it, and so I gave myself permission to appropriate it.

Later that night, after we had gone to bed, I was woken by the door being inched open. My sister and I were in the guest bedroom, as usual. It had twin beds and, in front of the window, a dressing table completely different to Mother's, this one shaped like a kidney with glass on the top and flowery fabric that matched the curtains that were so full and swishy they should have been swirling on a ballroom floor.

If you drew the curtains back – which you couldn't do by pulling them across, only by tugging on a wooden handle on the end of a piece of rope – you would see the tight lawn on which we learned to play croquet, neat and ready. To the right, the garden wall covered in roses. In the middle of the wall, the arched secret-garden, white wooden door. This led to the smaller walled garden of sprouting, spreading vegetables, which, in turn, led to the next garden with the swimming pool. Far to the left, the lawn loosened up and the trees gathered in clusters like old men chatting. Near them was the mini house we used as a Wendy House and the grown-ups used for outdoor chairs or tools. Straight ahead, marking the boundary of the formal garden, was a wooden fence, just two parallel pieces of crooked brown wood with a gap between them so wide you could pass a sheep through it. The green of the lawn touched the untamed green of the South Downs Way that came tumbling down to meet it. When I had walked on the Downs with Mother and Libra I was walking part of a trail that led all the way here.

The bedroom door opened more fully. I scrunched my eyes into sneaky slits and watched as the tall figure crept in and put half a leg on the end of my sister's bed and another on mine. Then back out it crept. My eyes, accustomed now to the conspiratorial dark, patted the giant's sock, a rough woolly thing rammed with hard objects all the way down to the toes. Excited, I put my head on the pillow and went back to sleep.

In the morning, we woke to the stockings we had never had with Mother. Not knowing when we were supposed to open them, we asked our father's first wife and she said, open them in your room, so we did until our beds were covered in toys and toothbrushes and knick-knacks. And then we went down for breakfast in the dining room that didn't relax, not even on Christmas Day, and afterwards we went into the drawing room. Every chair and sofa, the ottoman too, was piled with presents. Two chairs had stacks higher than any other. We didn't open the presents right away. That's not how things happened. It was church next, a little old thing of dappled stone that matched the walls of the Sussex house, and I didn't know what to wear. I thought I would wear my red dress and, not knowing if that was a good idea, I wanted to ask and knew I shouldn't, knew I should do things on my own and stop pestering the adults. I could hear my father's first wife in her bedroom next door to ours and so I went and stood by her open door and I called her name. Then I went in and I said, shall I wear this dress, and she didn't make me feel like I was a bother and an irritation on this busy morning, only said, what a good idea, your red dress, yes, wear your red dress. I walked beside her as we crunched our way down the drive and turned right out of the gate and up the lane and into the little stone church. The pews had cushions hard as bricks hanging on hooks and everywhere there were adults in fat furry hats and children just like us in their best coats. There were carols, the same ones I had sung the year before and the year before that, and in a sense everything was the same and also so very different that I wondered when it would ever go back to how it was before.

The two armchairs piled with the most presents were for my sister and me. There must have been a chair with a big pile of presents for my brother too, but it was my sister to whom I was joined like a branch to a tree and so I mostly saw things in relation to the two of us. Besides, my brother did things his way as he was old, fifteen already, and I was never alone with him, in a new bedroom, say, or a stranger's hall or back at boarding school, negotiating the new ways together or at least just being together in them, as I was with my sister.

Some time after Christmas we drove up to London again, to stay a night or two with Tamsin in her narrow house. My sister and I were in the back of the car and my father's first wife was in the passenger seat, her husband, the Major at the wheel. The sky was galaxy blue. Christmas tree lights sparkled in living-room windows. Carols were playing on the radio. We all sang along. It was cold outside and cosy in the car. 'The Little Drummer Boy' was the next carol and I sang up. It was one of Mother's favourites and I knew all the words. She must have sung it in America because I always thought it was an American carol, one that English people didn't sing. I was surprised to hear it, a sound from the old world. 'There's a lovely voice in the back,' said the Major. My sister was officially the singer, not me, and won all the school singing prizes. I was pleased to be praised. I got that happy feeling again; the glow of it took me off my guard.

When we went down into the basement of the narrow house, there was a list of what we liked to eat on the kitchen wall. Our overnight bags were in the dank dining room with the brown sofa that, it turned out, was also a double bed. We were staying.

7

BRIGHTON KNOCK

'How on earth did you find Tamsin?'

'We found her on the grapevine!'

'Oh, you are clever!'

I overhead the grown-ups' exchange and pictured the vine in Aesop's fables, the leaves hanging down, the juicy grapes just out of reach of the thirsty fox. A human on a vine did not make sense. I decided that Tamsin must have been hanging around like ripe fruit, waiting to be picked.

In a sense, I was right. Tamsin was not married and did not have any children. The chance to look after a clutch of orphans when all her contemporaries were married and her sister had a horde of children would balance things out. Also, she was from Sussex, as we sort of were, so there was no question of her upping sticks from somewhere far flung like Scotland or Devon, as some of the *Lady* applicants would have had to do, and she was Catholic. Perhaps, to outsiders, it seemed like a good match. She was the person my half-brother had had in mind when he was trying to sort out Firle Place. She wanted the job, he told me years later, and was a family friend.

Tamsin moved out of her dolly house and into a bigger one on the Brighton seafront, settled upon after the Firle Place option fell through. It was a tall white house in an all-white terrace that curved up a hill and had its mirror image in the crescent opposite. If you took a left at the top of the hill, you were in Kemptown and if you took a right, you would soon get to the gasworks that we could see from the back balcony of our old apartment in Marine Gate. The white house had black and white tiles on the stoop, a shiny big chessboard. Grandfather could have shown us some moves, no hurry, work out what to do next. The front door was a black solid ram of a thing, and on the other side of it was a clickety-clack hall leading to a wide staircase. Two flights up, there was a door on the right: in we went, into a flat that had its own staircase. Maisonette, the grown-ups said with a flourish, a maisonette in Lewes Crescent. But I knew *maison* was a house and that what we were living in now was a house cut in half, not all there.

Tamsin moved in ahead of us. She brought a big wardrobe with her and placed it, inappropriately, in the living room. I had been to Narnia many times in my imagination but that wardrobe was about as uninviting as an empty candy store and I never once looked in it. Nearly all the furniture was Tamsin's; most of ours had been sold, as had Mother's jewellery. Tamsin liked to sit opposite the big wardrobe in her undersized chair by the window and smoke a cigar – the occasional indulgence of an otherwise measured woman. She didn't have a record player. She put on the *Nine O'Clock News* and then, occasionally, she lit up, her knees to one side, her stiff body facing the fireplace and her head inclined towards the sash window overlooking the sea. If she were to raise the white roller blind and look out, what would she see? The coast road that took her east to her parents and to her sister, both living about half an hour away. The sticky black railings that kept non-residents out of the communal gardens and the gate opposite our front door that led into it, providing you had the special key to open it. The trees and shrubs and neat lawns within and, in the middle of the garden, an ivy hillock that concealed the entrance to the magic tunnel that went underneath the coast road and came out on to the beach. Did she venture down a rabbit-hole and see the three of us, me, my sister and her, ambling rather than dragging our way through the tunnel on a summer's day, one of her woven beach mats tightly rolled under our arms, picnic baskets and swimming togs as she called them and we didn't in our hands? Did she picture the ham sandwiches she had made and feel a rush of hope that the picnic would be different, that this would be the one where we laughed and swam and she, after everything was tidied away, would be able to call her sister to say that she and the Fox girls had had a *super* time at the beach?

When I looked out of my bedroom window, one across from the living-room window where Tamsin liked to sit, I too saw the coast road. The one we used to take with Mother. I saw the smaller road beneath it that flanked the sea, the same sea, maybe even the same brown and grey pebbles. It hadn't been that long since we'd walked on them together, she less than one year dead. Of course there had been storms since. I had seen what the sea got up to, how it reared up, lashed the shore, licked up the pebbles and the shingle, too. After retreating with its spoils, it came back and did the same thing all over again, spewing stones on the shore, dumping the rest on the sea floor. But supposing Mother had kicked off her shoes and edged her way, barefoot, over the pebbles, past the tar and black bladderwrack to the sea's edge; supposing she had curled her painted toes into the shiny shingle and let the lapping waves lick her feet before they made off with the shingle; it was just possible that some of that shingle could be on the beach now. If I crept out of the house and through the tunnel to the beach and took my own shoes and socks off, I could stand where she once stood, feel what she once felt; feel her. Feel her in my toes and in the sea spray on my upturned face. She was one year gone and I was ten now and she was still more part of my world than not part of it. But she was not tangible, and I was starting to lose the sound of her in my head.

So. Everything was the same when I looked out of my bedroom window. The crooked arm of the marina over to the left, the amber roofs of Volk's Railway, parked up at Black Rock. We used to ride the mini railway all the time, my sister and I, on our own, or with Mother and Grandma. Now and then we went to the Black Rock lido on the other side of the car park, too. It had a ladder you could climb down to get straight to the beach, and there were rock pools, shallow, the bright white water flashing with weeny fish shaped like apostrophes. Sea anemones stuck to the sides. For a dare, I would plunge my pinkie into the wriggly red, feel the squish of the squirming tentacle mouth. When the season came to an end, the Bathing Machine bar was boarded up and the water from the big pool and the paddling pool was emptied. The high diving board would bide its time and the flintiness in the grey air was just the way of things in winter and didn't make you lonely.

I don't think we ever went on Volk's Railway with Tamsin; I, for one, did not want Mother's memory contaminated, and riding the mini railway was something we loved to do together. My sister and I always tried to nab the very back seat of the second car, which faced outwards, and Mother and Grandma sat behind us, facing forwards, like everyone else. As my sister and I travelled backwards, the Seven Sisters cliffs pushed away into the distance until their chalk skirts blurred into a wall of white. Pebbles nestled alongside the skinny tracks on the beach side and a saggy mesh fence divided them from Madeira Drive, the lower beach road. When a car came alongside we cheered on the toytown train, willing it to speed up and outrun a car for once. But away it trundled, taking a break at the mini fun fair which had the worst Ghost Train on the south coast. Ten seconds in, the spider's spindly legs were on the back of your neck. All well and good. On a bit, and the Screaming Phantom lunged at you in the second before the wagon hurtled to the right. And then stopped. Every time. The trick then was to keep your fear up until the wagon got going again and the Cascade of Creeps fingered your face. But sometimes the lights came on instead and you had to not look at the peeling black paint or the Phantom that was just a toy mask on a stick and the strips of cotton that were the Cascade of Creeps and wait for the ticket man to push you through the double doors and into the daylight.

When we got down to the Palace Pier, we bought hot ring donuts and cotton candy that started out as a popsicle stick spinning on the inside rim of a metal pan and ended up as a puffy pink sugar cloud. Cotton candy, not candy floss. Popsicle, not lolly. We sat on the tiered benches in the aquarium that had the dolphin that jumped through a hoop, the same dolphin doing the same trick every time we went, the reward never the open sea. We went up to the window of Forte's the ice cream parlour and walked away with 99s or, in Grandma's case, just a swirl of vanilla, no chocolate flakes. She'd do her tongue-lip thing then: a lick of the bright white twirling tower and, when she came in for another, there would be a blob of undigested ice cream on the end of her tongue and on her upper lip by her black mole. I'd have to look away. Occasionally we went inside and sat at one of the shiny tables. Mostly we went to the Grand Hotel for afternoon tea, never the Royal Albion right on the roundabout, which was shabby and felt like a sinking ship.

Grandma loved ice cream. Mother and Richard Williams loved pubs, restaurants and, most of all, hotels. Tamsin loved – what? I don't know. Brighton in the early Seventies was in the vanguard of exotic culinary consumption from the Continent, as Europe was referred to. Wicker-bottled Chianti, avocado prawn, and cannelloni were the pinnacle of sophistication in a town that offered pockets of pleasure, not the saucy ones of its past, but boutiques, antique stores, bistros. The venues were small and the big fur coats and high hair that Mother favoured made them feel smaller still. My favourite was Al Forno, the Italian with the orange walls outside and the stone pizza oven and wooden tables inside. Mother's was Wheeler's, the tiny fish restaurant with bottled bow windows and fishing nets draped about the place and lobsters scaling the walls of their tanks. Mother always made a point of saying she wouldn't order any seafood. She said that shellfish did terrible things to her, which I thought was dramatic and heroic. Later, I would lie and say I was allergic to shellfish, puffing up with our shared secret yet to be borne out. I had never tried shellfish.

When Brighton's venues were exhausted, Mother tried further afield. There was a dismal place along the coast called Rottingdean. It had nothing but a windmill and Roedean, the Gothic girls' school on the cliff edge that Mother threatened to send us to if we were bad, and a hotel called The White Horse. It was painted the same pale yellow as Mother's car and was close enough to the sea to be pushed into it. Once, bored after lunch, my sister and I snuck upstairs and found a big room with different sized tables and tall lights with hourglass lampshades with their waists sucked in. We crawled under the tables, bringing the standard lamps crashing to the floor. A waiter appeared from nowhere, prodded us downstairs and displayed us in front of Mother like a brace of pheasants. He waited for her to reprimand us. Softly, she brought us round, and made us see we must apologise. We spent our last Christmas with Mother in a hotel, the Metropole in Brighton, a huge red building next to the Grand. During the day I fed coins into a glass box on a metal plinth filled with cuddly toys and steered a mechanical claw over

Tweetie Pies and mini gonks I never managed to pick up. In the afternoon I hung around the waiters, who knew me by name and let me help them put out the white tablecloths and lay the tables in the dining room. In the evening we dressed up and sat at a table in front of a stage where people in sequins did dances and sang and Mother and Richard Williams drank cocktails.

We didn't go out to hotels, restaurants or pubs with Tamsin. We were either with her in Lewes Crescent or visiting her family. Sometimes, when she was in her chair, I tried to imagine what it felt like, being her, this woman who smoked cigars and felt so impossibly huge and old. In fact, she was in her mid forties and only two years older than Mother. Her hair sat on her shoulders and flicked up at the ends like an upside-down candy cane. Sometimes she did tapestries, laying the canvas across her big knees and making zigzags with the wool. She made them into cushions. Hers seemed a strange life, a half life. We weren't her children and the house we lived in together wasn't, technically, her house. The maisonette had been bought with our money, and she still kept her house near Sloane Square. Sometimes I wondered if, as the advertisement in *The Lady* had suggested, 'she', as my grandma and my aunt referred to both Tamsin and my father's first wife, was being paid to live with us. I never asked. I hoped she wasn't, because then it was just possible she *wanted* to care for us, that she acted out of love, though of course she did not love us, since you cannot love three children you found on the grapevine. It was equally impossible for me, at any point, to get close to loving her; just liking her was hard enough. I never did manage it, and I am not proud of that. I was the peacemaker, the one who did not cause trouble, the one the grown-ups did not lose patience with, but I could not give her what she needed. I wish I could have done. She always felt utterly alien to me, and there was that whiff of need and dependence about her, and failure, too, all of which was a bit too *Jane Eyre* for my liking, a bit too close for comfort. In Brontë's novel there is that hideous scene in which the emotionless missionary St John Rivers, blinded by his determination to do the right thing, asks Jane to marry him as he needs a wife to accompany him on his mission to save souls in India. She does not love him, and declines. 'You might learn to love me,' he says, to which Jane replies: 'I scorn your idea of love.'

Before us, Tamsin had once been a paid companion to someone, travelling with them to Italy, or somewhere else in Europe, and that was very *Rebecca*, just without a future with Maxim de Winter. Paying for friendship, or being paid to bestow it, it was hard to imagine anything more pitiful – until she told us about her lap dog. The interbred creature, a Pekingese, slept on the end of her bed in the dolly house. One night, it fell off the end of the bed and died. Then there was the antiques dealer boyfriend, who died, and had in fact been gay. All of this she shared with us; all of this we stored up and used against her.

Paid or not, and I reckoned Tamsin must have needed money if she had gone to Italy with a total stranger, I tried to work out how bad a deal we really were. Tamsin got somewhere nice to live, somewhere her tribe approved of. *Maisonette*, they cooed. *Lewes Crescent*. Laurence Olivier, she would tell people, lives on Royal Crescent, just around the corner. I didn't know who Laurence Olivier was and, after discovering that he was a famous actor, still could not see any connection. He was certainly not a friend of Tamsin's. We were also away at school for most of the time, another fact that surely made us a good proposition. On paper, we were a win-win act of charity. But we turned out to be trouble. We didn't do what we were supposed to do, or like what we were supposed to like. When we refused to do something, Tamsin would lament, 'It's your funeral!', drawing the 'your' out into a wail before slumping on to the emphatic 'f' of funeral. We failed Tamsin by not behaving as we should have, and so her project, the orphan project, failed too.

Before we lived with Tamsin, *good eggs* on the grapevine had my sister and me to stay for exeat weekends. They put themselves out for us. And as we came up the drives of their country houses, I felt sure the whisper would have gone up: *They're here, the orphan Foxes are here.* When we stepped into the next new drawing room, the adults stiffened with resolve and the children we would shortly be sent off to play with eyed us up. Sometimes we pulled off the weekends, sometimes we didn't, though I tried to please as much as the adults who took us into their homes tried to please us. After we had been living with Tamsin for some time, a year perhaps, maybe two, the whispers changed. It was no longer a question of seeing what the orphan Foxes were like but of how we were *treating* Tamsin; we had agency now. How we were treating Tam? 'Tam' was the girlish diminutive her family used for her; it smacked of an unfathomable fondness.

In the holidays, Tamsin had started to yelp when an exchange turned viperous. *Don't be so beastly!* she would cry, stretching out the 'b' within an inch of its life. Her misery made me squirm like those squirming sea anemones. She made it seem as though my sister and I were ganging up on her whereas it felt as if she brought the misery on herself, a bit like Sheila Hemp did. Sheila was the other orphan at school. She arrived about two years after me, maybe three, and the pair of us were lumped together, orphans both and touchline tragedies too, she the dumpy unsporty one, me the skinny unsporty one. The team captains picked me second from last, Sheila last. She gave orphans a bad image. She wore embarrassing clothes and stood with her feet wide apart as though she were about to do a jumping jack. One day, a girl in the year above told another girl to give me her hamster. I had been admiring it in the pet room, so-called. It was a cupboard off the Science classroom. 'Why should I?' the girl protested. 'Because Genevieve lives with her grandparents,' the other girl said. But I didn't; Sheila did. Worse than people getting the facts wrong, which they always did, was the belief that, in other people's minds, Sheila and I were two of a kind, linked by loss and other people's pity. I envied Sheila: her parents were killed in a car crash. This was the expected orphan narrative and, growing up, I often wished I had it to fall back on. Parents die in car crash. Grandparents step into the breach. End of a clear-cut story.

Tamsin's presence in our lives was much harder to explain than a pair of whiskery grandparents in anoraks taking care of you. But we could see that *we* could be Tamsin's clear-cut story – and a success story at that – if only we could measure up to expectations. We failed, repeatedly. *Think of poor Tam, can't you?* an adult would say when we had *gone too far.* Sometimes, when something was *just not on*, they simply exclaimed, *Poor Tam!* Conversely, when they were praising her, her family would say, *Oh, Tamsin, you are such a brick.* A brick, I thought, used for creating and for destroying, for erecting walls and houses and for smashing windows. It was such an odd compliment.

Tamsin made great efforts to make us food we might like and to get us to eat food we didn't like. I don't think there was much on that first list on her kitchen wall in London, apart from ketchup. By the end of our time with her we were eating shepherd's pie and fish pie and grapefruit cut in half with white sugar sprinkled over the top. I already liked cucumber, frozen peas, frankfurters, Smash – a simulacrum of mashed potato made from dry powder that you mixed with water – and tinned mandarins. I suppose I must have eaten other things too. I loved gherkins, and peanut butter and jelly sandwiches, taken with a glass of cold milk. The nuns did not scare the word jelly out of me and to this day I won't say jam if the stuff is bedding down with peanut butter in a sandwich; it's an affectation, like saying popsicle instead of ice lolly, to signal an Americanness I otherwise show no signs of.

Before, at Marine Gate, the milkman delivered our favourite things, including milk and Tizer. Tizer was a bright red fizzy drink that came in glass bottles three times the size of the milk ones. Mother left all the empty bottles outside the apartment door and the milkman took them away again. She did the same with the sheets and the rest of the laundry, which came back in long, charcoal-grey boxes with metallic straps on. The milkman also delivered eggs, bread and butter. I have no recollection of Mother ever going to a supermarket or cooking a meal.

I do remember her taking us shopping, which she always turned into an outing. She took us to Hanningtons, the department store near Wheeler's, to have tea and buy tights. Hanningtons had aspirations. The outside was painted in the same old lady's knickers pale greeny-blue as the Victorian railings on the promenade and it flew navy blue flags from its first-floor windows. Two pillars formed its main entrance and it sat on the corner of two streets, North and East, its apex forming the prow of a proud ship. You knew you were going places if you shopped at Hanningtons.

Inside, all the departments merged into each other like the shop floor in the TV sitcom *Are You Being Served?* It had a caged elevator, operated by an attendant. From it you could look out over the counters as you ascended – one *ascended*, one never just 'went up' at Hanningtons – to the first and second floors. It was a *premier* department store, a destination. It had a Ladies' Powder Room and it had airs. Grandma, who liked to wear gloves with her hats and kept a golden powder compact in her clip-close handbag, liked that. A twirling staircase led up to the tea room on the mezzanine, which sounded prawn-cocktail exotic but mezzanine just meant another floor. The smell of hairspray on the saleswomen's updos mixed with the puffs of perfume from Cosmetics. Mother sometimes bought Grandma a bottle of her favourite perfume, Worth, which came in its own black, brushed velvet pouch, and she bought her Lily of the Valley soap, too. She said it made a change from the carbolic soap she and 'Dad', as she called Grandfather, had at home.

I avoided going to Hanningtons with Tamsin, avoided shopping with her whenever possible. To do so felt too intimate. I never noticed Mother's presence, or where she was in relation to me, whether she was beside me, at the other end of a counter, or somewhere in the distance. It would be like noticing the air. But with Tamsin, I was always conscious of her physicality, as well as her proximity to me. It made clothes shopping especially fraught, and when my choices did not meet with her approval, even more so. I did not want to have to seek her approval in the first place. But on one occasion, I selected a pair of denim dungarees from Woolworths decorated with red and white toadstools on the bib. She liked them too, and agreed to complete the outfit as I wanted, with a red T-shirt to match the stitching of the dungarees. I was pleased, and so was Tamsin. I was keenly aware that the shopping trip was a success, the usual friction giving way to contentment; enjoyment, even. But that's all it was: one successful shopping trip. It did not mean Tamsin finally had a foot in the door. The experience was not going to get banked.

The time spent on our return from America with Grandma and Grandfather did. They didn't have a television in their bungalow, which was near Worthing in Sussex, used open coal fires in small grates with tiled surrounds to warm the house, and kept the milk on the outdoor windowsill. The birds pecked at the silver foil lids and drank the yellow cream that settled on the top like poker chips. Grandfather listened to the radio and slept, alone, in the back bedroom. He is a snorer, Grandma said, as if snitching on a war criminal or a child-snatching neighbour. His snores pounded through the wall as my sister and I slept in the living room, and I wondered how this bony man with white whiskers could make such noises. He wore blue striped pyjamas and leather slippers and insisted on medicated transparent loo roll. Each perforated square had the brand printed on it in green. The squares did not crumple upon use, but crackled like greaseproof paper. Grandfather used to come out of his bedroom and cough on his way to the loo, a step or two across the hall, and cough on the way back. 'Stop coughing,' Grandma would shout, which seemed unkind. But he got the message. He was dead within a year, from shingles; not the ones you get on the beach, more like patches splatter-gunned on to his tracing-paper skin. Mother took us to visit him before he died. I hate hospitals, she said as we tailed after her down a lofty corridor. Grandfather's bed was in the middle of a row, like something from a war movie. On the first visit he was an angular, whiskered thing in his striped pyjamas and then he turned yellow, like dying people seem to do.

The doctor told Grandma to move straight after Grandfather's death, and to drink more Guinness. But she loved her pebbledash bungalow and she stayed put for as long as she could. Tamsin had driven us to stay with her once, opening the gate we all used when our world was Mother, the three of us, Grandma and Grandfather. She talked to Grandma on her own stoop, as if that were normal rather than an act of treachery. The house was stripped of its protective powers after that. Grandma's move to a seaside flat in a rectangular apartment block in Hove with no garden or any smell of Grandfather was just something else to get used to, and that included the central heating. Grandma kept it on high so that when we visited her on the bus – a straight line down the coast road from Lewes Crescent, past the public dog toilet as big as a sandpit with a little crenellated wall around it on the lawn of a Regency garden square – and sat on her new sofa and watched TV and ate cake, it was hard to keep awake, even when she was snoring.

Once she and my aunt took us to a summer fête up on the racecourse. I spotted Richard Williams in the crowd. His blazer and cravat and Clark Gable looks marked him out. Look, I said, my heart alert, look who it is! I wanted to go to him. Come this way, my aunt said, taking my arm and muttering something about 'that man' under her breath. They didn't take my sister and me with them the day they paid a special visit to Brighton cemetery, something sharp stashed in my aunt's handbag. They found Mother's headstone and gouged out her surname, Williams, and scratched Fox above it. It was their own way of preserving the past.

One afternoon, they met my sister and me at a tea shop in Hove. I don't remember it being cold but I do remember tiny Grandma standing on the pavement outside, a vision of pint-sized bling in a white fur coat. It was made up of horizontal bands of fur, with narrower bands of white suede in between, and was pulled in at the waist with a thick belt and a giant buckle. Topped with a matching hat, she looked like a show poodle. My aunt was in something dark and fluffy, teamed up with a matching handbag. They took us shopping. 'Have whatever you like,' my aunt said. 'We're going to spoil you.' Using money from the dead, I thought. My sister chose a long green velvet coat with huge lapels that flapped like elephant ears, and a pair of wooden platform sandals. I chose a tan raincoat and blue satin wedges. The coat was like a trainspotter's macintosh and the wedges were too high and not right for my age or my skinny legs. I wanted not to be allowed them. I knew my friend Louise's mother wouldn't allow her to have them. They marked me out. When I came back to Lewes Crescent with the new shoes, Tamsin raised a disapproving eyebrow. They are too high, she said. No, they're not, I snapped back.

Tamsin had a gun to her head. As my half-brother later wrote in a letter to me, once your parents die – whom no one can replace, everyone else feeling inadequate – there's an element of Russian roulette in terms of who tries to fill in even your day-to-day needs. Tamsin did her best, and never knew what her best would trigger. Then again, she might have guessed, given that she had overturned a law of nature, a law already affronted by Mother's death, by stepping forward to take her place. She did everything the wrong way, which meant not the way we were used to. Getting things wrong wasn't her fault, just as the fact of us living with her in the first place was nobody's fault. I spent a lot of time in my small bedroom, listening out for her, wondering what she would do next. My bedroom was at the foot of the stairs so I knew what she sounded like coming down them. One afternoon her tread was accompanied by a swishing sound. I was at my desk, adding a stamp of a giraffe to my half-baked collection, having decided to be normal and have a hobby, like other children. My fingers froze over the plastic mount. Swish swish. There was no mistaking the rustle of denim. I stuck my head round my bedroom door and sure enough, there she was, halfway down the stairs in a pair of flared blue jeans. She had new shoes, too: a pair of navy leather wedged espadrilles. What was she thinking of? Did she want to be modern, or *with it*, as she would say? Poor Tam, indeed. Now I look back and see she was cutting a dash.

I had a best friend from my Mother days called Helen Carden. She lived near Preston Park and you couldn't get there by bus so Tamsin had to drive me. I hadn't been to her house since Mother died. Helen had gerbils now. I had Tamsin. The gerbils climbed all over me and ran across Helen's bedroom floor, leaving tiny pellets. We played on her climbing frame in the garden. Then Tamsin came to collect me, a big tree of a woman standing tall at Helen's front door, chatting to her mum just like Mother used to do. I didn't like going to Mass with Tamsin either; I started refusing to go. 'But your mother would have wanted you to go,' she said, which I thought was a low trick.

In the end I acquiesced and we went, to the very church in Kemptown we used to go to with Mother. The three of us would sit in a pew, my sister, Tamsin and I, an ordinary family, just without the father. Not true, I wanted to shout. It is not what it looks like. She is *not my mother*.

Tamsin dressed us in Clothkits – folksy Seventies sew-your-own creations that made you look like something the Woodcraft Folk dreamt up. Suffice to say they did not sell them in Hanningtons. Clothkits were made and sold in Lewes, a market town less than ten miles from Brighton and the metropolitan base for Tamsin's set. They all loved Clothkits. The kits themselves came in transparent plastic bags with poppers and plastic handles. This was so you could re-use them, which I thought was a desperate measure and further proof of Tamsin's wretchedness. The patterns, made from cotton or needlecord with geometric motifs, were already cut out. In *a jiffy* you could produce an A-line skirt with a pinafore bib attached to it or a wrap-around skirt made out of cotton so thick it stuck out like a triangle.

Post-Mother, it was suggested that my sister and I choose an extracurricular activity offered by our school. My sister chose piano, which required nothing but clean fingernails. I chose riding, which required an outfit. The question of jodhpurs came up for discussion when we were still at the Sussex house. There was an old pair somewhere, which I could use. Somebody dashed off to the boot room, rooted around, returned triumphant, clutching an old-fashioned woollen pair that puffed out at the sides like whoopee cushions. Try them on, everybody cried. Wanting privacy, I went off to the loo; stripping off in public was something only hearty girls did. *Come on, strip off!* they would say as they jumped, topless, into a swimming pool or removed their clothing and put on a nightie for bed. I emerged, a midget in a cavalry officer's cardboard-stiff breeches, and stepped into the nursery. It was agreed that the jodhpurs *would do*, they fitted. Indeed they did, in a she-will-grow-into-them-in-a-few-years, thinking-ahead sort of way. What I wanted was a pair of normal jodhpurs, beige stretchy things that clung to your legs, jodhpurs that would not make me stand out. I needed a riding hat next. This had to be bought new, as there weren't any spares to be had. The shopkeeper measured my head with a tape measure, found the right size from the shelves behind him and handed me a black velvet hat with majestic blue silken lining. It felt just right. 'Oh, dear! Your ears again,' wailed Tamsin, poking the tip of them and looking at the shopkeeper. 'Look how they stick out.' She and the shopkeeper tucked the cartilaginous tips under the rim of the hat. They pinged out again, pinker each time. No hat would cover them without covering my eyes also. In the end, I got the right-sized hat for my head; the ears, it was decided, could be sewn back until they learned to stay flat against my skull.

Grandma had a sewing machine. You pushed your foot on a pedal and turned a handle and the needle went up and down. We learned sewing at school. Admittedly we had only done squares of embroidery and hemlines so far, but I knew about needles. I was forever ramming them into my finger when my aim misfired. The prospect of forcing one through the hard crescent at the top of my ear was only ever matched in horror by being told I had to cut off my hair in order to play Edmund in a school production of *The Lion, the Witch and the Wardrobe*.

In both instances, I chose my emergency strategy: tell Grandma. It was a last resort. She was like a protective tiger towards us, but a tiger without claws. Though she resented Tamsin, the outsider, looking after us, her grandchildren, she kept her counsel when she was with her. When she came to lunch at Lewes Crescent, very early on, it was awkward: usually such a chatterbox, she barely said a word, gave off a silent growl instead. But then she complained about her behind her back. Given her communication skills, what were the chances of her saving my hair, or my ears?

Tamsin thought sticking-out ears would look more unattractive the older I got; they would mark me out, just as I thought my high-heeled wedges marked me out. Like bad teeth that could be made presentable with braces, another cosmetic procedure my sister and I resisted, to my later regret, or poor posture that could be corrected by turning your palms out as you walked (also resisted, and since regretted), it was just a question of sorting the ears out. But to my grandmother, the very thought of pinning them back was an act of barbarism. With me sitting next to her in her Hove apartment, she got on the phone to Tamsin and said, Don't touch my granddaughter's beautiful ears. Then she squared up to my English teacher, albeit by letter, and said, Keep off my granddaughter's lovely long hair. I played Edmund in a hairnet.

8

DR DISH

The hairnet was not a good look. Forty years later, I am thinking the same thing about the blonde bob lying on the Macmillan Help Desk counter. It is prognosis day – at last. On our way up to Head and Neck to hear how my cards are stacked, a volunteer picks up the wig and pushes a needle through the mesh and out through the crown. A wig. I'm not sure I would wear one myself, and realise Mother never wore one when she was ill. I think I'd go for a hat, and then I see my half-sister in her woolly hat, her hair gone due to chemotherapy for the bowel cancer that killed her, how dreadful she looked, and how lost. The hat, a thick thing you would wear out hiking, cabled, the rim turned up, was plonked on her head. Her alabaster skin was chalky and drawn. She had no vanity to draw on, no well of self-love, no habit of primping and moisturising. I had offered to go with her to chemotherapy and she said, there's no need, you just sit there. And I said, all right, and I was relieved, coward that I was. As a result, I don't even know what chemotherapy entails. A revolving stand next to the Macmillan counter displays leaflets, like supermarkets do. Instead of a recipe for *Easy*

Aubergine Parmigiana, I pluck out *Understanding Head and Neck Cancers* and slip it into my handbag.

Upstairs, Annie, my specialist Macmillan nurse, comes over to Richard and me as we wait to be called.

'How was your Christmas,' she asks, 'given everything?'

A white dressing the size of an iPhone is stuck to the cheek of a white-haired man sitting opposite me. I've been watching his eyes, and they don't move. The skin on the dressing side slumps over his jawline. The other side of his face is taut.

A toddler next to me is tugging at her mother's skirt. She sits, head bent, Pietà. She does not raise her stone eyes to her son.

A Darth Vader rasp rattles the complicated air. It's a patient with a speaking valve checking in at the reception desk. She turns around and I see the circle filled with six triangles, like a completed Trivial Pursuit pie, in the middle of her neck.

Given all of this, I say: 'Yeah, you know. Good. The boys had a good time.'

'That's the main thing,' she says, sweeping up our agonies in her careful response.

'That's the main thing,' we mumble, nodding.

'Dr Carnell is ready for you. She's just down here.' Footsteps, Annie's, ours, and then I'm on a plastic chair, sitting opposite the consultant, who has pulled her chair away from the computer screen, just like Dr Dish did on diagnosis day. Richard is next to me. Annie stands behind the consultant.

'So . . .'

This poised stranger is about to tell me whether I live, or die, and yet I don't know anything about her. I haven't looked her up, as I do everyone else who provides 'services' – our dentist, my son's guitar teacher, my eyebrow threader, my dog's groomer. But not this doctor. I know only what I have been told about her, which is that she is a first-rate oncologist. What I see in front of me is a woman with long blonde hair and a mouth that is about to be busy making words I may or may not want to hear and is covered with lipstick the colour of lightly grilled salmon. I see her sharp black shift dress and her well-cut heels and the computer screen she can slide over to on her chair by pushing down on the floor with the soles of her feet. She is privy to knowledge about my body and what to do with it and is about to share a fraction of this, just the essential parts, with me.

'. . . Team meeting. Yesterday. Cut it out. Don't cut it out. Cut out the tumour.'

I focus on her, try to fix her words before they fly off, but I only catch the cusp of words and phrases. 'Why put you through it? No, we say, no surgery. Chemotherapy. Radiotherapy.'

I blank it all out. Until I hear a figure.

'Seventy-five to eighty per cent? Is that what you said?'

'There's a seventy-five to eighty per cent chance of success.'

'Sorry. You mean, seventy-five to eighty per cent chance of me not having cancer after the treatment?'

'Yes. We're going for it, Genevieve. We're going for a cure.'

I have a weakness for social kissing, I kiss too easily and inappropriately. I want to kiss my oncologist, smackers on both cheeks. Blondie! Oh, we're on nickname terms now. Let me whisk you round the room, Blondie! Let's have a dance! Instead, I smile, and she's off again, talking about the treatment plan. I should listen, but I don't really care what she says. I slip back in my chair and cradle my new pet word, the only word I've ever wanted: cure. And then I suddenly feel so tired. The floor looks tempting. I might lie on it, the word in my arms. I would like to go home now, would like everything to be over. But this is just the beginning.

'So, the treatment plan . . .' Blondie is saying.

A treatment plan. They're nice. I've had them before, in spas. It's a facial peel first, then a mask, then more unguents, and a full-body massage.

'Chemotherapy, radical radiotherapy, fatigue, white cells, blood transfusions, swallowing, not swallowing . . .'

Steady, Blondie, don't get carried away. I put my fingers in my ears. 'La-la-la-la!' She is speaking a language I don't understand, don't wish to learn and would rather have no need of. She's said the word 'cure'. Must she go on? Apparently so. And on she does go, until the words reduce to vibrations, a muffled drumming. Then someone turns up the speed dial. Turn it down, please. Blondie's Beckettian mouth moves to the rhythm, her words endless, her supply of them endless. On she goes, and then the drumming slows down, peters out, and I catch five wayward words:

'We'll give you a peg.'

A peg? As in peg it, peg leg, news peg, something to stop your knickers flying off the washing line and giving your neighbour a surprise. To lighten long car journeys when the boys were little, we sometimes played word association. I'll start, I'd say. 'When I think of sausages I think of pigs.' 'When I think of pigs,' Bassy might say, picking up the verbal baton, 'I think of snouts.' And snouts would lead to warthogs, and so to Africa, elephants, Dumbo, cages, fugitive hamsters, student antics and onwards through a maze of words and stories plucked from my life and Richard's and from the boys' limited worlds of limitless wonders. Words united our worlds. They were a plaything, a bridge, an educational tool, an embodiment of love. Never a weapon.

But cancer holds your psyche hostage, as well as your body, and it uses language to grind you down. Everyday words, and words you have never even heard before, wrong-foot you, set you fumbling through the fog which, in my case, descended on Diagnosis Day like a theatre's safety curtain – one that never lifts. Ordinary words turn sinister on you. Alien medical terminology erodes your already precipitately eroded sense of being in control.

Blondie is now holding up a piece of paper.

'This is the treatment plan. Would you like to take this away and think about it? You'll want time to think about the treatment.'

Time. That's a standout word now.

'Some people need time to think about their options.'

Options. I can only think of two:

1. I reject conventional treatments and set about shrinking the tumour myself with an alternative regime of my own researched-from-scratch devising. This could include mistletoe injections, biodynamic carrot juice, fever therapy, vitamin C boosts, organic enemas and pins for sticking into a voodoo doll made of sugar. And then I die.
2. I send in the chemical and radiation hit squads, with the surgeon's scalpel for backup – and I live, all being well.

I know which one Richard would choose. I don't need to ask him.

'It's OK. We'll sign.'

'Are you sure?'

'Yes!' we chime.

'Just one thing,' I say. 'To be clear. Did you say you are going to hit me with as tough a treatment as you think I can possibly withstand?'

'Yes. Some might say it's too much for you, too arduous.'

'I can take anything. Will it –' and of course I don't know what the 'it' refers to, short of a bullet that will save me, 'will it definitely be the most you think I can take?'

'Yes, it will. Like I said: we're going for it.'

I reach for the document in Blondie's hand, lean on the desk and sign the form. There's an expression for signing a document the contents of which you don't understand. Signing your life away. I am signing to keep mine. I am putting myself in the hands of the NHS's medical specialists. White coats. Drugs. Three cycles of chemotherapy, followed by six weeks of combined chemotherapy and radiotherapy. More chemotherapy, if needed. Surgery, if needed. Whatever it takes. Bring it on.

Two days later, I've morphed into a couch potato. It is 9.30 on Friday morning and I'm engrossed as Repo Man squares up to a defaulter's 4x4. I gawp at the screen, no longer a journalist, a daytime TV dropout now, all my plans and to-do lists discarded by the cancer wayside. I sit about, wanting nothing except for the phone to ring and to be given a date for my treatment to begin. It is twenty days since the diagnosis, over fifty since I found the Interloper. When I asked Dr Dish if the delays caused by the Christmas and New Year breaks mattered, he replied, 'To your outcome, you mean?' Yes, I said, to which he replied that a week or two wouldn't make a difference. Even so, the waiting is not easy. The owner of the 4x4 has just started giving Repo Man abuse for trying to tow away his car, when the landline rings. No one ever calls on the landline, except Margaret, my mother-in-law, and PPI snake charmers. My cancer has given it a new lease of life. Now it is ringing, pointedly, like a rotary phone in a 1950s drama. On cue, the heroine picks up the phone and, in clipped RP, says: 'Hampstead 2–3–7–9,' followed by 'A murder, officer?' and then the camera pans to her brooding lover, who is standing by the mantelpiece, a cigarette in one hand, a highball of whisky in the other.

In my own little drama, I answer and say 'hello' in my best, firm voice.

'Is this Genevieve Fox?'

'Yes.'

'I am calling from the imaging department . . .'

Imaging? I was hoping for Oncology.

'. . . I've had another look at your scans and, unfortunately, something has come up.' The man has a soft voice; it sounds no note of alarm, but his words do. 'I've spotted a shadow, just a faint one, on your right breast. It is probably nothing . . .'

Breast cancer, of course. I walk over to the sofa, the phone to my ear, and sit down. What made me think I could slip under its radar, even now? I took precautions: I had years of not being on the pill to avoid the associated risks and have had annual screenings over the last five years under a family history screening programme. I am my mother's daughter. Separated in life, we'll share the same killer.

'. . . Barely perceptible. You'll need to come in for another scan. Is Monday at 9.20 a.m. OK? The breast clinic has a slot.'

A slot. Such a breezy word. Hair salon receptionists use it. Hello, Just calling to say we've got a slot for you for your half head of highlights that you wanted. A client has just cancelled.

'Great. Yes. Monday is fine. Thank you.'

One phone call and now there is a loaded gun to my head: two cancers at the same time, one curable, and the other? Inside my head, the plates collide. There is lava everywhere and I am on the run, searching for safe ground.

Is it even possible to have two cancers at the same time? That's the million-dollar question. I don't know the answer. I can't do 50:50, since that would still leave one cancer, and I can't phone a friend since the first cancer is a secret and most wouldn't know the answer anyway. I contemplate asking the audience, by going on the Internet, but I won't get a straight answer. Worse, I'll stumble upon a medical research paper on the subject and, baffled by its findings, will decide the answer is yes.

Wrong answer.

The weekend passes in a fug of fresh fears and the decision to start telling people my news. 'News': the word also has a discordant energy about it. I don't know how to roll my news story out. I could do a Round Robin; people expect those around Christmas. Mine could be a New Year missive.

> *Dearest all, Happy New Year! Hope you've had a great Christmas. We've had quite a year! Pepper won best of breed at Crufts, the boys represented the UK in the Maths Olympics, Richard sold his start-up to Apple —and here comes the big news, I've got Cancer in, guess where, my head and neck. It's a cheeky squamous cell carcinoma stage 1b, with a 2 cm by 2 cm submandibular tumour and an unknown primary so it's a game of murder in the dark for the oncologists!*
> *All our love, Genevieve, Richard, Reuben, Bassy and Pepper xoxox*

A tweet might be better. I could channel Miranda Hart, the comedian whose hearty exuberance never ceases to amuse me: *'Have cancer – really got it in the neck this time. Such fun! #headandneckcancer.'* A text could also work. *Just to let u know, got cancer* ☺ ☒ ✒ *Will keep u posted. Gx.* In the end I plump for the old-fangled phone call. It's probably more crass than any form of social media, more like cold calling, really, because I'm in effect cornering the unsuspecting sods who pick up.

'Hi! Just calling to say I've got cancer,' I say, albeit after some warm-up. Whoever picks up wants to hang up, and can't.

'Yes, that's right, sorry, I've tricked you into picking up the phone – usually we just have a chat, don't we?'

And the person you call does not say, because they can't: 'Yes, and you are making me feel wretched. You are putting me in a position of obligation.'

'I know I am. I'm sorry about that. And I realise that you want to help, but don't know how to. I know you've got enough on your plate. You've just been a sickness buddy. You're a carer, as it is. All this is leaving you feeling awkward, inadequate, or feeling guilty. So sorry. I thought you'd want to know.'

The actual calls go something like this.

'Hi, It's me. How's everything? Oh, that's good. I am so pleased. What are you up to? Oh, good. Really? That's great. And the kids? Great. Listen, I've got some bad news. I'm not very well. The thing is, I've got cancer . . .'

At this point I find it helpful to scrunch up my nose and grind my teeth. Then I do the positive prognosis, I'll be fine bit, which makes me wobble because I don't know whether to believe I will be, or which side of the statistics I'll fall, or what cure actually means. Does it mean survive, as in you will be cured of the disease and then, after a number of years, it will come back? I leave out the breast cancer worry, which I don't want to vocalise, lest doing so makes it real. Uncertainty is the tick that bores into your flesh, hooks itself on to something soft, digs in.

Each and every precious friend responds by saying, 'Let me know what I can do. Anything at all.' They don't sound cornered at all. They mean it, they actually mean it, and you want so badly to think of something they can do, but you have no idea what is needed, what might be needed. A head transplant might be nice. The thing is, you are well. Never felt better. So you say, thank you. I'll let you know. And when you do know, you don't ask. Because asking is not what you do.

Unseemly sickness, like need, pushes people away. It pushes me away. But people are much nicer than I am and, as I discover over the next weeks and months, there is a lot of love out there. It will get me through my illness. Love alone doesn't heal me – I don't become that much of a space cadet – but without having been awakened to its healing powers I question *how* I would have healed. I question how any cancer sufferer truly heals, psychologically and emotionally as well as physically, in the absence of love.

I call my friend Debo, last seen in furs and thigh-high blue suede boots at the Christmas Eve carol service, while I am out walking Pepper round the block.

'Hi, Fox here . . .'

'How *are* you? Oh, gosh, it's non-stop, isn't it! I've just crashed on the sofa to watch a golden oldie. How was Christmas?'

'Oh, fine, yes, er . . .' Pepper has ground to a halt in someone's open gateway. Not on the pavement in front of the gateway. She's up on the path leading from their gate to their front door. She is straining her haunches and arching her back. '. . . No, no, no.'

'Sorry?' says Debo. 'It's not a very good line. Ours was exhausting . . .'

I yank, Pepper pushes, and the damage is done.

'We were sixteen for lunch. How we all fitted round the table I don't know, especially given how much I ate.'

I rummage in my coat pocket. Keys, an old Snickers wrapper, no dog bags.

'Oh that's great,' I say, sizing up a fallen leaf. 'The thing is, Debo . . .' I pause to pick up the leaf and wrap it around the ring of turds.

'Hello? Are you still there?'

'Yes!' I boom, like blokes do when their football team has scored. I've managed to get the loaded leaf in the palm of my hand and the lead shuffled back on to my wrist, leaving my other hand free to hold my mobile. 'The thing is,' I say, adjusting my tone to something sombre, and then I blurt out my news. Debo responds with noises and questions and wants to know about the treatment. I get to the bit about not being able to eat and having a feeding tube.

'A feeding tube! How marvellous. I could do with that. Shift a few pounds. You don't need to, but I do. The C-Diet. I am jealous.'

I laugh so much I drop the leaf. She's a human cancer antidote. I should lease her to the NHS. That night I overhear

Richard explaining the prognosis and the side effects of the chemo-radiotherapy to a friend. 'She'll live, but she might lose her capacity to speak. It's a good trade-off – in fact, it's a result.' The NHS can have him, too.

During her treatment for terminal breast cancer, Ruth Picardie crept up on a mutual friend of ours – Plato-reading Billy, whom she knew from university – at a party and put her hands over his eyes and whispered in his ear:

'Rumours of my demise are much exaggerated.'

She spent the rest of the evening holding court and dispensing anecdotes, the patient helping the frightened well.

When I was at university my brother drew me a cartoon strip inspired by a news story about a grandson who lived alone with his oppressive grandfather. Provoked one time too many at the very moment the old misery leaned forward to stoke the fire, the grandson whacked him over the head with a coal scoop. The blow killed him. The grandson chopped off his head, put it in a paper bag and sat it on the garden wall. Not everyone would find that funny, but we did.

My brother sent me another drawing when I was at university, this time of burning flames and a quote from the Quran: 'Verily, those who unjustly eat up the property of orphans, they eat up only a fire into their bellies, and they will be burnt in the blazing Fire!'

During the service at West London Crematorium following my half-sister's funeral I was seated next to my half-brother in the chapel. She was lying in the coffin, displayed on the catafalque. Not lying. Laid out. She was laid out in the coffin, the lid on. I was trying to get my head around her being inside when my half-brother nudged me and pointed to a button on the side of the lectern. Next to it, engraved on a small plaque, was a single word: Curtains.

Before my father-in-law's funeral, his body was displayed in an open coffin. I was dying to have a look. But Richard didn't want to, so I felt I couldn't either. I've never heard anyone in his family make jokes about death or dead people, and they don't believe in taking children to funerals. I'm all for it. It toughens them up, or so I used to think.

Indulging my fondness for the macabre, Richard once bought me *The Undertaking: Life Studies from the Dismal Trade* by the American poet and undertaker Thomas Lynch. This is my favourite line from it: 'Nora Lynch was a tidy corpse, quiet and continent.'

Slipped away, sleeping, passed away, passed, gone to meet her maker, gone to a better place, gone, popped her clogs, hit room temperature, bought the farm, croaked her last, moved on, kicked the bucket. You kick the bucket and then what? The bucket lands, Laurel and Hardy style, on your head, and then you suffocate?

One of Emily Dickinson's best images is the one of Death as a horse-drawn carriage. It pulls over to pick her up 'Because I could not stop for Death'. Now that the carriage feels all too real and might pull up for me any time now, the image, like death itself, has lost its romantic lustre. I'm never reading Keats's 'Ode to a Nightingale' ever again, for the same reason.

The next call is to my brother. I offer up my one-liner straight off the bat.

'Hi, It's me. I've got cancer.'

Boom boom.

'You'll be fine,' he says, straight in, barely pausing to hear a single detail, hardly drawing breath: 'You'll be OK it will be different to Mother that was a long time ago everything's different now so different it won't be like Mother absolutely not . . .' *Won't be like Mother.* Better not be, which I don't say, because I can't get a word in edgeways. My brother is James Joyce after a Guinness, he's unsettling me, he's talking too fast, won't stop, but his words stop me in his tracks, take me back to a time when I – we – had a mother, a state to which only we are privy and which feels, momentarily, real. And then is gone. The scabby loss-wound is picked open. He prods it with a hot poker, prods some more. 'It's not the same now you won't go through what Mother went through.' That's another rewind moment I could do without. 'That was the Seventies the treatments were harsh not like now it will be fine.'

Harsh. Mother died from breast cancer in 1973, just under two years after President Nixon signed the National Cancer Act in 1971 and declared his 'war on cancer'. Early the following year, the oestrogen-blocker tamoxifen was licensed for the treatment of advanced breast cancer in the UK. But this was early days for the pioneering 'orphan' drug – so-called because it had started out as a potential morning-after pill and, when its efficacy was discounted, had very nearly been abandoned by the pharmaceutical industry. Initially used sparingly for palliative treatment, it wasn't until the late 1970s and the 1980s that tamoxifen started to be used as a post-surgery, adjuvant therapy, or one designed to prevent the cancer from recurring. I don't know what my brother meant by harsh, what stage Mother's cancer was when it was diagnosed nor whether she had a radical mastectomy. I do know that radiotherapy at the time was unsophisticated and punitive, that it sometimes damaged other organs, including the lungs and the heart. Would she have had chemotherapy, too? I don't know. But I know that, back then, chemotherapy sometimes induced strokes and heart attacks, and that only 40 per cent of women diagnosed with the disease survived.

For this call I am walking around the house with the phone. I pause by the window in my bedroom and gaze down at the indifferent street. I am suddenly eight years old again, peering out of that common room window, waiting for Mother.

'It's true,' I say to my brother. 'You're right. It'll be different this time.'

When I call my half-brother he says some of the same things, and again it is hard being taken back in time when all your life you have tried only to go forward. He tells me of a journalist we both know who had throat cancer. And it was awful, he said, and very hard. But he is fine. 'You'll be fine. I *know it*. I *feel* it. I know you'll be fine.'

This bloody cancer business is like short, sharp regression therapy I did not sign up to. I'm face-to-face with a nine-year-old motherless girl and I don't want anything to do with her lest she curse my children. The breast shadow isn't exactly helping me break away from the fear that history is repeating itself. I feel a momentary fondness for the tumour in my neck, simply because it differentiates me from Mother. I get to Sunday, the day before the breast clinic appointment, and though I've tried to resist doing so, I surf the Internet. I look up my head and neck diagnosis again, and the likelihood of being able to have two cancers concurrently, and it has made me twitchy. It is possible to have two different types of cancer at the same time. It is not common, but it's possible. On the plus side, the combination of head and neck and breast cancer is not common either. More often, the cancer has already spread at the time of diagnosis, giving the impression that there are two tumours when in fact it is the spread of the same cancer type growing as a tumour in different locations. Glad that's cleared up.

In the afternoon Bassy and I cuddle up and watch the *Lord of the Rings* trilogy, and I find myself musing on how like the magic Ring the Internet is – both deadly and irresistible. I would like the Ring now, use it to disappear and come up for air when the danger has passed. But the cancer would sniff me out. Has already sniffed me out. Finders keepers, losers weepers. Bassy is very perceptive about Gollum: what a decent sort he is, underneath it all. I had forgotten how moral the *Lord of the Rings* books are and how similar Tolkien is to C. S. Lewis. When Frodo gets to Mordor and has to walk over the fiery Cracks of Doom, I hide my tears. He is so brave.

When I was eighteen, in my last term at boarding school, I sneaked into the study of the headmaster's wife, Judith Marriott, my confidante and rock, and nicked her copy of *A Grief Observed* by C. S. Lewis. I had spotted it on her bookshelf and did not want to admit to wanting to read it. I was amazed to find that Lewis had the same please-come-back yearning as me and that the grief following the death of his wife felt to him like suspense. 'Or like waiting; just hanging about waiting for something to happen. It gives life a permanently provisional feeling.' That's it, I thought, all these years have passed, and that's how I feel too. Fortified, I slipped the book back in its place on the shelf.

For my breast cancer appointment the next day, I'm on autopilot. I head straight up the spiral stairs of the UCLH Macmillan Centre to Head and Neck and check in. No, they say. You need Breast. It's over there. The receptionist points across the atrium. A minute later I am in a whole other world of cancer patients and staff. I will not be drawn by the person who does my scan and biopsy and refuse to talk or smile politely. I don't scowl, either. I am trying not to be here. The shadow, she says, is indeed a shadow. It can be caused by folds of tissue indicating misleading density. Or something like that. I don't know, I can't follow her explanation, don't care to. I do not feel relief at the news. I don't feel anything.

The next day, at an appointment with the Macmillan dentist to check that my gums and teeth can withstand the radiation, I am back on form. I feel rage, indignation and humiliation as the Macmillan dentist asks me to lie down on a couch. To open your mouth in an O and have a man tap and scrape, his face so close, his breath there, behind a flimsy mask, is a bizarre intimacy. To have a man excavate your mouth to see if he must order the removal of its contents is a new and exquisite horror. My mouth is a midden, revealing future decay rather than past glories. If my gums are in poor shape, he says, my teeth have to come out and bridges be built before the radiotherapy shoots the gums to pieces, making future implants – in other words, false teeth – impossible. If my gums are strong and healthy, they can stay.

I'm in luck. The teeth can stay.

I finally get the date for my chemotherapy to start and am cock-a-hoop. Treatment will start in late January, two weeks from now. It is a week later than I had hoped, but at least I've got a date. I can start planning. With two Saturday nights left before I go toxic, I confirm a dinner at Scott's in Mayfair for the first one, and a fiftieth birthday in Sussex for the second. The whole year is a fireworks display of fiftieths, including my own; the cancer's timing couldn't be worse. I'd have preferred next year. Except that's Reuben's GCSE year. Anyway. The first Saturday comes round and I am in the kitchen, doing my make-up. Our friends Laurence and Emma, Lu and Andrew are treating us to dinner at Scott's. I am feeling chipper. Not only am I keeping my teeth and my hair – 'Hair may thin, but won't fall out,' Richard wrote in my notebook when Blondie went through the side effects of cisplatin – but I've also got just the one cancer. My reprieved breasts are in a push-up bra, my here-to-stay hair is in rollers, and my teeth are where they should be: in my mouth, and my mouth is looking forward to a cocktail.

I'll be having an Old Fashioned. It's my Death Row snifter –
bourbon, Angostura bitters, twist of orange. I could do with one
now as I look at myself in the mirror and rub foundation over
my face and neck. Over the hump my index finger goes. Let's
hope no one has a pool cue in the bar; the lump has 'pocket
me' written all over it. Then I take a selfie. Why? To cheer
myself up? To post on social media? My hair is in rollers and
I've got a B-movie blob sliding down my neck. It's hardly
Facebook material, or Instagram. Do they even allow cancer
lumps on Instagram? The selfie must be something to do with
the impulse to make a photographic record before I jump over
the edge.

It's time to get going. We say goodbye to the boys. I am glad
they are seeing us dressed up. It's the old us, still here.

Mayfair is medicinal. The sidewalks sparkle. We slip from the
silent street into the crisp lobby of the Connaught Hotel's
Coburg Bar. The panelled room is rammed with one-per-centers
half our age. Red cords, striped shirts, halter-neck tops and
backless slip dresses and not a growth or a blemish in sight.
The Interloper and I have never, in our short time together,
been anywhere so glamorous and reassuring. We find our four
friends sheltering from the Mayfairati at a secluded table by the
window. Lu is in the middle of an anecdote about failing to
lose weight and Laurence, who is a combination of Jonathan
Ross and Clive Anderson, puffs his cheeks out and pats his belly
in imitation of Lu in a fat suit. She shrieks and slides off her
chair, tears of laughter rolling down her cheeks, and a beautiful
waiter comes to take our order. None of us can speak, we're
all laughing so much, and he discreetly withdraws.

We eventually order.

My Old Fashioned is a fireball, and the colour of dawn. We
down another round, then it's over to Scott's where I order my
Death Row dinner: Lobster Thermidor. Creamed spinach.

Skinny chips. Bottle of Saint-Véran. Springy white bread with a thin crust and French salted butter in ramekins. Crisp white tablecloth. Weighty silver forks with thistle-tip prongs.

During dinner we talk over each other and finish each other's anecdotes, we laugh so hard we fall sideways and I think, this is it, this is heaven on earth. Did I know this about friendship, BC, how much I love it? Yes. Did it feel this good, this rich, this *ample*? No. Laurence nudges me, I blink my from-nowhere tears away, and he whispers: 'Paul Whitehouse. Ten to two.' He says Whitehouse, I think Mary, and picture a lady with big specs who was anti-sex or swearing or having a good time, maybe all three. But who's Paul? If Laurence had said, Dolly Parton, ten to two, I would be with him. Any celebrity more subtle slips under my radar. It's why I mistook Colin Firth's publicity assistant for the man himself when I once interviewed him, at the time one of the most famous faces – and wet shirts – astride the earth. We all look. Then Andrew, perhaps prompted by the comedian's receding hairline, turns the spotlight on Richard. He wants to know how much he has spent on his new haircut, and repeats the question.

'Herecot like,' he says, grinning. 'How much did you pay for yer herecot?' This is his Liverpool accent.

'Twelve pounds,' says Richard, who is from Liverpool.

'Twelve pounds!'

'Plus £4. I gave the barber a £4 tip. Because he spent so long on it.'

'A £4 tip! But it's completely lopsided.'

We look, and it is. Richard's hair was so long when I met him he wore it in a ponytail. Now he's got a lop-sided bloke's short haircut and everyone's crying with laughter and I'm crying, for different reasons.

'Can you do something for me?' I say to Emma *sotto voce*, when we've finished dabbing our eyes.

'Yeah, of course.' She leans in.

'Can you, you know, look out for me?'

'Course I can.'

'The thing is, I think I am going soft.'

She raises an eyebrow.

'I told a friend cancer was a blessing.'

Her eyebrow pings upwards again, higher this time.

'I know!' I say.

'So, er, what exactly do you mean by that then?'

'Oh, you know. You get to live in the moment. That sort of thing.'

'Right . . .'

'I also said that cancer is a gift.'

'Oh, dear.'

I mean, really. Diamonds are a gift. Salted caramels are a gift. But cancer?

'Babe, wake up.' It is Richard leaning across the bed. 'Wake up!'

The phone has not rung, so no one is dead, myself included. What's got into him?

'I need your help.' His voice is shaky. 'It's Pepper.'

Now I sit up. 'What do you mean?'

'She's been hit by a car.'

Five minutes later, I've got my cowboy boots over my pyjamas, and we are driving to the emergency vet in Belsize Park. It is 1.30 in the morning, the night after Scott's. We've left the boys asleep in bed and fifteen-month-old Pepper is on my lap. She's not moving, she's not even whimpering, and we're not talking. All I can think is, she has to be all right. I start chemotherapy in a week. That's enough for the boys to deal with.

'She better not die.'

I don't mean to say the words out loud, but I do. There is censure in my voice. She got hit by a car, on Richard's watch.

The veterinary nurse asks for £500 up front. The vet won't even look at the dog without us paying in advance, she says. We try one bank card. It is rejected. We try another. The machine hums, out comes the receipt and Pepper is taken downstairs.

In the morning, after the boys have played an inadvertent game of hunt the puppy, we tell them Pepper is at the vet's because the cut she got on New Year's Eve has become infected. We think the boys can't take the truth, when it is the two of us who are shying away from it at every turn. This impulse to protect the boys from life's briers is more likely to make them weak in the face of them; panic is blinding me to the fact.

Before they get back from school, I manoeuvre Pepper into the crate I've prepared for her. I've folded up the fake fur throw from the sofa, and put her own rug on top of it, and put her toys in the corner. When she is settled, I wriggle inside as far as I can and rest my head near hers and stroke her head. It reminds me of looking after Libra as a child, after she was hit by a car. After Mother died, Libra had stayed with us for a bit at the Sussex house and then she was sent away. I had missed her and didn't want her to think I had abandoned her. We were told she was in a good home with Elsie, our cleaning lady. I wanted to visit her, but I didn't know how to go about it, and the weeks turned into months and the months into years and my missing her abated. It was different with Richard Williams. I always wondered if he was out there, and how it was that he simply didn't care about us. I wanted to find him, but didn't dare try. He might not have the Jaguar any more, or memories of us.

Years later, shortly after I had left university, my brother spotted an advertisement in *The Spectator*:

Lost contact with friends, old flames? Ariel Bruce – 'super-sleuth . . . perfection in detection' – finds them.

My brother, also a journalist, thought the super-sleuth would make a good magazine story, and had just the mystery subject for her: Richard Williams. He asked her to track him down. Bruce had started out as a social worker. Then one day her decorator, who was adopted, asked her to help him find his natural parents. She resisted, but he insisted that everyone has a right to know the story of their own lives. She duly found the decorator's parents and went on to find newswoman Kate Adie's birth parents. Surely she would find Richard Williams. I held my breath. When my brother called to say she had found him and that he was dead and, worse, that he had died only a matter of months earlier, I held back the tears.

Richard Williams's widow, for he had married again, told the super-sleuth that he had tried very hard to get in touch with us and regretted failing to do so. He felt he had been banished from our lives after Mother died, and it turns out he had. Apparently my grandmother and aunt had prevented him from getting in touch with us; he felt forgotten, a sorry twist for an acting major who had served in the Forgotten Army, as the British 14th Army, which comprised units from Commonwealth countries, was known. The irony of his banishment was that when we were living in Lewes Crescent, wondering why he didn't get in touch with us, he was living just around the corner. As my brother lamented, we could have bumped into him in the street. When his widow met up with my brother and the super-sleuth for cocktails in the Grand Hotel, one of our former family haunts, she was cross. Why hadn't any of us tried to get in touch with Richard before? But if I had tried, as I had fantasised about doing so many times over the years, I wouldn't have been able to track him down by his marriage certificate. It turns out he and Mother never married. She would have been disinherited by her mother-in-law, Granny Fox. Since Mother was dependent on

Granny Fox for her financial security, she changed her name to Williams by deed poll instead.

I look at Pepper, lying beside me with her broken leg just like my dog Libra had in the year before Mother died, and tell myself that history is not going to repeat itself. Pepper has a broken leg, and that's all there is to it. Even so, I don't want to tell the boys what has happened to Pepper. When they get home from school, she is in the crate, metal pins sticking out of her back leg and I still maintain the lie about the infected paw. They both look at me in disbelief, then Bassy climbs into the crate with her.

In the weeks ahead, looking after Pepper is a distraction from the Interloper. Perhaps it gives the boys something else to think about, too. The Interloper has spread out across my jawline, and it feels like it's got company. Whatever is under there itches like spiders on the march. The size of it worries me. I call Caroline and ask if a tumour can grow so quickly you can see it changing size from one hour to the next. I am beginning to understand why Mother's tumour stuck up through her nightie and why my half-sister needed loose trousers when her bowel cancer spread. Tumours take up space. I can't wait for mine to start shrinking. Richard and I have done our holiday chart. We'll be in Maine for the summer, in a house on our favourite lake, the tumour gone, chased off, zapped, the boys, my lifeblood, at ease again.

I take another selfie. I'm Morphing Zombie Mum now, the Interloper pushing out, mutating, metastasising. My cancer lexicon expands apace. So far I've got: CAT, CUP (Cancer of Unknown Primary Origin), cell, chemotherapy, choke, cure, decay, dentures, disease, dry, dysfunction, elevation, feeding, flaking, gastronomy, gland, hidden, immune, infertility, *in vitro*, jaw, killer, loss, nausea, nutrients, platelet, primary, protrusion, radiotherapy, retraction, saliva, scan, secondary, skin, squamous, surgery, swallow, system, teeth, thermometer, tinnitus, tube, tumour, unknown, xerestomia. Individually, each word is harmless, for the most part. Dysfunction might raise a puerile titter, and disease, cancer, chemotherapy and radiotherapy are hardly feelgood words, but the rest are all right, either prosaic or scientific gobbledygook. Put them altogether, though, and they are a mob out looking for trouble.

A few nights later, Bassy and I listen to a recording of Ian McKellen reciting 'The Rime of the Ancient Mariner'. Since we are a neo-Victorian, gather-round-the-fire-and-read sort of family in our dreams only, I have had to force him to climb on to the bed and listen to it with me. He's studying the epic poem at school. Not so long ago, I saw Fiona Shaw performing it, aided by a living prop in the form of a contemporary dancer, at the Old Vic Tunnels, near Waterloo station. I came away thinking, good old Coleridge, you can't beat a ballad, the form's forward-thrusting rhythm and hypnotic rhyme so spectacularly at odds with the sailor's cautionary tale. Listening to the ghoulish, Gothic story with Bassy, I'm enthralled all over again, and aghast at what the witless sailor has had to endure. There's the storm, and the ship hitting the mast-high icebergs with their 'dismal sheen'. Then the albatross appears through the fog, 'as if it had been a Christian soul', the wind returns and the stupid mariner shoots the bird, the bird that he has fed and which has been following the ship day and night. Why would he destroy the source of the wind, God's grace? So far, so par for the course. But then McKellen gets to the famous lines 'Water, water, everywhere/Nor any drop to drink' and I nearly choke on my own saliva, while I've still got it. The words feel so horribly prescient, it's as if the sailors themselves have leapt off the deck to throttle me. All the fabled side effects of the radiotherapy come horribly to life – the damaged salivary function, the perpetual thirst, difficulty in swallowing and talking, the risk of choking to death, the blistering tongue. 'With throats unslaked, with black lips baked/We could nor laugh nor wail.' The poem is a head and neck cancer patient's worst nightmare.

That night, I can't get that glittery-eyed mariner out of my mind. He shot an innocent bird, unleashing vengeful spirits. He was made to serve penance. Cancer, someone said to me yesterday in the cheery, thoughtless way that people do, is a curse.

Which begs the question: What did I do?

Cancer turns your home into a hotel lobby. People come and go, stay for a glass of wine or a cup of tea, use the bathroom, have something to eat, lounge on a sofa or perch on a chair, ask for a cab number, order a cab, ask for the Wi-Fi code, pick up a magazine, ask for directions. People 'pop in,' 'stop by', 'drop in' because they 'were just passing'. Pop, stop, drop; I come to dread these monosyllables.

I don't have a doorman, for a start. Funny, that. I don't have one of those wind-up relatives, either, the ones who appear in friends' homes when someone is sick or pregnant and take over the running of the house and answer the door to visitors. I don't even have a decent front door. The Victorian original on our terraced house has been replaced with something short and engineered. It has stuck-on panels. The panel of glass above it is puckered, which is up there with bobbly wallpaper on my Taste Crimes register. We've got that on the hall ceiling. I worry about these things, I really do. For as the Bible tells us, By what ye judge, ye shall be judged.

Now I've got cancer I'm a sitting duck. People who don't usually come to my house – colleagues with whom I've only ever met up in public places, occasional friends who have not yet had the invite to come round because the house isn't finished, parents from my children's schools, medical practitioners – start visiting. You would think, having cancer, I wouldn't mind about our reproduction front door, or the house being half-finished. But I do.

Our bedroom is a particular bugbear. It was getting to me even before I got the cancer diagnosis. It is oppressive and chaotic. Soon visitors will sit in it whilst I, presumably, am holed up in bed. Molehills of domestic detritus cover the carpet. Squash them, and another pile of discarded underwear, unread newspapers, old cables, and items for Oxfam spring up. Pictures and mirrors are stacked against the walls. I wish I were tidy and mature and lived like a fully-fledged grown-up. Better still, I wish I lived in a hotel like Granny Fox did in her dotage. Hers was called The Volney and it was full of elderly residents, including Dorothy Parker, who died five years before she did. I'd settle for the company of crinklies. At least I'd have staff.

Instead I'm stuck with an Eighties throwback of an unserviced bedroom, one entire wall of which is painted chocolate brown. There is a walnut-brown fan with silver propellers on the ceiling, vanilla walls and burnt copper silk curtains. We didn't inherit this colour scheme. I paid a colour specialist to advise me on it and this is what we came up with. Moody, she said. An interior to lose yourself in, completely different to the rest of the house. Well, she was right there. It is a Moroccan lantern and a few mouldy rugs away from an actual souk. This was her fantasy, not mine, and I bought into it, hence the 'colonial' ceiling fan.

The cancer brings me to my senses: the brown has to go. As colours go, it's a bit too earthy and shallow grave for someone about to be bedridden. I'll add 'bedridden' to the cancer lexicon, 'ridden' being the past particle of the verb to ride, as in: sit on and control the movement of (an animal, typically a horse): *Jane and Rory were riding their ponies* | [no obj.] : *I haven't ridden much since the accident.* I will be riding my bed, *Bedknobs and Broomsticks* style. Whoever comes to visit, however, will have to sit on the floor. In magazines, bedrooms have a little chair in the corner. We've got the molehills, but no chairs.

I add 'Get rid of brown paint' and 'Buy armchairs' to my To Do list, which of course no longer includes Compile Legacy for Boys but does include:

- De-register for VAT
- Check out Catholic burial grounds
- Call electrician
- Sort documents & will
- Invoices – any more?
- Buy blinds/shutters for kitchen
- Sort Bassy's outfit for David's bar mitzvah

Better get on with it all. There are only five days to go before the chemotherapy starts. But it's hard to focus. I've got that panic you feel in the final weeks leading up to giving birth for the first time. You've got so much to do, and flounder about, doing none of it, paralysed by everybody else telling you how your firstborn's early life puts your own on hold. You can't sleep, they say, can't make a sandwich, shower, get dressed, string a sentence together, read a book, go to the movies. Cancer is like that, too, just without the bonus of a bouncing baby.

I decide to call C-Diet Debo. She used to be a fashion designer and now she does up houses. She's a grafter. I propose my bedroom as a makeover candidate over a cup of tea, and half an hour later she is going through every room in the house, riffling through the unhung pictures and mirrors and eyeing up pieces of furniture that don't yet have a home. After the recce, she says that if I can get someone to paint the wardrobes taupe and buy some new bed linen ('You have got cancer, you do need some nice sheets'), she will sort the rest. A few nights later she appears with three bunches of sweet white roses, two square pillows and matching pillowcases, Italian *Vogue*, a bottle of

Chablis, a tape measure, a hammer and nails, and a scented candle.

'I thought you were more jasmine than figs. Am I right?'

I am working out the answer, but she's already moved on. 'Where's that ladder?' she says and within minutes she's on the top rung, ripping down the old brown pelmets and curtains. Up go some white silk ones, in come bits of furniture, and two hours later she's styled the bedroom into a louche hotel suite, complete with dressing table and *dressed* bed. All we are missing is the chair.

'Right, that's that. Shall we have a glass of wine now?'

There's a bottle of kale juice another friend bought earlier, now lurking in the fridge. If I wanted to connect to my body, I would say:

'Oh, no thanks. I'll have kale juice.'

But now, more than ever, I want to disconnect from it so instead I say:

'I'll get the corkscrew.'

9

LOVE AND LIGHT

Cancer is a journey. That's what people say.

Scott went to the Antarctic. Frodo went to Mordor. I've been up the Congo river, down the Yangtze, through the swamps of the Okavango Delta. I've been to Costa Rica, Myanmar, Vietnam, Thailand, Namibia and more besides. I've taken the ferry across the Mersey and the ferry to the Isle of Wight. All journeys.

Let's play word association. You say 'journey'. I say 'exploration', 'new frontiers', 'pilgrim', 'refugee', 'destination'. I don't say cancer. I might say: 'Piers Plowman' or 'Christopher Columbus.' I'd definitely say T. S. Eliot and quote that justifiably well known passage from 'Little Gidding':

> 'We shall not cease from exploration
> And the end of all our exploring
> Will be to arrive where we started
> And know the place for the first time.'

Life as a journey, bookended by birth and death, wisdom accrued on the way. Nice. The journey archetype is part of the cultural underpinning of Western civilisation. Think of *The*

Odyssey, The Iliad, The Aeneid, The Inferno. I haven't read any of these, but I've read snippets and watched the film *O Brother, Where Art Thou?* at least five times. Think of *Eat, Pray, Love,* which I also haven't read. But over ten million people have, and more still watched the movie. The point is, we all love a journey; that's why even marketing whizzes have appropriated the word. Brand specialists describe going to the supermarket as a 'consumer journey'. HR functionaries chart the 'employee journey'. Disneyland's Twilight Zone Tower of Terror, my favourite theme park ride, is described as 'a thrilling journey into another realm of sight and sound you're sure never to forget'. Dead right. Swap 'cancer' for 'Twilight Zone Tower of Terror' and 'journey' doesn't hold. Cancer does plunge you, with G-force ferocity, into another realm of sight and sound, but it's not a journey, and it's not thrilling either. I can say this because I've been to Disneyland *and* I've got cancer.

Name me one way in which 'journey' conveys, in an illuminating, accurate or arresting way, preferably all three since to illuminate is the function of metaphor, what it is to endure cancer. In his book, *Listening to Pain,* David Biro, a New York doctor, points out that overused metaphors become redundant; they no longer convey the essential nature of whatever is being described. Rather than shedding light on the particularities and essence of a phenomenon, the metaphor throws us back on the word itself. You say 'journey' in connection with cancer and I am none the wiser.

Cancer. One word, different experiences. Dr Suleman, the Macmillan clinical psychologist, tells me that the journey metaphor, like the phrase 'cancer experience', functions as shorthand; patients and those associated with them find it helpful. I don't. The word is a stooge, and a liar. Journeys take you somewhere. You initiate them and plan them. I didn't plan my cancer and now that I am apparently *on my way,* I don't know where I am going, despite being on a road most travelled, to misquote Robert Frost. This is not a pleasant feeling. I don't even have a starting point. Is it when the first healthy cancer cells mutated and mutinied? When was that, then? Months ago? Years ago? Generations ago, when a cancer gene took up residence? As for a destination, I suppose it is to move away, or back, to my starting point of good health and to no longer take it for granted, which is very philosophical and T. S. Elioty, but not helpful in the here and now. If I were terminally ill, what would the destination of my cancer journey be then? Death? Well, we're all heading there.

'It will be quite a journey, Genevieve,' someone said to me. No it won't.

And besides, how would they know? Who are they to say? If the statement is supposed to be helpful, give you a heads-up, it fails, especially for those who hate journeys, prefer staycations, get carsick, can't travel due to dizziness, are fearful of being in unfamiliar environments.

Dr Suleman listens to my ranting with an attentiveness I find overwhelming. He makes me feel that I am not going mad. He suggests 'experience' as an alternative to 'journey'. Yes, thank you, I'll take that instead. 'Cancer experience' removes the pressure on the cancer patient, the *voyager*, to have a good time. Or at least to bring back some interesting souvenirs, such as evidence of a change of character, or of transformation, which is the cancer journey's USP. That's if they make it back. Cancer makes you see the world with new eyes. That's something else people say. Which begs another question: What am I going to see? Pass the blindfold.

Richard and I were blindfolded once, on a pavement in Primrose Hill, along with Fliff and her husband Steve. We were bundled into a car and driven to Simon Drake's House of Magic. We knew that's where we were going, but we didn't know its location and therefore how to get there. On arrival, the driver led us to a door, whereupon he invited us to remove our masks. We did so, and entered a phantasmagoric garden, and from there a house full of curios and automata. Then we watched a beautiful lady having her head chopped off. Magic makes you see the world with new eyes. But cancer? Let's wait and see.

Today's mystery destination is the Nuclear Medicine department at UCLH. When I find the sign announcing it on a hospital wall, I pose in front of it and ask my brother, who has accompanied me for my CAT scan, to take my photograph. I know he won't find the request odd and will see the funny side of 'nuclear' and 'medicine'. It's a bit like 'cancer' and 'journey': an unlikely coupling.

My brother, sister and I have only ever made two journeys together: one was to Italy, and the other was to see Father's grave, in Southampton, Long Island, when I was twenty. The journey to Father's grave goes to show how you can set off looking for one thing, and end up finding something completely unexpected. I found Granny Fox lying next to Father. Even though Southampton is where she had her summer house, where she married my grandfather, a lawyer, and where Father was raised, I just wasn't expecting to find her there. Irrationally, I resented the two of them, bedded down like that, together, smug, back where they belonged, belonging. Later, researching Granny Fox's Southampton house, I discovered that she was what child-rearing experts today call a co-sleeper. The detail was hidden in an old-fashioned news story in a *New York Times* cutting of 1916 that explained how Granny Fox had all her wedding presents and wedding jewellery stolen. The headline is the vintage sort that swirls in front of the camera lens in a Hitchcock movie: $15,000 GEM THEFT AT LAWYER'S HOME. *JEWELS TAKEN AS MRS. LYTTLETON FOX SLEEPS IN HER HOUSE AT SOUTHAMPTON.* The diction is archaic: "'Mr Fox had gone to New York," said Mrs Fox last night in telling of the robbery, "and I was alone in the house with the children and the servants."' She then says: "'My small son was sleeping with me ... I left my jewelry on the dresser and some of it in the drawers. When I awoke the next morning I found it was all gone, except my watch. I heard no one in the room. We have had detectives from New York working on the case, but have not gotten the slightest clue.'"

Father used to sleep in her bed as a little boy. I didn't expect that. Granny Fox was billed as a forbidding matriarch. A mother who has her son in her room, or perhaps her bed, when he is seven years old must be in possession of tenderness. Which goes to show something else: family lore, like Chinese Whispers, changes as it passes down the line.

Granny Fox died a year after Father, so she must have requested to be buried alongside him. I didn't like the two of them interred side by side, with no room for the rest of us, including Mother. I didn't like the dates on the tombstones either. 'Genevieve Fox. Born 1878 – 1970.' That was OK. But 'Lyttleton Fox. 1909 – 1969.' I always told people Father was very, very old, offering this up as an explanation for his death when I was very, very young. But I never had the facts, the dates, to hand.

In one of my most precious photographs of him he is smiling, one arm on the mantelpiece where the collection of fox ornaments were laid out, his legs crossed, a bow tie round his neck. He doesn't look ancient at all; far from it. I told people he was old because it simplified things. Until that day in Southampton I never knew exactly how old Father had been when he died, and I made sure I never asked. Eliciting information about my parents from other people was something I took care not to do. Revealing that you don't know the basic facts about your own parents is like not knowing the capital of England or that night follows day. I kept my ignorance under wraps.

That day, standing in front of his grave, I did the sums for the first time. Father was fifty-five when I was born. Now, that is old. I felt cheated, as if I had never had much chance of growing up with a father in the first place. I was flabbergasted that he could be so selfish. The tears came then. Embarrassed, I did my best to hide them.

Then, when we were weaving our way out of the cemetery, we stumbled on a grave with my name on it, a name but no date. Just plain 'Genevieve Fox'. It was as if the grave were waiting for me. It was only natural that, in the spirit of an orphans' day out, I should sit atop it, smile, and have my picture taken.

That's why I know my brother won't think it's odd to want to take my picture in front of the 'Nuclear Medicine' sign. All my siblings like a bit of macabre. I do my default, toothy holiday smile. An elderly couple walks by, she with a stick, he looking grey and anxious. They do not stop to take photographs. When my brother presses the shutter, I say, 'Brilliant, thanks,' as if he's just snapped me with Leonardo DiCaprio. The photograph then languishes on my phone, along with the early selfies. If cancer is a journey, then these are postcards from the edge.

A week later I am off to the hospital to get a pick, as in axe. Pick. Pickaxe. Glaciers. Mountaineering. Harness. Losing your foothold. Falling. Losing control. Giving yourself up to the forces that have overtaken you. Actually, it's PICC, not pick. PICC is one of the many acronyms you encounter on Planet Cancer and it stands for peripherally inserted central catheter. Catheter. I know this word. As a child I heard adults whisper about old men using one when they couldn't wee. I've come for the PICC insertion on my own because I don't want to make a fuss; later, when my defences are down and I cannot bear to be on my own at all, let alone go to appointments on my own, I will see how deliciously in denial I am at this stage. The procedure may be straightforward, but its implications are traumatic. It would be quite reasonable to have brought a friend along for moral support.

'It's just a tube for the chemo,' I told Richard when he offered to come with me. Then I corrected myself. 'Chemotherapy. It's the little line thing, for the chemotherapy.'

I am going to use the full term. Me and the cancer-killing drugs won't be on nickname terms. 'Chemo' is an abbreviation, not strictly a diminutive, but it suggests a certain fondness all the same. What would 'Chemo' call me? Gen? Foxy?

All through my treatment, and afterwards, I resist the faux jauntiness of 'chemo'. I prefer to keep things formal. Chemotherapy. Radiotherapy, not 'radio'.

I affect a little hauteur, a little distance.

I sit on a chair in the basement while a charming Specialist Nurse wipes my left arm with disinfectant. I want to ask her to take a photograph of me and my arm, a Before and After. I should have brought my Nikon. I should be treating cancer as a project, be professional about it, use it as an *opportunity*. Way back, I fancied myself as an explorer. Aged twenty-five, I *journeyed* up the Zaire river, as the Congo was then known, in search of the truth about missionaries. I had a full kit: moleskin notebooks as favoured by Bruce Chatwin, my half-brother's old fishing bag, a tape recorder, a Nikon and a stack of lenses, a camping stove (but no gas), a Swiss army knife, a bottle of ketchup, library books from the Royal Geographical Society and the London Library and an Issey Miyake, squishable no-iron dress. I saw myself as the fully clothed answer to anthropologist-explorer Benedict Allen, whose naked antics up the Orinoco, and elsewhere, I greatly admired. Now look at me. I haven't brought a proper camera, let alone a camera crew, and here I am, calling myself a journalist. Or rather, I did, before the cancer made off with my identity. In the event, I worry that the Specialist Nurse will mistake me for a weirdo hospital addict so I don't ask her to take my picture. She inserts the PICC line into a vein in my arm.

'Having a PICC line,' I learn later from the Macmillan Cancer Support video, 'means you don't have to have repeated injections or needles.' To implant it, a needle is threaded through the vein and the line is threaded through the needle and into the vein. Then it's pushed all the way until the tip sits just above the heart. The heart. My heart. The needle is removed, leaving the PICC line in place and ready to send in my chemotherapy cocktails or someone else's blood, and somewhere on the PICC line there is a 'lumen'. I can't work out what a lumen is. Lumen in the gloomin. Sounds very Robbie Burns. There's a connector, a plastic thing a bit like a bicycle tyre valve, at the end of the PICC line, and fluids will go through that instead of straight into the flesh, and a bung goes into the end of it when it's not in use. The bung, as in bung me a tenner, why don't you, is held in place with a see-through dressing to stop it falling out, a thought I find utterly disgusting. How can something that has touched my heart, or sat close to it – whatever the hell that means – fall out? And what unguent would spout from it if the bung came unbunged?

After a nice lie down on a couch during a scan to check the PICC line is in the correct position next to my indignant heart, I leave for my next appointment, a metal triangle inside my left arm and a tube of plastic running through it.

My elbows are out, like Grandma taught me to do when getting on a crowded bus in curlers, as I zigzag my way down Euston Road. It is four o'clock on a Friday afternoon, the wide pavements are rammed and I am in danger of being late for my hearing appointment. No one looks at me. Were they to glance at me, they would not know that I have cancer. This is, momentarily, astonishing. And I wouldn't know a thing about them either. The man in the suit and dark coat who won't budge an inch as I try to pass him might just have lost his wife. I walk around him, feeling neither rage nor impatience. The tall woman with the ponytail just in front of me might be terminally ill. My eyes mist up, and I am only looking at the back of her head. *Her* head? Perhaps it's *his* head. She might be a transvestite. I don't know where this sudden concern for the human race has come from, but my head is filling up with it; it must be all this time spent in hospital. According to a former editor of the *Daily Telegraph*, the supermodel Naomi Campbell signs off her emails 'love and light'. Am I feeling the love and seeing the light? Is that why I am concerning myself with the identity of the stranger in front of me who is in my way and whom I would ordinarily hurry pass with pointed agitation?

I arrive at the hearing hospital near King's Cross, and take in the sign above the door. It says Royal National Throat, Nose and Ear Hospital (RNTNEH). People talk about Ear, Nose and Throat, not Throat, Nose and Ear. When I was a toddler, living in New York, I was 'an ENT kid', constantly in hospital for check-ups. In the end, when I was four, I had my tonsils taken out. The doctor sat with me and helped me do some colouring in. Then I took the tonsils home in a jar. So I know. ENT.

Before going in, I take a picture of the sign. Then I flag down a passer-by, worry he could be deaf (he is right outside the hospital doors), wish I hadn't, realise it's too late, and, exaggerating my lip movements, ask him to take my picture next to the sign. I smile, the village fool of Planet Cancer. Inside is George Orwell grim: grey, dirty-feeling. I've been spoilt by UCLH and its Macmillan Cancer Centre, both shiny, state-of-the-art. Moreover, the reception staff at Healing HQ, as I like to call the Macmillan Cancer Centre, and in every department I have encountered at UCLH, are engaged, alert, friendly, helpful. The receptionist here is like a cardboard cut-out that speaks. She's about twenty-five, probably a temp, and she's bored rigid by her job. Fair enough.

I descend a stone staircase, go through three sets of double doors, go to another reception area which turns out to be the wrong one. Extras from *The Living Dead* are slouched on plastic chairs. I find the right place. As I approach this receptionist, who is sitting, head lowered, behind the counter, I wonder if she is actually dead.

I am here for some hearing tests, I say, and hand her my appointment letter. She takes it, so is alive, after all, and asks me to wait.

I want to go home. Cry baby.

The hearing tests will provide the doctors with a baseline audiogram should any hearing problems emerge. Cisplatin was approved for use in humans in 1978. It's a molecule made from platinum, the shining metal beloved of brides and rappers, and it induces cell suicide. In other words, the cancerous cells can't divide and conquer. Its side effects include nerve damage and hearing loss, as well as kidney damage and severe sickness; its nickname is sickplatin. Radiation to the head and neck can also cause impaired hearing, such as tinnitus and the inability to hear high-pitched sounds. Since I am neither a dolphin, whale, dog nor mother of infants whose yelping I need to be able to hear through thick walls like the ones I am surrounded by now, not being able to hear high-pitched sounds seems quite agreeable. Low-pitched sounds, such as a human snoring, I'd also like not to be able to hear. Still. Loss of balance is another side effect. In short, you get the symptoms of old age before you've even got used to being middle-aged. No matter: the side effects are part of the cure; part of the trade-off. No matter if I lose my balance; I was hardly planning to take up slacklining.

A woman calls my name and asks me to follow her. She leads me down a narrow, dark, airless corridor into a cell. There is a glass screen dividing it from a cell on the other side. Initially, we both sit together and I peer into the other cell, expecting to see Hannibal Lecter gurning at me. He'd like it here. The audiologist puts a metal 'bone' on my head; it's a headband, only it goes across my skull, from the back of my head to the tip of my nose. I don't care if I have tinnitus or my fingers tingle for the rest of my life. They might. They might not. My swallowing may be permanently impaired. It may not. There's not much I can do about it. W. H. Auden would seem to agree; he's suddenly in my head with the lines 'Time will say nothing but I told you so,' and then Othello pipes up with his 'Destiny, unshunnable, like death' in his self-aggrandising voice. Was head and neck cancer always on the cards for me, is that what these two are trying to tell me?

'What do you think caused your cancer?' a friend asked me last week, suggesting that my fate is in fact in my own hands. Did I cause it, or was it predetermined? Is it a test? If it is, am I allowed to fail it? I mustn't think like this. Despair is forbidden. I learned as much from the nice old priest who came to Moira House with his stoop and his white hair every Wednesday evening at seven o'clock to give my sister and me and the few other stray Catholics catechism lessons. Despair is a mortal sin, he told us. *Mortal* sin. What does that even mean?

The audiologist ushers me into the adjoining cell. There is a machine on the table. Press the button when you hear the sound, she says.

The instinct is to do well, in any test, so I try hard to react quickly. But after a few minutes, I just press the button when I get round to it, after my mind has got back from elsewhere. The tests go on and on, I'm taken to another room, have some different tests, then I'm allowed to leave.

I get the best seat on the bus going home, the one on the top deck at the front, and feel an inane rush of excitement, and then of loneliness. Loneliness: it took root with Dr Dish's words, 'There is only one way to put this . . .' and now it is under my skin, along with my PICC line, and the voice in my head that never takes time out. I don't know what my brain was even doing, before. Lazing about, shooting the breeze. Cancer is an electrode on the temples, it's circuit overload, it's your thoughts and your terrors sparking off each other and the flames licking your loneliness. It's your loneliness pulling up a chair when you are sitting next to someone you love and who you know loves you back and that counting for nothing, you strung out in some godforsaken desert of a desiccated nowhere. If I knew how bad the loneliness was going to get, that this was only the merest hint, I might feel less lonely on the short bus ride home.

That night, when Richard comes to bed, he wraps himself around me and he tells me he loves me and then he puts out his light and he tells me again and then several times during our wakeful night. It's getting to be a habit.

In the morning I ask him to stop repeatedly telling me he loves me.

It's not normal.

10

CALL ME GINGER

I spot a bald woman my age on my first day of chemotherapy and feel a shot of cheer. That won't be me. She, poor thing, may as well walk around with a sandwich board saying 'I'VE GOT CANCER,' which is a bit like being heavily pregnant and everyone knowing your business, only without the coos and the 'when's it due?' In the elevator going up to the chemotherapy *lounge* (you say 'lounge', I say 'airport', 'hotel', 'living room', never cancer), Richard is pale. I am bright red, having been garrotted by self-disgust. Only an emotional freak would feel good about keeping their hair when other women lose theirs, and another part of their identity along the way.

Cancer is supposed to make you into a nicer person, smooth your edges. I have slipped under the net.

We step straight into the open-plan chemotherapy lounge and eau de cancer is all over me. Boiled turnips infused with mothballs, grief and dead cells, topped with a metallic nose. I'll be wearing it myself soon, but I don't know this; for now, while I am still allowed to wear perfume, I am wearing Rive Gauche, and I recoil at the smell of the place. Blinkers on, eyes straight, keen not to look at any patients, I head for the reception desk at the other end of the vast room with its spectacular glazed atrium that fills the healing space with light. There is one treatment bay to the right, and two main ones to the left. I make it past the big round table in the middle of the room and the cocktail-party clusters of pink chairs, some occupied, some not, and their side tables, when a Humpty Dumpty head catches my eye. It is protruding from a blanket in a treatment bay on the left. It is turned to the side, the visible eye closed and nearly obscured by the pillow that flips upwards either side of it. A tube is spouting from a hefty arm that lies like a fallen branch on the bed cover. Who loves him, this big man, reduced to this? What are his chances? I keep walking.

When I greet the receptionist, I go for a game-show delivery.

'Hi, my name's Genevieve Fox and I'm here to start chemotherapy.'

'Sorry, your name is . . .?'

I repeat it. As I watch the receptionist looking me up on his computer, the voice in my head goes all Tourette's on me.

What the fuck. Who'd have ****ing thought it: Genevieve Fox, yes, that's me, and I'm here to start chemo-****ing-therapy and I am NOT happy about it.

I need a punchbag. I need arms around me. I need the child that has sprung up from nowhere to back down or get a grip.

'Oh, yes. Take a seat. The nurse will be with you in a minute.'

We sit, side by side. Richard reads the paper, I look at the red and white linoleum floor tiles. I recognise the artist, the jubilant Rob Ryan. We've got a set of his blue and white plates at home. We serve canapés or cookies on them. Once the treats have gone, messages reveal themselves. On my favourite plate, a fairy-tale couple cavorts in branches festooned with bunting. 'We had nothing,' it reads. 'We had not much. We had enough. We had everything.' It's written for me and Richard. Someone calls my name, a question mark sounded at the end of it, sending me floating up into the medicinal air. Richard and I look over our shoulders. A nurse is scouring the room, eyebrows raised.

'Yes!' I say and I wave. Coo-ee. Over here. As if someone else will answer to my name or nick my place.

'Shall I come with you?' Richard asks. Neither of us knows what will happen next, so I say no.

I grab my bags, drop my jacket, pick it up, hurry over to the nurse. Behind her is a whiteboard and there's my name, right at the top of about seven names, written in blue marker pen. In my sessions that take place once a week over the next three months, it is always like this: efficient and punctual. I am never kept waiting for more than a few minutes.

'Take a seat,' says a nurse. I perch, teeth tight, on the edge of it. She wheels over a metal trolley, then tries to roll up my sleeve. She has to get the needle into my PICC line to take some blood. The PICC line is forgiven: I never have to have a needle invading my skin for the duration of my treatment. So is my fashionista friend, who asked: 'Have you thought about what you'll wear for chemotherapy?' to which I thought: funnily enough, hospital chic is not on my list of priorities.

It turns out she had a point. It is important to get your chemotherapy outfit right. The long-sleeved T-shirt I have turned up in is too tight; so are the sleeves of my sweater, which I end up having to take off. I'm then cold as another nurse takes me across the lounge to one of the treatment bays. I sit in a padded chair as comfortable as any in a de luxe beauty parlour. What I would like now is for a woman in white linen to wheel a trolley over to me and give me a manicure. I'm not complaining, I am lucky to be here, it could be worse. And so on. Richard sits in the chair next to me. One of the two treatment chairs opposite me, mercifully far enough away to preclude chat, is occupied by a woman dressed in loose flannel black trousers, scoop neck black top with three-quarter bell sleeves. She knows the ropes, then. Her outfit is offset by a turban and soft, kiss-me pink lipstick. She could be in *Vogue*. Maybe she works for *Vogue*. I should network. But no, she's too curvaceous to work for *Vogue*. And too stylish to be here.

The nurse does the name/date of birth routine in front of another nurse. This happens every time they change the drip, every time my blood is taken, every time I receive any treatment at all. No chance of being swapped, then. She hooks me up to a drip coming out of a plastic bag that hangs like an over-ripe mango from a metal hangman's stand on wheels. The bag is filled with saline solution.

'To flush out your kidneys,' the nurse says. I don't know what she is talking about. Have they been in hiding?

The drip is attached to an electronic monitor. It beeps non-stop, adding to the chorus of machines that chirp from every corner of the lounge all day long. I come to hate the sound.

'You'll need to pass one litre of urine before we can start the cisplatin,' the nurse says next. She hands me a grey cardboard bowl with frayed edges. Handy for boarding school, I think. I could pitch these to *Dragons' Den*, parents of young boarders with weak bladders the target market.

Richard gets coffee and snacks, starts the crossword. I drape around me the new blanket Vicky bought me, insisting I would get cold during chemotherapy, and instead of reading my magazine, just sit, eyes open but not seeing, like one of those upright dead people I saw in the ENT hospital. Twenty minutes later, I need to pee. Up I get, holding on to the hangman stand with one hand and the edge of the cardboard bowl with the other. I take a couple of steps, and then I am stuck. I flap the bowl at a passing nurse.

'You're all right,' she says, 'you've got batteries.'

She unplugs me from the mains socket and then I set off for the lavatory. I can feel Richard's eyes on me, so I do a skip, to show everything's all right.

'You're Ginger. He's Fred,' he says, pointing to the stand.

Someone is having treatment in a chair bang opposite the lavatory door. I'm glad I'm not docked there, I think as Fred and I lock ourselves inside the cubicle. There are three metal bins, handrails everywhere, a long red string with a loop at the end of it and plenty of space to spin Fred. It smells like the nursing home I had to visit for voluntary service at school. Fred is next to me as I undo my jeans. This is my first manoeuvre with a drip attached to my arm. I'm like the receiver attached to a rotary telephone. Holding the bowl beneath me and peeing into it is unspeakable, not least because I am expelling a giant's volume of urine with the force of a carthorse. I empty the thing, shutting my eyes as I do so, then Fred stands patiently by as I wash my hands with unprecedented zeal.

I open the door, to see the patient still there in her chair, her friend beside her. There is no hiding where I've been. I smile at them, trying to feel the love and the light. They glare back. I trundle off.

'Excuse me!'

Fred and I stop in our tracks.

'Shut the door, can't you?'

We spin around.

'Sorry,' I mutter, unable to look at them. 'Of course.' Really, I am thinking, you're a charmless pair. But then the love and the light find a chink to squeeze through and I imagine being stuck in the train of lavatory traffic myself and realise they've been rather restrained. Up down, up down, these checks and balances are hard work. Being nice all the time would be easier, but impossible. I do not know how the staff manage it, day after day. I shut the darned door, and then I am plugged back in. The nurse is swapping my saline solution for anti-emetics when Caroline whooshes in.

'How are you doing?' she says, grabbing the mango bag and reading the contents. 'Yes! That's the baby, you got it!'

Who knew a bag of anti-sickness drugs could light up a human being's face. She hugs both of us, flashing her TV-teeth grin, and asks how the day has been and talks us through how I might feel later on. She is a glory girl. She lifts our spirits up through the atrium and skywards. We had lunch with her and her husband, Hans, the oncologist and immunologist, yesterday. After she leaves us and dashes back to her own patients, I tell Richard how Hans hugged me hard when we were leaving their house and told me I would be fine. If it's coming from Hans, I say, it must be true, he knows.

We skip the offer of hospital food in favour of lunch from Pret A Manger. All hail their rocket and crayfish sandwich. All hail chewing, the tongue, swallowing: the triumvirate facilitating the first stage of digestion. The cisplatin makes me sleepy, or maybe it's all the adrenaline, and I snooze. Before I know it, it's four o'clock and time to go home where I'll continue with the treatment, courtesy of a plastic baby bottle with a golden balloon inside it. This is filled with another chemotherapy drug, fluorouracil, or FU, and is attached to my PICC line. FU. There's an acronym. The bottle sits in a blue nylon pouch with a handy shoulder strap. It comes with a belt loop, too, so I can wear it at hip level like a pistol. By Friday I'll be all out of FU, the balloon will have emptied and I'll have two weeks off before round two of chemotherapy.

When the boys get back from school I show off my pump, which elicits a modicum of curiosity. Reuben says he will graffiti the pouch with 'champagne on tap' and then they both get on with their homework. At six o'clock I am under a duvet on the sofa down in the kitchen, shell-shocked and feeling floaty and faintly nauseous, but pleased as punch at how the day has panned out. The doorbell rings, there's a loud hello and a ripple of laughter. It's Sue, queen of the Meals on Heels rota, which she's set up with our old Primrose Hill primary school posse. She bounds down the stairs, all red lipstick and sailor's top and blonde updo and she's carrying an industrial-sized tray bursting with food: Ottolenghi leek and potato pie on a china plate, salad, bottle of dressing, apple crumble, custard, flowers, a vase for the flowers, a card. It's a first-class service.

And about time. I've wanted staff all my life.

In bed, the chemotherapy pump lies under the duvet like a dolly playing hide-and-seek. I check my emails and see that Vicky has sent me a poem. She is researching gold for a book project and has come across 'Mrs Midas' by Carol Ann Duffy and thought I might like it. I do. It is spirited and funny and full of cracking images. When the narrator, the wife of King Midas, serves her husband corn on the cob for starters he is soon 'spitting out the teeth of the rich' because, of course, everything he touches turns to gold. A few minutes later, fearful of his touch – the Midas touch – she takes the precaution of putting the cat in the cellar. That night, her husband is banished to the spare room, promptly turning it 'into the tomb of Tutankhamun' while she barricades herself in the bedroom. She dreams she gives birth to his baby with 'perfect ore limbs, its little tongue/ like a precious latch'.

I picture that metal tongue as I take the various drugs that have appeared on my bedside table. One of them knocks me out. I don't dream. I don't dream for three nights. Then my subconscious breaks its chemical chains and I have one nightmare after another. In the first, I am wandering in a Boschian hellscape of a forest. Dead foxes, bears, stoats, cats and horses hang, distorted like Dali's clocks, from scorched trees. I worry that a bloodied tail or dripping gut will touch my bare scalp but I don't duck. Then I see Pepper, hanging from another tree, her little body twisted and disembowelled. The following night I dream that Bassy has been stabbed and I don't realise. He cries out for me. There is blood on his mattress.

I call the ambulance. I wake up before the ambulance arrives, the nightmare my waking reality, and I get up and hurry to Bassy's bedroom. I stick my head around the door, see him sleeping, shake my head at my folly. Then I creep in the dark down to the kitchen and make some tea, bring it up to the study and, sitting at my desk, turn on Radio 3. Violins are dancing, reaching, running. Bruch, I think, and then Bruch's Violin Concerto No. 3, Op. 58 in D minor flashes up in tickertape on the digital screen. Bruch, always so harrowing. Not tonight, not after that nightmare.

Four days into the treatment, I step into the shower with the pump pouch swinging from my shoulder like a naturist off on a beach walk. What to do with the thing? I squeeze it between the shampoo and the conditioner on the corner tray, the conditioner tumbles out, I bend over to pick it up. The pump's strap tugs taut. It has got itself wrapped round the temperature dial, leaving the pump suspended in mid-air like a Zeppelin. The golden balloon inside the pump itself has shrivelled up like an old man's bad dream, the FU now fully dispensed. I reach out to untangle the straps and water seeps under the freaky elasticated waterproof sleeve I am wearing on my left arm to protect the PICC dressing and which makes me think of incontinence. Which I'd rather not.

My social life is under threat, thanks to the Ancient Mariner side effects predicted for the combined chemo-radiotherapy: boils, ulcers, scabby neck, burning tongue. Some women like to wear a pashmina to cover up, advised Khalda, my new specialist nurse. Pashminas! I thought they were safely buried in a shallow grave along with the Sloane Ranger. Is cancer the death of style? Since the only alternative I can think of is my black feather boa, the answer would seem to be yes. I resolve to get my socialising in while I am still sartorially fit for purpose. This sees me negotiating

Camberwell Road in my puppy-chewed Prada heels the following night. We're off to have dinner with friends, only accepting the invitation at the last minute since we didn't know how the chemotherapy would leave me feeling. Bassy is on a sleepover and Reuben is at a party, so we're not leaving them on their own. Ordinarily we would happily leave them to fry their brains on *Call of Duty* and binge on Domino's pizza while we discussed, without irony, the cultural wastelands inhabited by twenty-first-century adolescents. Now I don't want to leave them on their own. I don't credit them with sufficient emotional resilience not to feel bereft in our absence.

Richard and I are on form. Ten minutes into the journey, we are arguing about directions. An hour later, we are lost in south London. I text, on behalf of both of us, to say we are close. Then we stop arguing and play spot the off-licence. All we can see are pound shops and newsagents. I end up standing in the middle of a busy high road, buses shaving my backside as I wait for a lull in the traffic. I secure a bottle of Pinot Grigio; it's hardly worth risking my life for.

I text again to say we are nearly there, then rumble us by texting to ask for directions. We arrive, late, and in the excitement all I want to do is sit back on the comfy sofa and let my sudden light-headedness settle. Our friends give us a tour of their new house. I follow our host up four floors of their Georgian terrace, each flight climbing, like Escher's stairways, into nowhere, with me headed straight over the top. I feel worse than light-headed, I feel like my brain is exposed, and have to grab the banister. Then, as is the way, we have to go all the way down again. The basement kitchen is cold. Or rather, I am cold. I sit down, an old lady in a bath chair, wanting a blanket and not having the wherewithal to ask for one. I feel so odd and disconnected I don't even trust myself to speak, and studiously avoid eye contact. I sit very still, anxious not to turn my head, which is now about to take flight. Soup spoons clatter. Edward Scissorhands blades tap my skull. My whole body is unearthed. I am like a tree without roots. If a tree were afraid, or under siege, this is how it would feel.

I sit, smiling, uneasy. I hear everyone discussing movies and the cross-dressing man from whom Helen and Nancy bought this house, how he had clandestine deliveries of yellow push-up balcony bras from H&M. I hear our friend Heidi saying Northumberland is beneath Shropshire and I think, no it isn't. Then Richard says it is beneath Scotland and nowhere near Shropshire. Shropshire is near Wiltshire, Heidi says next, and there's a bird cry and then another, it's everyone laughing, and then they talk about something else and I can't follow the conversation. I don't know Nancy nearly as well as I know her partner and I think she must think me very dull for just sitting here, this tree-human with an exposed brain. I want to be in bed.

The Primrose Hill posse's Meals on Heels menus are so elaborate, I come to suspect my friends are running a cash-prize competition at my expense. Highlights include: starter of home-made mushroom and thyme soup followed by prawn and coriander curry with an optional cashew nut garnish, served with tricolore salad. To finish off: apple pie with choice of crème fraiche or vanilla custard. A tray of salmon fishcakes is accompanied by a side of green beans with shallots, in an oven-ready dish. Afternoon tea includes banana, honey and nut cake, so good it would make Mary Berry quiver. Some cook on site, and even lay the table. For a main: salmon on rough mash with honey and mustard dressing and lightly boiled egg, served with green beans and a bottle of Saint-Aubin. To follow: chocolate pudding. The deliveries come with cards, flowers, potted orchids, pouches of fresh herbs, notes about how to heat the food, wine, champagne, juices, supplements, medicinal tonics, vitamins and, since we are pescatarians and the boys are not, meat options for them as well.

Sometimes, though, the deliveries don't come at all. My friend Jules texts me to say she is in the country and is worried that she won't get back in time to make her scheduled early evening delivery. I tell her not to worry. Half an hour later I get another text: *Sorted. Salvino's are doing a delivery for me.* Salvino's is the local Italian deli, and they don't do deliveries. Jules, who I know has used them to cater for her in the past, is clearly a favoured customer. Goodie, I think.

Come early evening, Richard and I have to go out for a couple of hours. I tell him about the Salvino's delivery and we run through what might be coming our way: their ravioli stuffed with mushrooms and chestnuts, perhaps, or roasted aubergines with sun-dried tomatoes, or a tomato and mozzarella salad made with their silken burrata. Then, half an hour before we get home, I get another text:

Thank you so much for the Salvino's supper. So thoughtful of you. You are too kind. All our love. S and I. xxx.

It's from our neighbour, who is ill with a very severe stomach condition. But they do like their food, even now.

I check the time. 7 p.m. Too early for supper. Surely they won't have eaten yet. There's still time to get our hands on the delivery. If I had only told them I had cancer in the first place, and not been so English and restrained, this would never have happened. Trying to be selfless always backfires.

I compose my text. *Woops. Not meant for you. DO NOT EAT IT.* That sounds rude. A prank might work. *What delivery? Must be a hoax. Probably a bomb. On way. Don't touch.* Then I try being nice: *You're welcome.* Which they aren't, followed by *Hope you enjoy it,* which I don't.

In the end, I go for: *That's good to hear. Was it delicious? Hope you are feeling better,* and press send.

Other deliveries put *Come Dine with Me* in the shade. Eco-Debbie, our gardening friend, seems to be taking notes from the reality TV show. She's got the part where the camera films guests arriving at the host's front door in fancy dress off pat. For her first delivery she comes as Hiawatha in braids, kohled-up eyes, miniskirt and plum suede wedge boots.

'Plaice!' she says, thrusting a tray in my hands like an ice-cream usherette doing a runner. 'All fresh! Fifteen fucking quid!'

I grab it. She steps into the hall, whips off a sheet of aluminium foil. Four fish fillets lie on a baking tray, a lemon slice on each, a sprig of parsley. There's a bowl of mashed potato, another filled with leeks, sliced and ready to cook. A large pot of swirly organic fudge yoghurt. I've watched Eco-Debbie cook, seen unidentifiable foodstuffs fall out of the oven on to the kitchen floor, only to be tossed back in. I've seen the home-made blinis that look like they've been fired out of a splatter gun. Something's shifted. Suddenly she's like someone off *MasterChef*. I stagger downstairs to the kitchen with the tray while she and her partner, Steve, make themselves comfortable on the sofa in the living room.

'If you think you've had a bad week,' she bellows down after me, 'wait til you hear about mine.'

I come back up with cups of tea and trip over her coat, dumped like an art installation in the middle of the living-room floor.

'. . . We're talking thousands of pounds here . . .'

She's close to exchanging on a property deal and a few hundred thousand pounds have got lost in the ether, apparently. I'm about to offer her the fifteen quid back to tide her over when she segues from solicitors to the piles she had a few years back and how evacuation – my word, not hers – was like shitting a hedgehog – her words, not mine. It's her way of saying: How are you?

Shortly after she's disappeared in another puff of profanities and eccentric love, fairy dust floats through the house in the form of Howard, a musician friend from school and Reuben's godfather. He asks me, in his quiet, gentle way, if I see myself as waging a battle against cancer. Is the battle metaphor apt, he wants to know. A battle is what is expected, we both agree, it comes with the territory, along with 'journey'. *She is battling cancer,* people say. I am not. I realise, talking to Howard, that I have accepted the fact of my cancer; I am not fighting it, have not turned it into a tangible foe in my mind or felt the need to turn it into a metaphor. As with the journey metaphor, the battle one does not hold: I don't have an army to send in, for a start. It's too late for that. It would make more sense to say that I've been ambushed, taken hostage. A battle suggests forces, pitted against each other and, putting aside the possibility of a truce, one outcome: a victor and a loser. But whether I prevail isn't up to me. I don't have any weapons. The disease, on the other hand, has ground troops, already deployed, and psychological warfare, also deployed, drawing me into a minefield of mind games which, much further down the line, will truly put me on my mettle.

If anyone is fighting a battle, it is the oncologists and their teams, armed with their drugs and their scalpels, their machines and their expertise. In my case, their deadly weapon is a combination-therapy two-drug missile. Each drug, the cisplatin and the fluorouracil, has a unique destruction mechanism which goes for head and neck cancer cells, no hostages taken. The cancer cells try to change to escape obliteration. One drug only, and it is relatively easy for a cancer cell to escape and then grow as a drug-resistant cancer cell. Send in two drugs, though, and it's much harder for any cancer cell to become resistant to two different killing mechanisms. Impressive. A dove myself, I like my oncologists' hawkish ways.

But what arsenal have I got to offer? Hope, herbal teas and turmeric. Oh, and determination. All of these might help a tad, but they alone can't defeat my cancer, nor anyone else's. To suggest they can is illusory: mind alone cannot conquer matter. Which is just as well, since cancer turns the mind into a cowering thing.

Are you angry? Howard asks next, and I, who am habitually enraged by the slightest thing – from overpriced 'fresh' smoothies and my children not coming down for supper when they are called, to privately educated university graduates who live in council flats and friends who shop at Primark – reply: no, I am not angry. Frightened, yes, but not angry, not in the slightest. I've got something close to inner calm to draw on. I've got something else up my sleeve, too. A secret weapon. No one knows about it, except Reuben and Marjorie, the boys' Church of England primary school vicar who I went to see in that limbo between diagnosis and prognosis. I haven't told Richard or Bassy about it. I haven't told Richard because the secret weapon is a dream. I did once tell him about a recurring dream I used to have, hoping that, in the spirit of playground reciprocity, he'd then tell me one of his. In mine, I've just left the newspaper where I work and am driving, naked, up Kensington Church Street, quite unselfconscious. Then, when I get to the traffic lights on Notting Hill, I come over all Adam and Eve, but have nothing with which to cover myself up. I cast about on the floor, on the back seat. Nothing. Meanwhile, the lights fix on red.

Ever had a dream about driving naked? I asked Richard when I'd finished. Nope, he said, never have. So I keep my big dream, which I had two months before the diagnosis, largely to myself. Until now, when I test it out on Howard.

I was high up in the sky, I tell him. It was very bright. The sky was baby blue, the clouds fluffy. I was aware that I had never been so high up. One minute I was contemplating my vertiginous position and the next I was falling, fast. The shock was terrifying. It was like being pushed out of an aeroplane door, only this wasn't skydiving and I didn't have a parachute or a burly instructor attached to me. I was shooting back down to earth, like a rocket in reverse. I knew I was going to die. I had never, until then, known terror, in my subconscious or conscious life. In the moment of that realisation, a moment of profound sorrow, a hand reached out, a Michelangelo hand, large, its creased fingers extended. With fine timing, it stretched beneath me like a net and caught me.

What struck me then and when I woke up in the morning, elated, the dream foremost in my mind, was the kindness of the act. It wasn't about power, or the showing off of power, as in I (whoever or whatever that 'I' denotes) have the power to catch you and I am going to leave it til the last moment before I do so. That way, you will be very afraid and then pitifully, desperately grateful and indebted. No, it was a benign act, as automatic as a parent taking their child out of danger. I only experienced a split second of terror; the conviction that I was safe, loved and not alone was, by contrast, enduring. It was my moment in the rose garden. What I didn't tell Howard was how, for the next few days, I felt joyful. I wanted to tell everyone about it. *Guess what happened to me. You'll never believe it.* But I couldn't tell anyone, because I'd sound like an intellectually challenged God Squad groupie or a card-carrying Christian having a moment. That's not me. I only get to church a dozen times a year, tops. I am not a God person. The dream would give people the wrong idea about me. Besides, I needed to make sense of it myself, decide if it was an intimation of a truth and something, as the vicar suggested, to be trusted, which she would say, or just a dream. Either way, it had short-circuited my consciousness. I *knew* I was safe, whatever happened to me. Safe, I think, is another word for love. Howard, who comes to most things with an entirely open mind, and an open heart, likes the dream, is taken by it. The hand of God, he says, and then he smiles.

I take a nap on a razor's edge. Mother used to nap, and look what happened to her. As I lie in bed trying to recharge before the boys get home from school, my mind rewinds to Mother and that last day I saw her in the hospice. It's hot, I'm in my summer uniform, carefree in cotton dress, long white socks, sandals. I leave my school friends doing French skipping on the lawn. The cab pulls up outside a red-brick Victorian building with gables, a pointed roof and white window frames, like a smaller version of one of the boarding houses at school. The air inside is tight; it makes you feel as though it is wrong to make the slightest movement. When a nurse shows my sister and me upstairs and into Mother's room, the adults who surely must have been with us vanish. My sister, always by my side, vanishes too. I run into the room on my own and the air tries to ground me, the nurse tries to slow me down with her eyes. I can't get to Mother's side, only as far as the foot of her bed. The woman with the backcombed hair and the song-bursts and the laughter has gone. In her place is a jagged bird, wingless. No more round cheeks, with their hint of bone. Everything in the room is white; it is pressing down on her tiny frame. The light from the window pushes into the whiteness. The bed frame is white and on it are white sheets, with part of Mother there, underneath them. She is dressed in a white floral nightdress; it floats around her body, reluctant to settle on her skin. There is so little flesh. She does not seem to be occupying her body; does not seem to be connected to the bed either. Beneath the sheets and the nightdress, where I cannot see, is the cancer bump, the mound of distended organs that says what is so hard to say, what she does not say to me, perhaps does not know: it is all over.

'Hello, darling.' The voice that used to belt out arpeggios and a string of clee-clee-clee-clee-clee-clee-clee-cle-clars as she practised at the piano is scarecrow scrawny now.

'Hello,' I say, approaching the bed. The narrow translucent plastic band on her wrist shuffles up and down the bone like a bracelet.

'There is no need to whisper, darling, just because I am.'

'Of course not,' I whisper back. I cannot make myself speak any louder, and feel stupid for it.

That visit did not last long; we were soon back in the cab. I never saw Mother again. It was years before I stopped waiting for her to come back for us.

It is nearly half past three now. My cheeks are wet. I will dry them, swap my tears for wings, big, golden annunciation wings with tips and arches that reach above my shoulders. I will spread my wings, keep them open, give my sons something to lean against.

An hour later I hear Reuben's key in the front door and I hurry to the landing and take up position. In he comes, followed by Dan, Toby, Seb and Mish, all here for the Super-bowl party, which Richard lays on every year. I start walking down the stairs and casually say hello as the boys file past me and go down to the kitchen, all of them so tall and handsome in their black blazers, their big feet like flippers. I've known two of the boys since they were two, another since he was seven, the fourth just for a couple of years. My heart tumbles. Life-lust catches in my throat.

I hear their deep voices jump an octave as they fuss over convalescing Pepper. Cupboard doors crash, the fridge beeps, plastic boots kick the table football, shouts go up. Bassy comes home, I reappear, but he is too intent on hugging Pepper to hug me. I sneak back up to bed. When Richard gets home from work he makes platters of nachos and they all watch the game and I think of that afternoon two years ago when

I visited Cassandra Jardine in her family home. She had stationed herself on a sofa in the living room. Her sons and their friends were sitting in their TV room in the basement, watching a football match. When I excused myself to use the bathroom she, no longer strong enough to go up and down the stairs, asked me to check on them. I duly went down and stuck my head around the door and said hello. They were sprawled on the sofas, engrossed. I came upstairs and reported back. Then a roar went up from downstairs. She put her index finger to her lips, then said:

'A goal!' She smiled, her head cocked. After a minute or so, she added: 'I love to hear them. Happiness!'

One of the perks of being ill is getting to see more of your friends. There is an intimacy, too, and a change in tempo. You get beneath the surface. Estèlle, the pin-up of the Meals on Heels rota, rocks up in vintage Chanel jacket and shorts, her long hair pulled up in a ponytail, showing off a face that should be on the side of a bus. Too rarefied to drive, she has travelled by taxi carrying army rations of vegetarian lasagne. It feeds us for two days. I let slip my anxiety and she says: how could you not be anxious? You are living your worst fear. She helps me see past it: her father had very nearly the same cancer and punitive radiotherapy as me. He had a mask, she says, and they strapped him down and buckled him in and he had to put a bit in his mouth to stop him from biting his tongue.

My friend Lu takes me to a warehouse designer shoe sale in Notting Hill. The sale is a scorcher: the shoes are about £20 a pair; they're usually six or seven times that. I buy five pairs: clogs, snakeskin brogues, pink suede boots, two-tone cowboy boots, high-heeled brown boots. Lu does not bat an eye. Indeed, she buys me an additional pair of cowboy boots, with a four-inch Cuban heel and a wine-red and cream colour scheme as a birthday present. The rest of the stash is my birthday present from Richard.

Over lunch, Lu grills me on how I feel. Queasy, I say, thinking she is talking about the shoe binge. But it's the chemotherapy she wants to know about, and I explain how it is so much better than I expected and what a relief it is to be able to be out and about. I try to explain the low-level nausea and the discombobulating feeling that I might float up into the air at any minute. Then I run through the Meals on Heels menus so far, thinking she will find this particularly encouraging, her prime pleasure being food, the second being planning what she is going to eat. It's love on a plate, I say, and I see a flash of fear in her eyes.

'I wonder if my friends would do the same for me,' she says.

The trouble with me, I realise, is that I portend ill. This is the year in which most of my friends turn fifty; adults aged fifty to seventy-four account for just over half of the new incidences of cancer in the UK. I am a living statistic, the spectre at the life feast.

11

FITTING IN

One of the many good things about boarding school is that you're all incarcerated together: children of divorced parents, children of perfect families, of exiles, diplomats, the miscellaneous, orphans. At Moira House some of the parents lived in their native Nigeria, Pakistan, Kuwait. Others were stationed in exotic places like Gibraltar. In the absence of relatives or hired guardians, many pupils stayed at school during the exeats. The parents might as well have been dead, for all their children saw of them. I liked that. It created a level playing field.

Regular letters home kept the parental flames alive, including mine to Mother. On Saturday mornings we filed into a ground-floor reception room with big windows, our writing cases under our arms. Mother had bought me a black leather one. It had a gold zip with gangster teeth and when you drew the zip round, it opened flat on the table like bat wings. A pad of white Basildon Bond writing paper slotted over a flap and rested against a blotter. The pad came with a sheet of thick-set lined paper to keep your hand straight. There was a leather loop in the spine of the case for storing a fountain pen. The left flap had a slot for envelopes, and three smaller ones. I kept strips of stamps in one of them. We each carried our own pot of deep blue Quink.

I liked writing home, until home went AWOL, after which I wrote to Grandma instead or, when I felt it was cruel not to and couldn't stand the guilt, to Tamsin. On her instant replies, the sight of her emphatic handwriting on the envelope made me wince. Poor Tamsin.

I was proud of my writing case, and kept treasures in the side pocket, including a sketch of Sydney, my ursine husband, sprawled on his back. The recumbent pose was the touch of a bohemian English artist called Adrian Daintrey who knocked it up on a visit to the Sussex house. He liked bears; he did portraits of his friend John Betjeman and his bear Archibald, too. Louise, a new boarder, pitched up with a red leather writing case of briefcase proportions, not to mention a mother and a father, two brothers, a Labrador and a kidney-shaped swimming pool. Her writing case had a handle and her initials engraved on the outside, and when you opened it there were flaps that ran the length of the lid for different sizes of paper. Louise, who was half Swedish, also arrived with a duvet – a sort of fluffy eiderdown you wrapped in a giant pocket of a sheet, sealing it up with poppers – and tubes of fish paste that oozed out like sugar-pink toothpaste on to the giant pieces of crispbread she kept in her tuck box. The duvet, which got her out of the hospital corners for which I always got a black mark during daily room inspection, was the first one in the school, and so was the luxury triplex cage that housed her hamster. Its three floors were connected by transparent tubes. Louise was the talk of the pet room. I started to stay with her family for exeat weekends and, sometimes, for half-term. Luckily for me the weekly boarding we had done with Mother had been phased out. We only had to go 'home' for two exeat weekends and one week-long half-term holiday per term. When Tamsin collected us from school, I watched as her mustard-yellow Fiat pulled up and saw her flicked-up hair and her big fingers on the steering wheel. There was no choice but to get in and drive all the way from Eastbourne to Brighton, my body rigid for the full 40 minutes. My sister would not speak, in what I took to be an ongoing and justifiable act of resistance, so I had to. It felt mean not to talk to Tamsin, as if we were sticking pins into her. But when I did talk to her or, worse, chat, it felt like another act of heresy. What if she thought I had overlooked the fact that she was not our Mother?

The Lord, they say, loves a trier. Well, Tamsin was certainly that. She did her best, and when that was seemingly thrown in her face, she did her best all over again. Once, I came back from school to find a nightdress laid out for me on my bed. It was a white, sleeveless smock with pink flowers, the cotton thick and stiff. I could see at a glance that it would stick out like a tutu. I hated it, on sight. It didn't look like a regular nightdress. Worse, it was home-made; it was fine when Grandma made me clothes, like the cat costume she made me for a fancy dress parade and the Holy Communion dress. But for Tamsin, different rules applied: no hand-me-downs, nothing home-made, no gestures of effort or care.

Novelties were also on the unspoken list of no-no's. One day, Tamsin produced a terracotta pot moulded into the shape of a chicken. It is a brick, she said, clutching the head and the tail before putting a raw chicken with its legs tied up like a criminal inside it and then loading the whole thing into the oven. When she brought it out, the chicken was crispy. She ate some and I thought, she is eating herself. A brick.

The first time we visited Tamsin's sister and her family in their rambling house in Sussex, we went in through the front door. After standing around in the entrance hall, awkward orphans on parade, we went into the drawing room. We all sat down. Children of various ages appeared. These were Tamsin's nieces and nephews, come to see the orphan Fox girls. I felt like Jane Eyre on her stool. I was paired off to play with a niece a year younger than me, and my sister was paired off with a girl a year older than her. Later, we compared notes. I liked my playmate. She was friendly and full of suggestions about things I might like to do. We became friends, and wrote to each other. My sister felt less well matched. Here was another betrayal: I had let my sister down by enjoying myself. From then on I was cautious, I held back; I did not want either of us to be singled out.

We were a liability on the house weekend circuit all the same; we constantly needed to be told what to do. Unpack your clothes and put them in the one empty drawer in the chest of drawers in your room. Eat in the nursery at 7 p.m., not with the grown-ups at 8 p.m. If you want your shoes polished, leave them outside your bedroom door before 9 p.m. Don't ask me, ask Nanny. Stand up when adults come into the room. Don't sit down to eat until everyone else is sitting; stand behind the chair! Next time, ask other guests if they would like a bath first before you just go ahead and run one for yourself. Help with the washing up. *Muck in*. Once, at a Christmas house party, I was told off for staying in the drawing room when the other children were helping with the washing-up in the kitchen. 'Princess Margaret's children help with the washing-up. Why shouldn't you?' Quite what the Queen's sister had to do with me I did not know, and I could make nothing of the reference. My policy, when nervous or sick with dread that I was doing the wrong thing, was to stay put, and that's what I had done. I looked back at the grown-up, played mute, felt mortified. My default, dead-ant strategy had backfired.

We were terrible company, a drag, a drain, shy, quiet, louring. I could feel the effect we had on people every time we walked into a drawing room. Fearful, frangible, we exasperated. Buck up, girls, buck up, Tamsin used to say. But we couldn't buck up. I am not a horse, I said once, in a moment of defiance that startled even me. The thing is, I knew we shouldn't be in any of those houses in the first place, so I shrank into myself instead. I longed to fit in and made myself stand out. *Weed! Weed!* That was the taunt we used for drippy girls at school. If only they could see me out here, in unsafe territory: outcast, unwanted, weed.

There is a photograph of me sitting on the edge of the swimming pool at the Sussex house aged nine, shortly after Mother died. I am hunched up, shivering in the yellow and orange towelling top Mother had bought in America. Libra is nearby. Sometimes, when I look at that photograph, I want to shake that little girl and say, warm up, open up, charge about. Stop being *a drip*. Buck the fuck up. Then they'll stop being on your case and let go of their pity and their resentment and their contempt. Then you'll fit in.

At Christmas, the country houses we visited came spectacularly to life but none was more magical than Firle Place. You went down the long drive and then into a courtyard like the one in Narnia where the petrified centaurs and satyrs are brought back to life. Once through the big front door, a towering Christmas tree reached up towards the impossibly high ceiling in the huge Little Hall and it shimmered with real candles just like the tree at the Sussex house. In all the houses, sideboards were piled up with chocolates and boxes of ginger, and family traditions were rolled out. Charades was the killer. We played it in the house in which I was told to wash up like Princess Margaret's children. When it came to my turn I stood up, face blazing pink, feeling the adults' eyes and the children's eyes on me. I stood still, a frozen faun, willing myself invisible. Come on! brayed the children. We hadn't played Charades before, and I didn't know about signalling the provenance of the title, whether a book or a musical and so on, with a single gesture. I stuck up six fingers. Then I did four fingers for the fourth word and made big arcs with my hands. Words came at me, all wrong. Six fingers. Sixth word. I put my head to one side, my clasped hands beneath one ear, and shut my eyes. And then my time ran out. I revealed my title: *Joseph and the Amazing Technicolor Dreamcoat*. 'And' was the only word guessed correctly. What a wasted opportunity. Tamsin had taken us to see the musical and I had loved it. I had my chance to fit in by pulling something off. I could have made Tamsin happy, too, and I blew it.

One day Tamsin brought a phial of urine with her into the car. We were going to visit her sister. She laid it on its side in a transparent plastic bag on the front seat. 'It's for the hospital,' she said. When we got to her sister's house, the bag was waved about and admired. There were hoots of laughter. I saw then that her family was rallying around Tamsin, and I was glad for her. They were supporting her, their laughter the buffer between the urine in the little glass bottle and whatever illness lurked inside her. Here, with her immediate family, she felt comfortable, safe.

With us, she was on the outside, waiting to be let in. For that, I pitied her, and wanted none of her.

12

THE GREAT ESCAPE

Tamsin had a biblical little house on the island of Malta and she took us there on holiday. I loved the heat and the foreignness, the short old people with olive skin who smiled and said hello on dusty streets, the donkeys, the leather, the bright, blue-blanket sky and the sea that was a mermaid's tail of blue and green. All of it was new and exciting. Tamsin's house sat right on the street, no pavement in between it and the road. The house had a flat roof and a yard of a garden to the side of it with prickly green cacti swollen like butcher's toes bulging over the top of the wall. It was dark inside the house, and cool. Outside was hot. It was a dry heat, and it determined everything, changed the pace of our days. It was my first taste of languor. I lay on the low wall and fed lizards dried egg yolk saved from breakfast. We went to a lunch party with a flamboyant and, to us, unlikely friend of Tamsin's, a whirlwind in tight white trousers and flouncy shirt. He lived in a big white house that had a magical garden full of lemon trees. When I cooed at them, he reached up and picked one for me. Then he cut it in half, added sugar and showed me how to slurp the sweetened juices. He made Tamsin sparkle and laugh, which was a revelation.

For another outing Tamsin took us to the sixteenth-century castle on the far side of the island owned by her sister's family, and it had a glamour to it that made everything, even doing nothing, feel intoxicating. The girls had long hair and the boys had floppy hair and tanned skin. Once, we joined them for a picnic overlooking a cove. They did that English thing of whisking off their clothes as they stood right by you, and then sat about in their swimming trunks and their bikinis. We kept covered up. Two of them, a boy and a girl, aged seventeen or eighteen, sauntered to the edge of the cliff. The rest of us watched them, and I sensed that they knew it. The boy raised his ankles and, arms outstretched over his head, feet tipped to the sun, out and down he went, plunging into the mermaid sea. When his head popped up we clapped and then the girl dived into the bay. Together they swam to the water's edge and clambered up and came and sat back with us as if diving from that height had been nothing, as if their display was not needed to keep their place in the tribe but something accidental. We stayed at the castle into the evening, without Tamsin, and there were drinks and mussels and, heady from the sophistication all around me, I thought, I'll try them. One of the older teenage boys drove us back to Tamsin's house. He drove fast, windows down, the warm night all over us. And then I had to say: Stop the car, please. I threw up against the wall. Further down the road, I threw up again. None of those perfect, pretty people back at the castle would ever have done anything so uncool.

A few days later Tamsin was driving one of the teenagers to catch a ferry. Time was short, and she, too, drove fast and with daring, overtaking cars, beeping, laughing. I willed her on. We made the ferry. The teenager was grateful, and impressed. So was I. It was a good holiday moment, very good. But there were others where my sister or I were tricksy and drew unfavourable attention to ourselves. We looked odd on the beach, wore layers of clothing in the hot sun, woollen socks, floppy straw hats. We lowered ourselves on to the sand, stayed put: no running into the sea for us. We were not like Tamsin's nieces and nephews, fluid as the sea, connected. Poor Tam. I could see her getting upset, could feel her willing us to be normal and to fit in, and then of course she kept trying to make the next thing right. There were arguments. We scowled, sulked. Were we rude to Tamsin? I suppose we must have been. We certainly antagonised her. I think, looking back, we all did our best, and no one more so than Tamsin. On our return word got out that the Fox girls had been difficult. Shortly afterwards our father's first wife picked us up from school in the middle of the week and drove us into Eastbourne for dinner. 'You must be nice to Tamsin. Do you see?' I did see, but I couldn't see how, neither sitting in that Italian restaurant with its white tablecloths and nobody else in it, nor when we'd played happy families in Malta or when our father's first wife said it again in the car on the way back to school either.

It was a relief to get back to school. It always was. Some people are scarred by boarding school; psychotherapists treat 'survivors' for Boarding School Syndrome, addressing the part of them that felt rejected as a six- or seven-year-old child, their attachments with those they loved abruptly, inexplicably severed. Others have been victims of systemic and institutionalised bullying or abuse, of acts of criminality and cruelty that scar deep. I was lucky, and found school a place where I could relax. But what is wretched about boarding is the absence of an emotional safety valve, an adult to turn to, talk to, trust, when another adult, or a child for that matter, lets you down or behaves in a way that is unsound. Once, at the end of a general knowledge lesson, my teacher asked the class something about mothers, as in, how many of your mothers regularly clean the house? or something equally mundane and mundanely sexist.

All the children umm-ed and aah-ed until someone put up their hand, then another followed suit, and another, until all the kids had put up their hands. She came up with three or four questions of this nature. Each time, my hand remained on my lap and all the while I had Mother in my mind. She was in a coffin, it was her funeral and I was trying not to cry during the service. And then I did start to cry, right there in the classroom. What a spectacle I made of myself; I felt singled out, displayed. After the class had disbanded, the teacher, who knew my recent change in circumstances and had comforted me on previous occasions, said, Don't worry, you'll make a beautiful bride one day, and a fantastic mother and have a family of your own. Something about her conduct wasn't right; she had reduced me to tears and I sensed it was deliberate.

I was already in tears the night I crept out of bed, unable to sleep from sorrow, and stepped into the forbidden territory of the landing after Lights Out. The duty housemistress's door was ajar, her light on. I knocked. Miss Rado was in her armchair. She ushered me in, pulled me to her, hugged me. Safe in her arms, I cried even harder. Many minutes passed. Then, abruptly, she dropped her arms, withdrew, declared that I was not really sad. In fact, she went on, I was glad that my parents were dead; I just wanted attention. Out you go, and she sat me on the sofa on Blue Landing. Sit there until you've stopped crying. I wasn't there for long. I decided she had a point: I should cry less, and from then on, I did.

At the beginning of every term we had a medical. We formed a line outside the 'surgery', an unused bedroom between the walk-in airing cupboard – which housed an iron mangle to which we fed our hand-washed 'smalls' – and the lavatory (the one I didn't make it to on my first night boarding). The doctor was waiting inside the room. We knew the drill. In you went, tongue out, say ah, pants down, do a twirl, pull your pants up, everything all right? Yes, doctor. I was at that school for nine years, from the age of seven. I don't remember being asked to drop my pants aged fifteen or sixteen so let's assume that this part of the 'medical' stopped when we were thirteen and no longer compliant. In a school of 500 or so boarders aged seven to eighteen that would still have left 250 girls per term dropping their knickers.

Every night I went to sleep with the spectre of the doctor hanging over me. 'You need to wear fresh underwear,' the housemistress used to say, 'in case the doctor comes in the night.' We laid our dressing gowns on the end of our beds and tucked our slippers beneath them for the same reason. Every morning before breakfast and every evening before supper the boarders lined up in the corridor by the staircase that led down to the dining room. Next to it sat a big brass gong. Whoever was the first in line, and it was often me, got to whack it three times, following a signal from one of the teachers. Then, our imaginary books balanced on our heads, we walked in single file up to the duty housemistress waiting in the formal entrance hall, curtsied, shook her hand and said 'Good morning Miss So-and-So' or 'Good evening, Mrs So-and-So'. Some of the women weren't even housemistresses; they were sub-housemistresses, with no title or official position. Miss Rado was one of those. She had fingers like my knitted rabbit's arms, long limp tubular things with no articulation. Then we continued out of the hall and, as soon as the hall carpet gave way to the lino of the corridor, broke into a run, rounding the corner before pounding down to the dining room. There was no need to rush. Reconstituted scrambled eggs, tinned tomatoes and white sliced bread awaited us, but Rose the cook was something to wake up for. She had a Wife of Bath smile, her white chef's overalls pressed her breasts down to the same level as her belly and her pink cheeks shone like the sun, day in, day out. We pulled the middle out of the white bread and rolled it into balls and flicked them at the ceiling, or we toasted it and slathered it with butter wrapped in golden rectangles of foil. The discarded wrappers had to be put in their own dedicated plastic bucket that sat on a trolley at the end of one of the long tables. Those of us who had misbehaved had to rinse each wrapper by hand with soapy water. 'For the blind,' the teachers said of the cleaned wrappers. An old man with a bald head who smelt of urine loaded the kitchen's industrial dishwasher. One night after Lights Out me and Louise let ourselves out through the tradesman's entrance and climbed up the fire escape of the school building opposite. Somehow we knew this was where Dishwasher Man lived. A window was open. I peered through. The room was bare save for a single bed, a table and a chair, and reeked of neglect and of adults not treating their fellow adults properly. Seeing his quarters offered a glimpse into our adult rulers' world we didn't know what to do with.

At the weekends we hung out, not doing much. We were like dogs that sleep for a bit, then get up and walk around, only to come and lie down again in a slightly different position. On snowy winter nights we suspended each other from the gabled bedroom windows by the ankles so we could reach down and collect snow from the roof and make slushy drinks. In summer we did French skipping and played Kick the Can, Camp and British Bulldog. As we got older, we got bored. Daytime games gave way to twilight dares, Grandmother's Footsteps to Flasher's Footsteps. The main lawn, dug out of the chalky landscape, was flanked by sloping paths that climbed up to the South Downs where we used to play Sardines on Sunday afternoons with the teachers. For the rest of the time a high brick wall and a bolted and padlocked blue door kept us away from the outside world. But the outside world was curious.

One summer evening I was hitting tennis balls in the half-light, thumping the ball against the practice board in the small tarmacked play area in front of the Downs wall. Camp HQ, the clearing in the undergrowth where we kept prisoners by day, their backs up against a tree, was a few metres away. The bolted Blue Door was directly behind me and the shed where the gardener kept his stash of *Playboy* magazines was tucked away behind the overgrown bushes. I lobbed my tennis ball over the wire fence into those bushes. As I went to retrieve it, an older girl ran out of the prisoners' hovel and shot past me.

'A man!' she gasped like Shakespeare's Miranda, only more in fear than wonder. 'A man!' I caught up with her outside the pottery room at the bottom of the slope and formed a two-girl huddle, itself forbidden under the No Smoking, No Drinking and No Physical Contact rule, subclause: No getting closer than two inches to another girl.

'A man,' she said, 'there was a man. Sitting on the wall!'

Word went round about a bogeyman and the insolent summer evenings became charged with purpose. We had a new game and, unlike Grandmother's Footsteps, it was played solo. The aim was to get as far up the path as you dared before you chickened out. You won if you got as far as the Blue Door and saw The Man. One girl did see him, said he looked up, looked down, did something with his raincoat and something else with his trousers and she, triumphant and afraid, ran down the hill to share the alleged sighting.

I had no fear of bogeymen the night I disguised myself as a boy – the disguise trousers, a sweater, hair pinned up – and tiptoed on to the street clutching my white vanity case. I was part of a band of three: me, my sister and Sarah Crompton Heath, and we were running away from school. We should have been four, but the fourth girl, who always did have the whiff of toeing the line about her, had bottled out. Even when we were planning our great escape, huddled in the cloakroom opposite the staffroom, monitoring our supplies amassed from weekly tuck shop purchases and running over the route, I could tell her heart was not in it. Our shared realisation that boarding school was a prison and therefore something to be escaped from as a matter of self-respect no longer bound her to us. We took the road to the town centre, but veered off down a left fork into a tunnel of trees and a footpath running parallel to it that gave on to the golf course. Heads down, we kept in close to the trees on the edge of it, pausing only to rub soil on our faces to act as physical camouflage and to make us look poor. My white vinyl vanity case shone like the moon at my side. I had assumed a boy's name. We all had, and we used these to call out to each other, speaking 'common' as part of our disguise. I was Peter. Articulating our feigned social status seemed more important than moving across the terrain in silence. We left the golf course for the open road and arrived at Eastbourne train station at about nine o'clock. We bought three one-way tickets to Brighton. That, I thought but did not say, since my position as tagger-on rather than ringleader precluded it, was where our plan was weak. Escaping to a place you liked less than the one you were leaving didn't make sense.

Forty-five minutes later, as the train pulled into Brighton station, the need for an onward destination presented itself. I had fancied we might try a bus shelter on the promenade, and regroup from there, Lewes Crescent being a no-no, obviously. Sarah had said we could stake out at her house. It was too late for all that now. We needed to make it out of the station. We walked, three abreast, down the platform. As we neared the ticket barrier, two police officers and a station official took up riot positions, legs wide apart, shoulders almost touching. Sarah and my sister broke ranks and walked right up to them. They gave themselves up. I charged at them and then, in a cunning dart to the left, slipped past the officials and ran across the station concourse towards the exit.

'Where do you think you're going, then?' A hand grabbed my arm. 'You're coming with me, young lady.'

The police had an office off the concourse and it was there we were interrogated. My vanity case was opened.

'What's this then?' asked the police officer, pulling out one of three transparent plastic bottles held in place at the back of the case with elastic. 'Eh?' He shook the liquid. 'Vodka, I suppose.'

'Water.'

'Water!'

He dabbed some on to his finger, licked it, put the lid back on and threw it on top of the Opal Fruits and orange Club biscuits.

An hour later, a hot red lobster head sitting atop a squat human body exploded into the police station. It was Mr Crompton Heath, Sarah's frothing father.

'Out! All three of you!'

We sat in the back of his saloon car, listening to adults talking on the radio. There was no music. The voices, and Mr Crompton Heath's fury, made me giggle.

'What's so funny?'

It was one of those adult questions you weren't supposed to answer.

The headmistress was waiting up for us as we filed up the steps of the front entrance used only by visitors. Without ado, she ushered us straight up to bed, indicating we use the main staircase. We only got to use this at Christmas when the Salvation Army came to play carols in the hall. We'd sit on the stairs in our long dresses and platform heels while men and women in black bonnets with red trim blew their cheeks out and thrust brass instruments about. Mr Crompton Heath followed the headmistress into her study. After she had finished with him, the headmistress came up to say goodnight. She was sorry I was unhappy, she said, and wanted to do what she could to help. Grandma had told us that Mother had asked the headmistress to look out for us. Once, we stayed in her mansion flat overlooking Hampstead Heath for the whole weekend. How to admit to her now that I had run away only because my sister and Sarah had hatched the plan and my sister, then my Juno's swan, wouldn't countenance running away without me?

13

HELLO, DAD

On the rare occasions I am in a building I know Father has been in himself, I spin in a split-second fantasy in which he is alive, and I am with him. The boundaries between the living and the dead rapturously blur. Everything has led to this moment, all the yearning, and the grieving; this momentary reunion is the pay-off.

The buildings in question are mostly in America. In the UK, there is Farm Street Catholic Church near Scott's restaurant in Mayfair and the American Embassy in Grosvenor Square where Father met Mother, and that's about it. I know of other places he lived, or visited, but they are not places I have been, or have access to. Cliveden House in Berkshire is one of these. Father had stayed there during his first marriage as a guest of Nancy Astor, the society hostess and first woman MP to sit in the House of Commons, who was his first wife's aunt. Cliveden, which had been a wedding gift to Nancy and Waldorf Astor upon their marriage in 1906, is now a luxury hotel with a very good tea shop in the National Trust gardens.

For one of our very first dates Richard suggested a day trip to the stately home made infamous by the Profumo affair of 1963. I thought, I'd rather not. Father used to stay there and what a complicated story that is. I didn't want to go into it with my very new beau so, to avoid having to explain why I didn't want to go, I agreed to the visit. Then Richard's ageing Hyundai Pony wouldn't start. It was a glorious day and we had already made the picnic so we borrowed my half-brother's car, loaded it up, and off we went. Peter, a friend, came with us. We had our picnic on the lawn, just beyond the parterre. After we had eaten our bread and cheese, the two men lay in the sun. I sat up and scrutinised the building and speculated about which rooms Father might have been in. I decided, arbitrarily, that his bedroom was the one just to the right of the middle window on the first floor and imagined him looking through the sash window, across the gardens, to where I was sitting. Suddenly, I wanted, very much, to get up and go inside. If I couldn't go upstairs, I could at least look for the visitors' books and see for myself that Father had been here. But what right had I to be stalking lives that had nothing to do with me? Father wasn't married to Mother then, obviously. His Cliveden days aren't part of my history. That chapter of his past isn't a chapter of my own. I felt like an intruder, even contemplating the idea. Going inside would mean stepping into a past for which I had no room plan, no guide. It would also be an admission that I missed the father I never really knew and wished, even now, that I could make real to me. So when Richard suggested, a bit later, that we might go inside I said no, we're better off out here – here in the knowable, manageable now, enjoying the sunshine.

Since then, Richard and I have visited Cliveden a few times. We've walked by the river and had tea, or visited

Cookham village where the painter Stanley Spencer lived; there's an eponymous gallery there, in an old chapel. I love Spencer's paintings and '*The Resurrection, Cookham 1924–7*' (housed in Tate Britain) is a particular favourite. In it, the artist's dead friends, family and neighbours burst back to life in his local churchyard. Spencer is there, naked, taking in the scene, and so is his fianceé, the artist Hilda Carline; three times, no less. Some of the villagers are examining their own names and inscriptions on their headstones and everybody seems quite calm and ready to pick up where they left off. What a lovely thought. I may have grown out of the promise of heaven, but the energy in Spencer's anticipated reunion captures that thrill I have known in my own fleeting fantasies.

Much of what I know about Father is anecdotal and therefore undermining; I have so few first-hand experiences to connect me to him. Once, a couple of years after university, I took the train down to Lewes with his first wife; we were going to an opera at Glyndebourne. We chatted, and I told her that I was deciding whether to take up a friend's offer to share an apartment with him in New York. Go, she said, you might fall in love with a nice American and get married. And then she said, I loved your father, it was the alcohol that destroyed us, and I thought, you've had a whole life full of complications and look what you've done for us. I thought about Father then, too, had a glimpse of him as an ordinary man rather than a fairy-tale figure. I thought about the alcohol, didn't know what it meant for liquor to destroy love. All I knew was that Father no longer drank by the time he met Mother – or so I've been told, and so I want to believe.

I do have a few of Father's books, but they are esoteric, and do nothing to flesh him out. Having no use for the likes of *The Life and Times of Abraham Lincoln* or *Rudimentary Geometry*, before we moved I kept his books on the top shelf of my old study in Primrose Hill. Once, in an act of deadline-dodging, I decided that the cobwebs that had been up there for months, years probably, had to come down that instant. The newspaper piece I was writing could wait. I stood on my desk and, brandishing a feather duster modelled on a retro Zoom ice lolly – tiers of yellow and red and orange – lunged at the spectral threads. My study overlooked the artists' studios once occupied by the Pre-Raphaelite painter J. W. Waterhouse who, in 1888, had posed a live model in a boat he kept in the cobbled courtyard. The painting would become *The Lady of Shalott*. I went at those cobwebs with such vigour I lost my footing and very nearly fell through the window and joined the Lady of Shalott's ghost. I grabbed a shelf to steady myself and a fat book caught my eye. *The Epic of America*: the title was wonderfuly ambitious. The spine had a reference number, 970A, daubed in white Tipp Ex on the red leather spine in Father's rounded hand. He marked many of his books that way. Curious, I took it down. Inside, Father had rubber-stamped his name and Manhattan address. Beneath it, in pencil, someone had written, 'From Nancy Astor, Cliveden, Taplow, England'. I am not even sure whose handwriting it is, but it is energetic and rounded and takes up the whole frontispiece. I think it is Father's but it might be Nancy Astor's. I decided it was Father's, imagined him writing it, and then I closed the book and put him back on the shelf, out of reach.

Growing up, I used to copy Father's habit of putting his name in his books, and the date of receipt. Mother did the same, and sometimes they inscribed the books they gave each other. In *The Complete Works of Shakespeare* Mother wrote, 'To

Lyttleton, From Thelma'. I love to see her handwriting. I see from the date that they had been married less than a year. By writing his name and her own, Mother writes out their love, locking them in an eternal embrace. This is another orphan perk: you get to idealise. I've always liked the phantom footprint of the signature. Visitors' books are good for those and, before my diagnosis, I had begun looking into why the British keep them and what they reveal about our social history and mores. In my research I came across Holker Hall, a vast estate on Cumbria's Cartmel peninsula which has been owned by just three families and passed down the family line during its 400-year history, ending with the Cavendish family. Another estate in the family collection is Chatsworth House, home to the late Duchess of Devonshire. Family members include Georgiana, Duchess of Devonshire, whose *ménage à trois* was eerily mirrored by her great-great-great-great-niece Diana, Princess of Wales more than 200 years later. I felt sure Holker's visitors' books would have some stories to tell as a result. I duly wrote to its owners, Lord and Lady Cavendish, to ask if I might have a look. Hugh Cavendish invited me up for a taster. There were stacks of the books, he explained, and I couldn't possibly get through them in a day.

Up I went a few months later and after lunch in the dining room of the Jacobean wing of the house, Hugh and his wife Grania, a photographer, left me alone in the panelled Brown Hall, one of the drawing rooms in their private quarters. The rest of the house is open to the public. Grania's four sepulchral greyhounds lay supine on the flagstones on the other side of the door. The fire was blazing, and dozens of books were stacked on a window seat and a side table. They were more like scrapbooks than traditional visitors' books, which customarily contain nothing more than a name, date and possibly an address. These books were packed with sketches and watercolours, photographs and aphorisms. After a romp through the nineteenth century, mindful that I only had a few hours before I had to catch my train back down to London, I abandoned my chronological search and picked up books at random, switching centuries and decades. It was quite a social whirl. In the Seventies I spotted Prince Charles and, during the same visit in December 1973, a photograph of newly-weds Camilla and Charles Parker-Bowles. Idly flicking back to see if the love triangle had made an earlier appearance, I found my half-sister's signature instead. There she was: 10 September 1972. I knew by now how aristocratic tribal links worked, how everybody is related to each other one way or another. My surprise turned into that rush you get in a dream when someone you have loved, and lost, is alive again. My half-sister had been a constant source of love to me. It was a Stanley Spencer *Resurrection* moment. I would have been eight years old when she signed her name. She would have been twenty-three. I imagined her staying here, in this magnificent house, and wondered what her emotional state had been. As a schizophrenic, there was much loneliness in her adult life, and anguish, too. Psychiatric wards, halfway houses, those cruel voices in her head that played havoc with reality.

A few minutes later Hugh Cavendish came in to see how I was getting on. I told him I had spotted my half-sister's name. He looked at me and said, 'Are you Lyttleton Fox's daughter?'

No one has ever asked me that, before or since. Mother, by seeking refuge in England after Father's death, pulled up the drawbridge so that by the time she died the links to relatives and friends which could have connected us to him were no longer current. I did not go back to America until I was thirteen so the adults I met in England who knew him were, by and large, linked to him by his first marriage. That, to my young self, was humiliating, which is one of the reasons I hadn't wanted to visit Cliveden. Over the years, I came to feel that Father had only been a father to his first two children. I had no claim on him. Only when I was an adult did I compute that Father had spent more years with us than he had with my half-brother and half-sister, and that they had had to endure the absence of their father and considerable adjustments of their own. Hugh went on, to my absolute delight, to talk about the last time he had seen my father. It had been in Eaton Square in London around the time of his divorce, and he noted how sad he had been. I realise that a personal pronoun has crept in. I never say 'my father'; plain, Victorian 'Father' does the trick, something people frequently remark upon, but since Hugh's question I have felt on more intimate terms with him. My father, Hugh said, was funny and clever and eccentric. He painted a vivid picture of him once donning a green wig at a smart dinner. He would have approved of those Egyptian boxer shorts on my head, then. Hugh also mentioned that he and my half-sister had once dated, and I thought of the photograph of her as a ravishing debutante and imagined what she was like before the fairies – and the voices – got her. 'I always thought you'd marry a lord,' she once said to me when she and I were visiting a National Trust property together. At the time, it struck me as an extraordinary comment, and I couldn't see why she would make it. Now I think she was talking about herself.

Waiting at Cark's two-track railway station for the London train, I called my old school friend Kate and told her about Hugh Cavendish and his question to me. We lost our signal, but a few hours later, she texted me. *Amazing to have had that conversation about your dad.*

'Your dad.' This was another first. No one has ever said 'your dad' to me.

In what would turn out to be the autumn before my diagnosis, feeling something like my father's daughter, I finally decided to see if I could find Father in the Cliveden visitors' books. Nine of them are held by the University of Reading in their Special Collections department, housed within the idiosyncratic Museum of English Rural Life. I made my way past poles, ploughs and smocks to the small library where a metal trolley awaited me, stacked with dark, leather-bound books marked CLIVEDEN in gold lettering.

On top of the pile was 'Cliveden Jan 1910 to June 1914'. I wasn't going to find Father in there, so I skipped that one, plus six more spanning 1919 to 1940, though I would have found Charlie Chaplin amongst their pages, as well as the members of the so-called Cliveden Set, the allegedly pro-appeasement cabal which met at Nancy Astor's home. I hesitated before going through the next book, dated July 1941 to Dec 1945; I needed to look up the date of Father's first marriage on the Internet first. Married 1943. Divorced 1950. Right, so he could be in here. But it did not look hopeful, the number of signatures dwindling during this period – proof that the war years turned the social lives of the nation's country houses upside down. I pass royal lovebirds Princess Elizabeth, aged seventeen, and Philip of Greece, twenty-two, who signed the book in November 1943, and Kathleen 'Kick' Kennedy, the American socialite and younger sister to future US president John F. Kennedy. But why was I letting myself get sidetracked? It was another ghost I was after. I heaved July 1941 to Dec 1945 back on to the trolley and brought over my last chance, Cliveden Dec 1945 to Aug

1951. I skipped past plenty of familiar names I had seen in visitors' books up and down the country, but when Kick Kennedy's name stopped appearing I cross-referenced online. She died in a plane crash in France, aged twenty-eight, along with her married lover, Peter Wentworth-Fitzwilliam, 8th Earl Fitzwilliam, in 1948. Kick's mother is reported to have said: 'That airplane crash was God pointing a finger at Kick and saying NO!'

I grew up wishing I had a mother, and then I read something like that and I think, mother love is not always what it is made out to be.

I noticed a big Canadian contingent for Christmas 1946 and several Americans in the autumn of 1947, but no Lyttleton Fox. His father-in-law signed the book, and I thought, foolishly, given that his name appeared all the time, that I might be hot on Father's trail. His father-in-law signed again in May 1948, but there's still no entry from Father and his wife. I didn't even know what Father was doing in 1948, or where he was living. Indeed, if I had to offer up twenty facts about him, what would I say? I grabbed a piece of paper and started a list: lawyer, law professor, in US Navy – admiral, Catholic, Irish, alcoholic then on the wagon by the time he met Mother, funny, went to Yale and Harvard, wrote poetry and short stories. That was it. Hardly intimate stuff. Tearful now, I humiliated myself further by seeing what I could find about him on Google. First up was an obituary in his old school newsletter, St Paul's in Concord, New Hampshire, at the time an Episcopalian boys-only boarding school.

Archive Name: Alumni Horae
Volume 49, Issue 2,
Page 134, Obituaries 3
Originally published: Summer 1969
Obituary: Lyttleton Fox, Jr.,

1927-Lyttleton Fox, Jr., associate professor
at the Seton Hall University School of Law,
died in Newark, New Jersey, March 11, 1969.
A gentle, amusing man, with many friends,
he was deeply versed in the legal aspects
of international transactions and government
contracts. His first seven years as a lawyer,
following graduation from Harvard Law School
in 1934, were spent in general practice in
New York City but then World War II took him
into service in the Navy from 1941 to 1946
and he became deputy director of procurement
for the Bureau of Aeronautics, with the rank
of commander. He continued in government
service for another twelve years, chiefly
in London, England, with responsibilities for
United States defense [sic] purchasing, and
finally in Brussels as counsel to the United
States Commissioner General at the Brussels
International Exposition. After five years
as counsel to United Aircraft International
and four years of private law practice in
Manhattan, he joined the faculty of Seton
Hall Law School in September, 1967, continuing
in that position until his death. He was a
member of the Baker Street Irregulars and
was a Latin scholar, fluent in several modern
languages, who had written and lectured widely
in international law. A native of Hampton
Bays, Long Island, he was born August 23,
1909, the son of Lyttleton and Genevieve
O'Brien Fox. School friends remember the
place he made for himself at St. Paul's where
he was an assistant editor of the Horae, winner

of a Williamson Medal, secretary of the
Cadmean (as well as a notably witty member
of the Cadmean debating team) and winner of
the English Composition Prize in 1927. He
was also a member of the Old Hundred track
team. He graduated cum laude in 1927 and
went on to a distinguished career with the
Class of 1931 at Yale . . .

So that's 'my dad', parsed from a school obit, virtually
every detail serving, once again, to make him less real to me
and setting me off on yet another trail. Now it is his connection
to the Baker Street Irregulars I'm after. Father was invested
in the BSI in 1969, taking the title The Gloria Scott, from
Arthur Conan Doyle's eponymous short story, and he made
a speech too, according to digital records. I find nearly 100
BSIs in a photograph taken in 1969 at the BSI annual dinner
to commemorate Sherlock Holmes's 115th birthday. I scan
the black and white photograph, taken at Cavanagh's, an old
Irish restaurant in Lower Manhattan. There is a man in a
deerstalker, another brandishing a deerstalker on his clenched
fist, men in lounge suits or black tie, and several men in
severe, black-rimmed spectacles looking like members of the
CIA, rather than of a jovial literary and dining society.
They've got ice cream sundaes in front of them. Father is
slap bang in the middle of the picture, smiling at the camera,
his mouth open – the way I smile myself. I click the magnifier
on my computer screen, click again. He looks younger than
I've seen him for a while, and so well. Two months later, he
is dead.

My fellow researchers in the library probably assumed
I was a scholar, like them. But I was a shadow, chasing a
dead man's shadow. Forget long-dry signatures – it was time
to get out of here. I stood up to close the book, wheel back

the trolley and let a gust of autumn air blow some sense back into me. And then I saw him, at the very bottom of the page I was about to turn before shutting the visitors' book. I am left-handed so the palm of my hand invariably obscures the left-hand corners of large books. I lifted my hand and there it was, his beautiful, friendly signature, so full and rounded and perfect. Lyttleton Fox. July 24 1948. I scrutinised it, even, I confess, ran my index finger across the thick, wide loop on the capital L, watched the 'y' fall, saw the fulsome crossing of the 't's. I liked this man, my father, just by the way he signed his name. I studiously copied his signature on to a scrap of paper; if I'd had tracing paper, I would have traced it. For a long time I kept this facsimile of his signature in a pocket inside my handbag. It looks as though he has just penned it at the end of a note, the top part of which has been torn off.

I arranged that long overdue tour of Cliveden House hotel for the following week. I wanted to look at the visitors' books they had there and, more than anything, to have a snoop. The hotel manager agreed to show me round. 'Visitors' books capture the essence of a person being left behind, don't they?' she said as we went upstairs. It was the East Wing I was after, since this is where guests used to stay in Nancy Astor's day. Inchiquin, Canning, Garibaldi, I looked inside various rooms named after former guests, each of which has its own visitors' book for hotel guests. It turns out I wasn't the only one chasing ancestors. 'Great-uncle Harold enjoyed Cliveden and so did we!' writes an H. Macmillan of the British premier Harold Macmillan, staying in the Henry James suite. I had no idea which room Father had slept in. It didn't really matter, not like it had all those years ago when I sat on the parterre and looked up at the mansion and felt I had no right to explore his connections to it. I looked around the room and pictured Father in his pyjamas (striped, I decided) and dressing gown (ankle length, blue tattered silk), looking out over the gardens towards the river Thames beyond, pondering his future.

'Hello, Dad,' I mouthed, and then I followed the hotel manager out of the room.

14

WHAT IS THE UNIVERSE TRYING TO TEACH ME?

Two weeks into chemotherapy I go round to my friend Tim the Buddhist's flat for a bit of slap and tickle. Tim is a craniosacral therapist and meditation teacher and when he offered to tickle my aura, I thought, why not? I'll have anything tickled if it will do me good. The slap was never on offer. I added it to cheer myself up. I get my laughs where I can.

As I walk into his bright living room up on the third floor of a converted warehouse, I notice a row of dense treetops almost bang up against the windows, like a flash mob coming to a party. A long black handle protruding from the ceiling also catches my eye. The treetops may have been there before, but the handle hasn't. It's a bit S & M, I think, which is not a thought someone with cancer should have. Tim explains that it is for hanging from when he walks up and down clients' backs. It alleviates the pressure on their spines.

My shoes are off and, doing what I am told, as I do nowadays, I feel my feet, feel the texture of the rug and all the while I am loving those trees and the leaves and the fecundity of them, and feeling a little self-conscious about the imminent tickling. Tim the Buddhist believes in his treatments; I am open to them, but can't for the life of me see how tickling my biomagnetic field might work. Then again, I believe in angels. I can't have it both ways.

So, here I am, bending my knees, but only slightly – any more and my posture is at risk of simulating evacuation – and taking deep breaths. Tim starts rubbing the air around me in broad sweeps, as if he's shining a window.

'What are you doing, Tim?'

'I am buffing your magnetic field.'

Buff away. He comes in closer to my face, then bends over and rubs my ankles and feet before crouching down and, just as I've started to relax, he presses on my toes, hard. I don't care what Buddhists say about the body doing the suffering and the mind being free of it, my big toe hurts and my brain says, ow! Heroically, or should that be stoically, I merely wince and keep shtum. He finally stands up and starts pinching the air, his thumbs and index fingers clicking like a hungry chick's beak as he pulls his arms back, as if teasing out strands of spun toffee. All the while he moves around me like a sprite, plucking at the air at shoulder height now, then at waist height, then everywhere. His fingertips alight on my shoulders, and there is more tickling of air. I stop watching him, shut my eyes and hear the sound of birdsong outside the window with my sharp new cancer-ears. That prompts a heart-surge-weep-cry-love-this-life-this-earth-don't-let-me-leave-it pang, and I open my eyes. My biomagnetic field has been extended, my aura fluffed and tickled. Forget the Virgin Mary's mega halo in the Wilton Diptych, I've got a shiny energy around my whole body, or so I am hoping.

We chat about the Buddhist take on suffering – I have never warmed to their bleak belief that to be human is to suffer. I don't mention my toes, but do mention the treetops and nature coming into sharp focus and how I am wondering whether everything really could be interconnected. Tim grabs a Post-It and on it he writes, in green felt tip: WHAT IS THE UNIVERSE TRYING TO TEACH ME? and I think, oh, the universe, how rich to be part of it, me, the trees, everything living one sacred whole. Exhilarated, I slip his note into my handbag and practically float out of the building. On the bus, I text Fliff to say where I've been. *V jealous*, she replies. *Would love to have my aura tickled.* She, like most people, is too busy leading a civilian life for such existential forays. I, however, appear to be on a roll. I dip into the William Stafford poetry anthology Tim has just given me, along with a pair of snazzy headphones. I don't know who Stafford is and flick through the book, stopping at 'How to Regain Your Soul'. I didn't know a soul was something you could lose. You can lose your hair, or your peace of mind, but not your soul, surely. I presume this must be a hippy poem about death and skim through it until I get to a line about white butterflies dancing 'by the thousands in the still sunshine'. What a wonderful image, I think: a sky filled with butterflies. 'Suddenly anything/Could happen to you. Your soul pulls toward the canyon/and then shines back through the white wings to/be you again.' *To be you again.* Is this a poem about reincarnation? I can't work it out. I seem to have lost the stomach – or the brain – for metaphors and abstract thoughts. The butterfly may be a concrete image, but I can't nail its meaning.

By the time I am back in my bedroom, the universe, energy fields and souls in sunshine have deserted me. I stick the Post-It note on the framed prayer about courage being silent on my bedside table. My mother-in-law has lent the prayer to me – 'just for now,' she said, 'I'd like it back. It's got me through the dark times.' That's what I feel now: dark, and deflated. What is the universe trying to teach me? No fucking clue. The question suddenly feels like a recrimination. Have I offended it in some way, brought the cancer on myself?

I think I've been found out. I make out that I like nature, but it's a stretch to go from liking some trees through a window to embracing the concept of a sacred, interconnected universe. To do so feels hollow, and a bit bipolar and extreme, rather like my mood dip now. I do like nature, and I love rivers and streams, mountains, the wind, the rain. But I am rarely *in nature*, to coin an odd phrase popular amongst Americans; I prefer to be in restaurants. I love nature more when I am reading about it. I could read Auden's 'In Praise of Limestone' til the cows come home, and that moment in the first book of The Prelude when the young Wordsworth rows across Ullswater and is filled with numinous awe is a transcendent one on every reading, his precocity notwithstanding. But I hate nature programmes and all that up-close cruelty. I frequently squash ants, despite proclaiming that one shouldn't in the Words To Live By legacy I am no longer leaving for the boys. I even lay down poison for mice. I am, in short, all talk. If cancer throws you back on your self, I would rather dodge mine. I'd rather not have the cancer while we're at it, but that's not an option. As for the self I am now spending so much non-quality time with, it's riddled with inconsistencies. Having them rammed home whilst negotiating a chronic disease is not helpful. And, if more truth is to be told, I don't even like butterflies, fond memories of my grandfather also notwithstanding – and don't even get me started on moths.

Once, at boarding school, I reached for my cup of water in the night and something woollen with edges fluttered on my lips and I screamed and flicked my tongue in and out and jumped out of bed and then jumped on the spot, too and woke up my room-mates, one of whom turned on the light. The offending moth hurled itself into the overhead light bulb.

If I had swallowed it – the moth, not the light bulb – the sacred universe might be inside me now, and I might be loving the universe and loving the cancer. I have a book that tells me to do just that: Love your cancer. As I say, I get my laughs where I can.

The trouble with cancer is how needy you become and how much you want to take control of what's happening to you. It explains the attraction of both positive thinking – the idea that the mind can heal the body – and alternative healing to the habitually rational. Whether it's the belief that you can move energy around inside the body, surround your self with more positive energy – which is what I understand one's biomagnetic field to be, hence Tim's attempt to extend mine – or tap into positive energy to heal disease, these approaches become hard to resist. Several years ago I read Helen Garner's novel *The Spare Room* about a woman who lets a friend with stage 4 bowel cancer come and stay and then is scandalised by how she squanders money, and time, on peroxide drips and intravenous vitamin C. What a foolish woman, I concurred. But I had never endured chronic illness, didn't know what it does to your brain or how fear is the death of rational thinking.

I now understand why even the most cynical let the healers in, or at least let them get a foot in the door. Consequently, when a vortex healer-friend I once dismissed as end-of-the-pier offers to give me life-force energy healing and to put me in touch with 'the divine source', I let her do her thing. Healers are, by and large, a well-meaning lot, and pay you attention, which is welcome when you're out there, alone on a still glass sea. Who cares if you've got nothing to show for it after they've gone. As the weeks tick by and you get weaker, you become increasingly disconsolate in the face of acute loneliness and you'll take anything on offer that makes you less so. It is a dangerous position to be in, particularly if you were emotionally vulnerable before you got ill. But if, like me, you were both emotionally robust BC and grew up with a faith system, when mortality takes you by the throat you are open, as never before, to the possibilities that faith offers, possibilities which, however fanciful, can ground you when you feel anything but grounded. There is an instinctual repositioning of your self within a bigger picture of benign design. I even try to define heaven, as if such a thing existed, and am keen to pin down the human soul. Is it an energy particle that joins a greater mass of positive energy when we die? If so, how can it be that our soul exists within our bodies when we are alive, and leaves it when we are dead? What contains it?

Is God cellular, and we become part of that cellular loveliness? Is that it?

I need to know about heaven and my soul because, if I do die soon, I have to be able to connect to my boys. It's not about teleological conceits; it's about practicalities. I will need to watch over them, as Mother and Father watched over me. This may sound juvenile, but I've got cancer. It goes with the territory.

Meanwhile, I've got some temporal concerns to deal with, chiefly Bassy's chemistry project, which he is starting with a friend this afternoon. Talk about stressful. It's one of these hideous projects, done in pairs, which the children have weeks and weeks to complete and which we – note the choice of pronoun – get done at the last minute. Should I peg it, I will at least be spared Bassy's school projects. This term, he and his friend David have chosen to make a cut-out animation about the life of Joseph Priestley and his discovery of oxygen in 1774. I'm tempted to get them to switch to Friedrich Sertürner, who discovered morphine in 1804, but think that might spook them. Determined to keep things normal, I stick my oar in and edit their script, despite my non-existent grasp of chemistry, a state of ignorance compounded by chemo-brain fuzziness.

I set my alarm so I can have a proper snooze, and am up when the boys come home. After much lounging about, they eventually set about cutting out characters and props from black card. I point out that the Bunsen burner is the same size as the baby (it's Priestley – his moment of birth is to be included in the footage). Bassy hands me the scissors, saying: You do it, then, which of course I do and they, exhausted, take a break and refuel on mini rolls and on-screen violence. Helicopter parenting isn't all glamour and prize-givings.

Then we go upstairs to film the biopic, me hauling the stepladder. Sebastian climbs up it, but can't tie the thread – it's too fine, I couldn't find any string – from the sheet of A2 paper to the chandelier. This will form the screen. Down he comes and up I go. I feel a bit dizzy and can't tell if it's the chemotherapy that's to blame or a fit of over-parenting vertigo. The other end of the thread is attached to the hook on the back of the door – the door that I then open on my way downstairs to get the six-foot floor lamp for the backlighting. The thread I've finally managed to tie snaps. Suddenly I don't want to do this any more. Frustration and impatience bubble up inside me like one of Priestley's concoctions. I want to abandon the boys and their stupid school project but I think, you can't do that, you've got cancer, what kind of mother are you? I come back up with the outsize lamp, *Eine kleine Nachtmusik* starts up (the period touch was my idea but now worry that Mozart is a bit of a giveaway and the parental intervention will be spotted) and the camera rolls as they perform the script and jig their cardboard cut-outs on kebab sticks. Oh, this is lovely, I think, it's like that moment in *The Railway Children* when they put on that play. Cut. They stop filming. David asks what's happened to the script. He says it's now got factual errors in it. I was only trying to help, I bleat, then flounce out of the door. They, relieved to see the back of me, wind up the filming and de-brief over four hours on the PlayStation and more mini rolls.

Back on my bed to rest, I wonder if everything feels normal for Bassy, normal being relative, and how often he forgets I am ill or if he's aware of it round-the-clock. With Mother, I carried a weight around with me, not heavy, but always there. I hope he does not do the same.

Friends and family send me cards and flowers. I don't read the messages or put the cards up; not for weeks. I put the flowers in vases, then leave them to it. It's Mother again. I remember all the cards and the flowers she got. I won't be fooled.

But the cards and the flowers and the gifts keep coming. The boys want to know about each one, who sent them. One day a huge bouquet of flowers and a box of beauty treats arrive on the same day and Reuben says, 'Wow, you're really milking this cancer thing!' I lighten up after that. The cards go up, the flowers get sniffed and my professed acceptance of my illness becomes more of a reality. The messages are heartening and, along with the flowers, they cheer the house up. Too busy being haunted by the past, I haven't thought how important this show of support is for the boys, how it supports them, too. Three weeks into the treatment, I get another gift, this one in the form of Peggy O'Hare, a primordial sound meditation guru. Peggy is a close friend of Jeannie, my one fellow orphan friend and one of Peggy's meditation students. Peggy runs her meditation weekends in Bedfordshire and has condensed one of these into a day's workshop especially for me, which she will conduct in my house. I don't know what primordial sound meditation is, but I've wanted to learn meditation for some time. I readily accept Jeannie's gift. When things get bad – whatever 'bad' means – I might be able to use meditation as a distraction.

On the day of the workshop I dress in white in an attempt to look enlightened. I don't have high hopes for Peggy's look. I fully expect some dread hippy vision in brown hessian and seaweed hair as I open the front door. But Peggy O'Hare is working a contemporary guru aesthetic: cropped hair, good bone structure, glossy lips, plum wide-legged trousers and a stylish coat-cardigan. Her elegance is uplifting. So when, later, she mentions that her friend Deepak, as in Chopra (the bestselling author, fellow guru and director of the Chopra Centre in New York), has sent over my personal mantra, I suppress the thought that it is not really personal and that this Centre of his must make a lot of money. Equally, when she talks of how we all need to caress our amygdalas and of how we all make 'our transition' – as if we were Martians – I bear with her. She's not a phoney. She is a friend of Jeannie, whose judgement I trust and, like Jeannie, she has a magnetism mixed with kindness that immediately puts me at ease.

The sunlight streams in behind her as she sits in the window and talks through the principles of primordial sound meditation. Your mantra, she says, is a sound or vibration the universe created at the precise moment of your birth; you use it to get back into the silences, or gaps, between thoughts. I told her in advance where and when I was born, but left out the time, which I don't know. This detail does not seem to matter. At her prompting, I bring out the little card that looks like a place name for a table setting and read my mantra to myself. Then I shut my eyes and say it over and over in my mind, rolling each syllable, as instructed (there are only two), while Peggy tells me to keep bringing my thoughts back to the mantra.

And so it goes, for ten minutes or so. And then something happens.

To my astonishment, I experience what those in the spiritual business call, I think, a moment of clarity and cynics call baloney.

Out of nowhere, unbidden, I have the conviction that my parents did not abandon me, that they were – and are – always with me, and are mine to call my own. Since I've never consciously felt abandoned, this comes as quite a surprise, as does the simultaneous conviction that I am not an orphan in the fullest sense because I have parents who loved me when they were alive and love me still.

Love, like heaven, shifts.

It is some time before I open my eyes and when I do, Peggy is sitting up straight, eyes closed, her hands on her knees. She opens her own eyes. Tentatively, I tell her what happened.

'Divine intervention,' she says quietly.

Perhaps. Or wishful thinking. A moment of susceptibility, or another moment in the rose garden. Does it matter? After all, if I feel supported, I can support my children. I am better able to cope with the fear of being lost to them.

We break for lunch. I leave Peggy to chew on her rice cakes or dried figs or whatever it is gurus eat and go downstairs to watch an introductory Primordial Sound Meditation DVD. It is a presentation by Deepak Chopra. He sits on a chair, wearing well-cut trousers and a white shirt with the collar open (in my ignorance of this cult figure, a man in a loincloth sitting on a mat would not have surprised me; the regular-bloke look does) and, addressing an audience I cannot see, talks through the different stages of consciousness. He does the lot in forty-five minutes.

To finish off our time together, Peggy would like to teach me to walk mindfully so off we go to Parliament Hill. I once ate a chocolate mindfully with no less a tutor than Professor Michael Williams, director of the Oxford Mindfulness Centre, whom I was interviewing for a newspaper piece. Walking mindfully should be a cinch.

'Heel toe, heel toe,' Peggy says, and I think, do some people walk toes first?

It is a cold, sunny afternoon. The Gherkin and the Shard are shining in the distance. A little girl is flying a kite with her dad on the top of the hill. Dogs are all around us, running, defecating, urinating.

'Good. Now, as you are walking, say thank you. To your knees, perhaps, your bladder, your bowels.'

I stop in my tracks. I turn to Peggy, who I like, not least because in her presence I suspend my instinctive mistrust of the mind being able to heal the body, and I think, you're losing me. You're seventy-five, so you may have good reason to be thankful for your knees and those unseemly organs. But me? No. My knees are fine. As for the B-functions, there is no way I am even thinking about them, let alone talking to them.

She looks at me quizzically. I come up with a ruse. I decide to thank my whole body, cunningly avoiding the visualisation of an individual body part or vital organ.

'OK,' I lie, 'I'm all set.'

'Good. We will walk then, in silence, for twenty minutes.'

Up the hill we continue, heel toe, heel toe, walking in mindful silence, my mind filled with the thought of a big bottom, old and crinkly, squatting on a lavatory.

In New York six months later, debilitated by a liquid diet of milkshakes and morphine and only able to walk five blocks before having to dash into the nearest McDonalds in search of a lavatory, my B-functions have the last laugh. Does the universe keep score?

That night, following Peggy's departure, a friend takes me to the ballet at the Royal Opera House. It is a last-minute invitation. We see three contemporary pieces. The bodies fall into each other, over each other, they fold and they pull back. They lift, they fall, they come back to the centre, to the still point, and then they are off again. Yes, I think, yes, yes, these are the pauses

Peggy was talking about. My crash course in higher consciousness is already reaping dividends; the timing seems providential.

Or it could just be happy coincidence. In my excitement I forget that I have always been quite taken by the pause as a metaphor for the breath of life, and that I discovered it through the poetry of Emily Dickinson many years ago. My excitement is just another bipolar thrill on the cancer rollercoaster, a heart-surging, mood-swing high.

It is good while it lasts. I feel so in tune with the universe I'm practically the Dalai Lama.

A few days later it is mask-fitting day. The Dalai Lama couldn't be further from my mind. All I can think of is Tutankhamun in his tomb mask and Estelle's father biting on a wooden bit and being pinned down with four-inch buckles. Reluctantly, I ask a hospital orderly for directions to the radiotherapy 'mould room'. I should be able to sniff my way to it. You say mould, I say: white velvet on red jam, blue veins on yellow cheese, grey fur on the sour cream we forgot to throw out. I also say: keep it off my face. When Richard and I eventually find the right room, I hesitate outside the door. I would defy the most curious, even Alice from Wonderland, to want to know what is on the other side.

We are welcomed by the mould technician, a quietly spoken man whose warm spirit meets my newly fearful one head on and says, it's OK, it's all OK. He introduces his assistant, who also has some magic about her. Neither is even slightly peremptory or rushed, both make us feel like they could not care more. Richard and I sit side by side on plastic chairs, me in my baboon gown, wishing I had asked Estelle how her father was able to breathe through the mask.

The mould technician shows us a demonstration mask, a duck blue, perforated thermoplastic shell in the shape of a human head, neck and shoulders. Then he shows us the sheet of perforated plastic that will become my own mask. It will be heated up first in a sink of boiling water and then spread over my face. His assistant gives me some toggles and tells me to put my hair in bunches; high ones, she says. Paired with the baboon gown, it's quite a look, until the gown comes off and on goes a towel across my chest, as though I am sitting for one of those head and shoulders portraits designed to look as if the sitter is wearing a strapless dress. I should have worn a string of pearls. I lie on a couch, again, and this time I am getting a tiny freckle of a tattoo on my chest; the radiographers will use it to position the mask in precisely the same place for every treatment – 65Gy to my oropharynx and bilateral neck in 30 factions – which translates as zapping the **** out of the middle of my throat behind my mouth and a dissection of my neck in thirty consecutive sessions of radiotherapy. The zapping area is huge because the primary tumour's lair is unknown. It could be on the back of my tongue, the walls of my throat, anywhere: hence the radiographers' decision to execute a blanket attack.

The assistant lowers a pre-cut piece of perforated thermoplastic mesh into a stainless steel box containing warm water, heated to 149–158° F. Three minutes later she wipes it dry so I don't get hot water dripped on me. It has turned into a large square of flattened quince, buttercup yellow, about 3.75 mm thick. The plastic is full of holes. She and the technician drape it over my face and shoulders, a hot face flannel, too hot. Click click click. Foam handles at the extremities of the warmed plastic are fitted into the baseplate. There is a bit of patting, first around my nose, where there is a hole, and then around my neck. Just a few minutes, says the technician, gently, his assiduous explanation of every step of the process saving me from fear. I wonder when they will cut the holes for my mouth, nostrils and eyes. I feel the two of them near me and then they are removing me from my own head and shoulders. Ta-da, your own custom-made mask. We will leave it on the shelf for you in the radiotherapy room, he says. It has your name on it.

I've had some more gifts, including a consultation with a healer so highly reputed her fans call her a white witch. The boys had a white witch for a nanny once, but the only actual witch I've encountered was a witch doctor in the Garamba National Park in what was then the Republic of Zaire. I went to see the witch doctor out of curiosity but he expected me to have a problem to solve and so I invented one on the spot. I said I was unmarried which, given that I was twenty-five, was an issue, at least as far as the people of Zaire were concerned. He prescribed dried snake and palm oil and, scalpel poised, he readied himself to make an incision on the top of my right hand before rubbing them in. I lost my nerve, made my excuses and paid up (in dollars, in lieu of a cow) and, accompanied by the ranger who had acted as a go-between, retraced the narrow path through the moonlit savannah to my lodging. There, I pitched my sorcery against his, chanting myself to sleep with Hail Marys.

Healers are no longer exotic in Western societies. In London they are like personal trainers and therapists: part of an affluent lifestyle package. As with Peggy O'Hare, I am hoping this healer might make me feel better although, as with the witch doctor, I don't know what she actually does. I have tried to find out. When I rang her to arrange my visit, I asked her.

'It's hard to explain,' she said. 'You have to come and see for yourself.' She also said: 'I can make sure the cancer does not come back.'

Bold, I thought at the time, and not entirely appropriate.

Cindy gets booked up several weeks in advance and her fee is £150 an hour. I am early for my appointment, so sit in the car and wait. I am in good spirits. I've worked at the *Guardian* earlier in the day, which makes me feel normal, and after the consultation, I am having tea with my friend Lu, who does a very good chocolate cake. From the car I can see the Indian fabric store where I bought the silk and lace for my wedding dress. I grimace. A very close friend's mother, a full-time housewife who had trained over thirty years earlier as a fashion designer but, to her regret, never worked as one, offered to make the dress for me. Offered, and I accepted what I thought was a gesture of love, a gift. The day before my wedding I stayed at her house, as I had many, many times over the years. On my return from the rehearsal dinner, I found an invoice for her dressmaking services on my pillow, which goes to show two things:

1. Weddings are a minefield.
2. Our own needs can hurt others.

As I get out of the car, I hope that when the boys are older they will learn how to follow love through and to steer a path away from selfishness to selflessness. I've gone soft again. I am a hundred years old and sentimental as spent blossom.

I ring Cindy's doorbell. She opens it and rushes me down her narrow hall.

'Shoes here, please, then you can wait for me downstairs.'

She's sorting payment with her previous client – I can see the back of another woman's head in the kitchen directly ahead – and hasn't left any buffer time between us. She is relaxed by the time she comes downstairs, and leads me into a consulting room fashioned out of a small back room. Grainy black and white photographs of a younger Cindy and magazine-beautiful children cover one wall. Her ego is very present. I start thinking about her life story, whether she is married, what led her to being a healer. Next to the photographs there's a shelf with ethnic artefacts on it and a few books and framed photographs. In one, Cindy is sitting between two men

in feathered headdresses and tribal attire. Opposite the shelf
is the massage couch. Cindy asks me to undress to my
underwear, lie on the couch and slip under a blanket. For some
reason, I do. She now explains how she works: she uses a
mixture of techniques, including acupuncture. Not the kind
practised by peasants, she adds, but something more rarefied,
practised by ancient Chinese aristocracy. I am partial to a little
VIP treatment, but this detail makes me feel uncomfortable.
I didn't know acupuncture was socially stratified. Then,
standing over me, she asks me about myself.

'Where is your cancer?'

Such a direct question.

'My neck,' I say, putting my hand on the Interloper's patch.

Then there's another one: 'What do you think of when you
think of your mother?'

'Oh, you know . . .'

And another: 'What do you think of when you think of your
father?'

'Well . . .'

I do my best to be vague. I do not want to talk about my
childhood. I do not want to tell her, this stranger, intimate
biographical facts. Once out of their trap, they change everything.
Avoiding her questions does not relax me. She is persistent, and,
after another question about my father, which is based on the
assumption that I grew up in his presence, I have no choice but
to put her right. The only way I can do so is by spitting out a
biographical bone: my father died when I was five. Cue a response
I did not see coming.

'Oh,' she says, putting her hand to her own neck, 'I know
why you got cancer. I know why you got cancer there, on your
neck. You could not speak to your father.'

For a fraction of a fraction of a second, I think: oh, right,
gosh, yes, that's it.

'How would you describe yourself as a child? Were you quiet? Shy?'

Er, yes.

'Did you want to scream, make yourself heard? You did, of course you did, but instead you kept quiet, always good, and quiet. But really you wanted to scream and say, listen to me, what about me?'

'Well, I'm not so sure about that . . .'

'So what happened to you? Who brought you up?'

I need her to stop asking me intrusive questions. She is cutting me open. It is my half-brother who has lovingly gifted me this consultation; the gift is backfiring. I should get up and leave, make my excuses, but I have lost dominion over myself. I lie there, infantilised, tears streaming down my face. Later I think, why the tears? I've always held loss at bay.

'It's complicated,' I reply.

She massages my feet, inserts some acupuncture needles and pinches the air, like Tim the Buddhist did. But this time it is a discomfiting experience. She finishes off by pinching the air right up around my head. I picture black crows, circling, hear them cawing. Then a bell sounds, or perhaps it is the clash of mini cymbals. I merely register a high sound, and recognise it as the traditional way some healers and meditation instructors end a session. Not before time.

'How do you feel?'

Strung out. Pummelled.

'Light,' I reply, saying what I think she would like to hear.

'Ah, yes, light.'

'Tingly.'

'Yes, tingly. Good.'

'Who is with you in that photograph?' I ask, pointing to Cindy and her befeathered friends, feeling considerably more tetchy about this display of cultural appropriation than I did before the treatment. Shamans from Brazil, she says, and she adds something about one of the men being her teacher, or guru or wise man.

Before I leave, Cindy takes me up to her kitchen where she shows me her NutriBullet, the Prada of juicers, and urges me to start a juice-only regimen to boost my immune system. The suggestion is entirely at odds with the recommendations of my oncologist and my Macmillan nutritionist, which is to bulk up while I can still eat, and to maintain my weight. If I lose weight, the mask won't fit, which will hamper the precision targeting needed during radiotherapy. You get a lot of advice about nutrition when you've got cancer; for non-experts, it can be overwhelming.

Out on the street, I vent my anger at Cindy but also at myself for throwing myself on the mercy – or mumbo-jumbo – of someone I don't know or trust. I should have just had another massage at Healing HQ; at least then I would be in the safe hands of alternative healers, including acupuncturists, reiki practitioners and reflexologists, who work with cancer patients and understand their vulnerabilities.

The next morning, back at the *Guardian*, I throw up for the first time since my treatment started. That evening Lu informs me that she has spoken to her 'hippy friends' on my account. They are 'ecstatic' that I threw up. 'It means the healing has worked and the blockage has been removed – who knew!!'

What blockage would that be? I am not a sewer.

Three days after the session with Cindy the healer, I attend a workshop on silence at the Jesuit Centre, attached to Farm Street Church. Father, who became a Jesuit before I was born, used to go to Mass here when he lived in London; the building has a hold on me. I only wish I could warm to its Gothic interior, often wish it wasn't so oppressive and smug. I had booked the workshop before my diagnosis, back when I was keen to learn about the practice of contemplative silence. Now, living so much in my mind, no longer able to read, listen to music or watch movies, the cancer has forced silence upon me. In the early weeks, alone in bed, I had binge-watched *The Good Wife* and the American series of *House of Cards*. Then, five weeks into my chemotherapy, I lost my reality filter and believed the stories were real. I fretted to the point of anxiety about Alicia Florrick, the compromised state attorney's wife played by Julianna Margulies in *The Good Wife*, and became convinced that the evil embodied by Kevin Spacey's character, Frank Underwood in *House of Cards*, would contaminate the world. I watched the film *Eat, Pray, Love* to calm me down. I had never read the book but had absorbed the hype, hence my (misguided) adoption of the title to signify my own spiritual equanimity. I was expecting *Odyssey* lite, a sort of romcom travelogue meets spiritual awakening and just what the doctor ordered. What I got was an ill-travelled, emotionally infantilised American goes abroad, eats new food (which, because she is ill-travelled, she finds 'exotic') and has no-strings sex. It was the last movie I watched on my laptop. After that, I spent hours just lying, or sitting, in silence. Wanting to explore silence now through the discipline of meditation and reflection feels like wilful masochism.

Still, I've signed up for it, and off I go into the crisp, cold March morning, Mayfair so majestic and me chuffed to be walking through it, feeling fine and only one week to go before my third three-week cycle of chemotherapy ends. I can't wait to get this phase behind me, much as I am dreading the next.

There is a morning discussion about the nature of silence and what we associate it with. Quite a few people in the group associate it with school punishments, as in, the whole class will now sit in silence after that appalling behaviour. For others, it brings to mind solitude, boredom and escape. We turn to the practice of chanting in the afternoon. Our workshop leader gives us a biblical passage to read, one about Jesus dropping in on Mary and her sister, Martha. I have never come across it before, and it's decades since I have even read the Bible. We are told to choose a word or phrase that stands out, for whatever reason and, if it is a phrase, to reduce it to a word or two, and, with our eyes shut, to repeat them.

In the passage, Mary sits at Jesus's feet, listening. Martha dashes about, doing the equivalent of putting the kettle on and rustling up some sandwiches for their guest. When she suggests to the young rabbi that he might tell Mary to shift it and help out, Jesus says: 'You've got your priorities wrong.' Which is a bit harsh.

Unspoilt for choice, I plump for the phrase 'sat at the Lord's feet', then don't know what to reduce it to, 'sat' or 'feet'. They are hardly spiritual firecrackers, either of them. I try 'sat' first, and immediately start smirking. I am back at St Andrews University. An English lecturer with a messianic weakness for Shakespeare is exhorting the wonders of Enobarbus's sparkling paean to Cleopatra's beauty. He recites it from memory, not needing to refer to the text:

'I will tell you . . .' he begins. A tremor in his voice alerts us to how moving he finds the speech. The lecture hall is silent.

'The barge she shat in . . .'

Titters gather into guffaws.

'. . . I mean, sat in – like a burnished throne.'

'Feet' is no better. I don't like feet, and have never got over my horror at discovering that Jesus voluntarily washed the stinking feet of strangers.

'Feet, feet, feet, feet.' I say it over and over, trying to be serious and spiritual, but now Dr Seuss is chipping in. 'Slow feet quick feet./Trick feet Sick feet./Up feet Down feet./ Here come Clown feet. Small feet, Big feet./Here come pig feet./ His feet,/Her feet.' *The Foot Book* used to be favourite bedtime reading for the boys. I've just got to 'Fuzzy fur feet,' a deliciously visual image, when we are invited to open our eyes and share

our experiences. A few admit to finding it hard to get going
on the chanting because the story itself got in the way; they
can't understand why Jesus was so hard on Martha. As for me,
I'm picturing Jesus's feet in a pair of those brown leather
sandals men wear with socks. Only Jesus isn't wearing socks,
which is how, spiritual mollusc that I am, I find myself
imagining his grimy toenails.

15

CANCER ETIQUETTE

Is it acceptable to do karaoke until 4 a.m. if you've got cancer? I wake up the morning after my friend Lu's fiftieth birthday party, concerned that I might have overstepped the don't-get-out-much, might-never-get-out-again mark. It's all very well doing mindfulness, meditation and abstract healing, but it's the coalface of cancer etiquette that I am now up against. *Debrett's* doesn't cover it. Myself and my Scottish friend Donald – owner of the Egyptian boxer shorts – hogged the mikes for a good two hours, he in a gold diamanté dinner jacket and matching bow tie, me in Doulton blue hot pants and a gold chain-mail top. The dress code, in our defence, was Gold and Bold, and I, in my defence, was celebrating getting through my nine-week chemotherapy treatment as well as making the most of my week off before the chemo-radiation treatment began. Nevertheless, the memory of me taking up a lunge position and then belting out 'I Can't Get No Satisfaction' is particularly vexatious. The fact that I had one glass of Prosecco – one glass, all evening – is also worrying me. It's not the quantity, which is a sorry pass, but the possibility that the guests who know I have cancer – and there was a fair share of them – may have thought: what a bad cancer person she is, drinking like that. Plus, I chatted and laughed, which is also improper in someone with cancer, and I gave the party bores and the moaners short shrift. I usually hear them out. One man went on about his nonagenarian uncle being stiff and immobile. It is very upsetting, he said. Just so-o-o sad. Really? Is it? The man is ninety years old. I made my excuses and swivelled. If you have cancer and you are at a party and find yourself talking to a moaner, make your excuses and swivel too. I'll put that in a Cancer Etiquette Handbook. There's surely a gap in the market, given how many people now get cancer and will survive it. In the How to Behave at Parties section I shall add:

- Dress up and wear make-up if you feel like it. Having cancer and trying to look attractive is not indecorous.
- Don't hold back on the dance floor; you are beyond judgement for once, so make the most of it.
- If eye contact makes you feel exposed or vulnerable, avoid it. Ditto conversation.
- If guests are standing and you need to sit down, go ahead. Just get someone to sit down with you so you don't look like a lemon.
- Remember: no one wants to have to ask you how you are, so get in first with a tactical conversational gambit and keep bringing the conversation back to your interlocutor.
- If someone does ask you how you are and you feel good, say so – without clarification.
- If someone asks you how you are and you suddenly feel grim, doomed and overwhelmed, either say, I feel like death warmed up, or, better still, say, fine thanks. Whatever you do, don't answer truthfully. You may have cancer, but at parties, civilian rules apply.

- Give the terminally dull short shrift; excuse yourself and go for the bright sparks.
- If you fancy a glass of wine and feel up to it, then have one. High morale is precious. Boost it while you can.
- Do a recce on arrival to locate the nearest bathroom.
- If you're about to throw up, abandon your conversation mid-sentence and leg it to said bathroom.
- If you enjoy karaoke, go for it. Just don't hog the microphone.

Four days after the party, it is PEG-fitting day. It's eleven weeks since the prognosis when Blondie first mentioned a peg. Or rather, PEG. I now know that it stands for percutaneous endoscopic gastrostomy. I've got 'percutaneous' off pat by breaking it down as you would if it came up in a game of Charades. Which it wouldn't, obviously, unless you were a medic who didn't get out much and I don't think they exist. Perk, as in job perk: free parking, for instance, or expense account. Cute, as in puppy, or Russell Brand on Valium. Anus, as in *anus* [*sic*] *horribilis*. Perk-cute-anus.

The Macmillan pamphlet says: 'When oral intake is impossible, a PEG feeding tube is fitted . . .' Fliff takes me to hospital. In the waiting room, she suggests it might be helpful for me to think of myself as a Royal Marine on a Commando course. Her dad was a military man. That way, she says, whatever comes my way won't seem too bad. I haven't brought an overnight bag because I will be home in a few hours, but the straightforward surgical procedure doesn't agree with me and I am hospitalised for two nights, during which time I writhe in agony. The abdominal spasms are far, far worse than labour contractions, my unsuspecting stomach protesting at the foreign tubing and plastic disk that stops the tube from being pulled out. I hold on to the sides of the bed and scream, no stiff upper lip for me. In between, I spew diabolic green bile into a succession of cardboard hats. I have injections of morphine, first, in my leg and, when the pain is pretty much unbearable, orally. At two in the morning I am wheeled down to the imaging department for an X-ray, but they find nothing awry. All night and the next day, the spasms persist. And then, on the second morning, they stop. I go home with a second belly button and a plastic triangle with a pixie's neatly coiled miniature garden hose sticking out of it, an adhesive dressing over the top.

An Abbott homecare nurse comes to my house to show me how to look after the PEG.

'It won't fall out,' she chirps, enteral nutrition, or tube feeding, being an Abbott nurse's speciality. *Come on up*, I don't say, as I lead her to my bedroom. We sit side by side on my bed. My T-shirt is pulled up.

'May I?' she asks.

She tugs at the tubing before I can say: no, obviously not. Don't touch me. Better still, go home.

'See?' she says. 'Doesn't hurt, does it?'

No, it doesn't. She's right there. But I still want to cry.

'You need to turn the tube 360 degrees every day, at least three times. To stop it getting stuck, you see, and the skin growing over. Have a little twizzle.'

Twizzle as in turkey, if you add an 'r', which I do.

'Would you like me to demonstrate?' she says.

'I can't think of anything I would like more.' I don't say that either. I treat her inquiry as yet another rhetorical question; I encounter so many of them on this so-called cancer journey. When I don't answer, she smiles and, very gently, puts her hand on the tube. I look away. She twizzles. I can feel the wall of my stomach.

'Oh, gosh,' I say, shutting my eyes. I am going to faint.

'There you are, you see. Easy! Would you like to have a go?'

Have a go? As in, have a go on the trampoline, have a go at the wheel of a sports car. Yes, to these two, no to the twisting of a tube going from the outside world into an organ I would rather not be associated with. We try out the syringe next.

'Have you got a cup of water?'

I get one from my bedside table. The water has been there all night.

'You must flush the syringe out with water before you draw up any feed,' she says, 'and afterwards. Like this.'

I know how a syringe works.

'Only use very thin liquids. We'll be delivering you some supplements. Milkshakes. What flavours would you like? There's chocolate, vanilla, strawberry and plain. Plain is sort of neutral.'

'They all sound good.'

'Just remember, never anything thick. I had one man who tried to feed himself porridge through the tube. Porridge!'

'Really? Porridge?'

We both laugh. How could he be so dim?

Radiotherapy starts the next day. 'Treat it like a day job,' I remember Blondie advising as I walk from my chemotherapy session in the Macmillan Centre over to the main hospital. 'You turn up day after day, at about the same time. There's quite a bit of waiting around. It gets tiring, you've got to get there and back and, later, there will be the side effects to deal with.' She says patients come to rely on the routine and that afterwards, when the treatment is over, some struggle with the lack of structure to their days.

'Morning Genevieve!' The lady on reception greets me like a new employee come to save the day. 'I'll let them know you are here. Take a seat right over there.'

Her warmth and friendly Canadian accent take the edge off my nerves. I sit, and I make sure I do not think and I certainly don't let myself look at anyone else. It's unnerving, waiting, when you don't know what you are waiting for. Just a few minutes later a young woman in hospital gear and sneakers comes to get me. Down the corridor we go, making small talk, and the small talk works: it stops me imagining what's coming next. We go through a second set of double-doors and she says: Sit here, please Genevieve. OK, I will. It would be rude not to. Besides, what help would doing a runner be now?

Inside the radiotherapy unit a stack of steel shelves is lined with blue masks. I see the smaller ones, and flinch. I strip off down to my jeans, wrap a giant blue tissue across my chest and walk over to the plastic couch. *Lie down*. Righto. *Keep still*. Will do. Then my bespoke Batman mask is over my face and I've got no choice but to keep still. Two radiographers are standing either side of me and they clamp me in place. Two plastic catches, not the four-inch buckles I had imagined, pin my right shoulder down. Snap, snap; the boys have let off a stink bomb, right by my ear. That's how loud it is. Two by the right side of my neck. Snap, snap. Two behind the back of my head. Snap, snap. It's getting weird under here. The feeling of the mask on my face is not how I remember it from the fitting. It does not feel like plastic any more. It's hard. There's no give to it. Two to the left of my head. Snap, snap. The radiographers are fast. Only two more to go, though I don't know this yet. Two more, by my left shoulder. My heart is a stallion caught in a stable fire, kicking down its door, jumping the yard gate, running for its life. My lungs, meanwhile, have forgotten how to rise and fall. The mask is pressing against my nose and throat. It is punctured with holes, 2 mm in diameter, but my brain won't give this information to my lungs. Myself, my lungs and my heart, we are all in a state of alarm. We think: we can't do our jobs.

But the mask is porous. There are two more holes, smaller than Smarties, over my nostrils. There is a mouth hole, as big as that of Munch's *Scream* man, but the hole is horizontal, rather than vertical. It measures 60 mm wide and 30 mm high. If you look at the mouth when mine is not there, it looks like a mouth frozen in mid-holler. The mask follows the hollow of my neck and the indent of my eye sockets. I peer through the perforations and see pale latticework and light. The shell is pressing on my eyes, so I shut them. Pinned down, I can only listen and wait. But I don't know what to listen out for.

I hear a high-pitched bleep. It sounds three times.

'We are going to leave the room now, Genevieve. We'll be watching you through the glass screen in the control room. Remember, if anything's wrong, just raise your hand.'

The radiographers have got sixty seconds before the radioactive rays get them too. A month after the Chernobyl disaster of 1986 I went to Krakow, 760 miles away from the nuclear power plant explosion, to study Emily Dickinson under a Fulbright scholar at the Jagiellonian University; the Soviet hotel I stayed in on my first night served radioactive lettuce on a platter, there was no food in the shops, and sinister figures roamed the streets clutching Geiger counters. Emily Dickinson owes me.

'We are starting now, Genevieve. Remember, just put your hand up if you need to.'

I picture the blue beams from *Star Wars* light sabres, only finer, going into my head and neck. The beams will go in heavier on the right side of my neck, obliterating my right salivary gland and damaging the left. The mask is smothering my neck. I visualise my skin, not only what lies just beneath it – blood vessels and lymph and who knows what other hideous viscous membranes – but how it stretches around my neck and up over my skull and my arms and legs and the points of my fingers, joined in one seamless body bag. In just five weeks, salt pans will crinkle across my neck. The concave crusts of burnt skin will be tiny at first, no bigger than the nail of my little finger and will rupture into wet wounds, before weeping and oozing into each other, forming one single bloodied, suppurating land mass. Leper. At least I will know what it feels like.

The machine goes backwards. I want to twitch my nose, but don't know if that counts as moving. I slide backwards, into the tunnel of the machine, or the whole machine comes forward and covers me. I am not sure which. There is a banging sound. Boom, boom, boom, boom. At the same time, high-pitched noises start up, eerie and other-worldly, like a dolphin's cry. It's too bad my hearing is not already damaged. There is the stampede of hooves again, more than one horse now, several, and everything louder as my heartbeat speeds up. More banging. More beeping. I am in a sci-fi movie. They'll turn off the machine, remove the mask and I will have superpowers. I open my eyes, see the grey of the machine, close them again. Then I remember. Peggy gave me a mantra, the one Deepak sent her from New York. It's just a pity I can't remember it. 'Fuck' would do, but it's only one syllable. I could say it over and over: the objective correlative incarnate. You're just being juvenile. You've got thirty-three sessions of this, so think of something. I rewind to my retreat on silence at the Jesuit Centre. Lying inside this machine, I need to chant in a way I did not need to then.

Heal me, Lord. Let me live in your light.

This is what I come up with. It is not very catchy, but in a game of verbal Ten Green Bottles, I knock off each word one by one as the light whirrs around me, alighting upon phrases within phrases.

> Heal me, Lord. Let me live.
> Heal me, Lord. Let me.
> Let me.

'Let me' turns out to be the most dizzying of all the verbal couplings, more so even than 'heal me'. When I am out of here and back in the world I have left behind, I must use it. 'Here, let me.' It's what you say to a child, or to someone in need. 'Let me help you.' When Jesus washed those dirty feet, he probably said, 'Let me.' I am flipping now, getting excited about all the good I will do back on Earth. I've gone soft, delusional, which is what I worried about that night at dinner at Scott's in Mayfair. It's the Cancer Effect, corroding my Not-Nice-Person-with-Cancer self. Something is shifting, and it's very disconcerting. I can't claim to be suffering, but the old cynicism is giving way to a more compassionate outlook that already leaves me raw. Love, I'm all over it. I genuinely, laughably, think that when all this is over I will put myself out for others, connect with them, help them. Here, let me.

Saint Genevieve. Look out for her in N19. And keep looking.

I take my mind back to the chant, and I break the words down again. 'Heal me, Lord' reduces to 'Heal me' and then I alight on the single word 'heal'. Simply by removing each word, one by one, I come to the miracle of the first and last and most important word: heal. The brilliance of it is that the word isn't about me, nor is it only for me. It is a word for everyone – patients, medics, everybody.

During the four minutes of the radiotherapy I say my chant over and over. Then, without warning, the noises stop, the couch and I go forwards and I can sense the arm of the machine moving away. The radiographers come in and the couch comes down, lowered with just a faint whirr like my half-sister's coffin in the crematorium, except there's a living me on top instead. Snap, snap. Snap, snap. Snap, snap. Snap, snap. Snap, snap. The mask is raised off my face and shoulders. I sit up, clutching the giant blue tissue to my chest. My neck isn't burning, everything is fine. I realise that not knowing what to expect is what had made me afraid. I get dressed behind the screen, say thank you, take the tube home, hug the dog, climb into bed, set my alarm for thirty minutes hence, get up five minutes before the boys arrive home from school, hug them, smile to myself.

It wasn't that bad. This radiotherapy thing is going to be a breeze.

16

TONGUE-TIED

What an unsung organ the tongue is. What wonders it performs. But I only give it its due recognition when it malfunctions. The taste buds go down first. There are eight to ten thousand of them scattered across its surface. Ordinarily taste buds are replenished with new cells every ten days but the radiotherapy disrupts this replenishment and therefore eliminates functional taste buds within ten days. Chemotherapy also affects taste, and from the moment I started on it, my sense of taste became distorted. Even that first evening, when Rota Sue delivered her Ottolenghi vegetable pie, I couldn't get at the flavours. I had been warned about a change in taste sensation; it's known as dysgeusia, and is typically experienced as food tasting metallic, but for flavours to be distorted this early on came as a surprise. The chemotherapy made me hungry, though, and in the weeks that followed this helped me push past the emerging taste barriers. I could still taste some foodstuffs, but what I could taste kept reducing – this is known as hypoguesia – until I could only taste sweet things. What you can't taste, you don't want. I duly morphed into my late grandmother and my mother-in-law, and packed away ice cream and over-sweetened supermarket apple crumble. I became puffy.

When I get further into the combined chemo-radiotherapy I will lose all sense of taste – a condition known as ageusia – and make the necessary mental adjustments. Not adjustments; handbrake turns, more like. I will resign myself to never being interested in food again, and I will mourn the loss. Later still, when I can't swallow, let alone taste anything, I will see for myself what it is to shut off from food, to acknowledge it and reject it as irrelevant. It is a shutting off from life, and it affords an insight into the death wish of the anorexic I could do without. Rejoining the eating club will be the most momentous challenge, harder than the radiotherapy and the loneliness.

For now, two weeks into the combined chemo-radiotherapy and twelve weeks since my treatment began, my mouth is merely dry and sore and my tongue is beginning to stiffen up. Wine is out of the question. The tiniest sip goes down like paraffin poured across its surface, a lit match chucked into the middle of it for good measure. It shrieks at anything acidic. I've become partial to very cold Mars Bar milkshakes, the super-sweet ones you buy in plastic bottles from supermarkets and newsagents. Or don't buy. Because they are junk. I do, despite various self-anointed cancer buffs continuing to tell me that sugar feeds cancer, as well as the NHS website telling me as much. It's a bit late for that, I scoff, but secretly I panic and think, what if I am killing myself with sugar? I can still swallow, but hard, jagged, dry foodstuffs such as bread or pastry squat on my tongue. It's as if I've scooped up a mouthful of bits of card whipped up with wallpaper paste. It's my beleaguered salivary glands. Instead of the one and a half to two litres of saliva they usually produce every day, mine are on a go-slow. Soft food – what a cheerless phrase – still goes down the hatch, but I am beginning to resist it. It offers nothing – no flavour, no texture, no pleasure, no returns save nutritional value. Even fish pie no longer slips under the net. I'm down to fudge yoghurt, vanilla ice cream and the Mars Bar milkshakes. I've got the Ensure medical ones, crates of them, in the larder. But I am not prepared to go there. Not yet.

I had forgotten, or probably never even knew, that we have more than one pair of salivary glands. There are the parotids, the largest – absolute whoppers, in fact. Imagine a triangular blob sitting beneath your ear and stretching down to the jaw. The submandibulars are a sixth of the size – more like one of those pink prawn sweets you get in a pick 'n' mix line-up – and the sublinguals that lie in front of them are about the size of an almond. It's the submandibulars, the ones that are home to the Interloper below my jawbone, that are being damaged the most by the radiotherapy. Eventually, the right-hand one will be destroyed altogether. I'll miss it when it is gone, as is the way of things, but not nearly as much as I miss all three pairs when I get further into the radiotherapy and they are producing no saliva at all. By that stage, my mouth will be a desert in a drought, a freak sandstorm blowing in dead roots and uprooted cacti that catch and scrape the insides of my mouth. Only then do I salute my salivary glands. If I had my time again, which I would rather not, obviously, it's my tongue and my salivary glands I'd give thanks for on a mindfulness walk with Peggy O'Hare. You live and learn.

I also learn to listen to my oncologists. They told me the side effects of the radiotherapy were coming, and I ignore their warnings, as well as their instructions for how to minimise them. Which is why I decide we should go back to Vicky's house near Bath for Easter, fifteen weeks since coming down for New Year's Eve. Near Bath, but actually in a hamlet. Some distance from a hospital. Anyway, Vicky and Martin are away and all we have to do is feed the dreaded cats, Chilli and Basil, who remain holed up in the study-turned-cat-suite next to the guest bathroom on the ground floor. I have invited friends to stay and a few more for Easter lunch, to jolly things along. I love Easter – it goes back to my sister and me dressing up in lemon coats and white gloves to see the giant chocolate egg in the lobby of the Plaza Hotel in New York and Mother taking us out to lunch. I've always marked it. I don't want this year to be any different. Or rather, I choose to overlook the fact that it is different.

It is just the four of us on Good Friday and in the evening we are playing poker by the fire when, out of nowhere, popcorn starts going off inside my mouth; my tongue doesn't know what's hit it. Over the next couple of hours the discomfort intensifies and it feels like someone is dripping acid on my tongue, and flicking it on to the insides of my mouth and lips for good measure. I keep sipping water, but the sensation intensifies. In the end I make my excuses and slink off to bed. Four hours later I am woken up by my tongue: it's now in a vice. The bolts on either side are being tightened and a blade is skimming the surface, bursting minuscule molten boils. I can't swallow and it's hard to breathe. The consultants and assiduous speech and language therapists have told me to expect all of this but, forgetting their warnings, I panic. Hospital may be necessary, I think, annoyed at myself for embarking on this fantasy of a normal, convivial Easter. I cannot fathom why, in the middle of combined chemo-radiotherapy, with a battered immune system, I would cut myself off from UCLH. I try to focus on whether the shortness of breath is a panic attack, but I've never had one before so don't know. Richard is sleeping beside me, his six-foot-four frame that usually stretches down the length of any bed curled up, tight as an ammonite. He sleeps fitfully nowadays; it is 2 a.m. on Easter Saturday. I am reluctant to wake him, but I do. He pings upright. Hospital, he says, better go, slurring his words and moving his limbs about in an attempt to show willing. Now that he's awake, I stop crying, take some deep breaths, check my temperature. I am supposed to go to A & E if I have a fever. I have a fever. But we don't know where the hospital is and agree that we will get lost. We decide to wait a bit. I take some Nurofen, can't sleep, get up and go to the bathroom to examine my tongue. The bathroom is next door to the study, where the cats are. I realise we have not fed them. If they are dead, who gets priority? Me, with a trip to A & E, or the cats, with corpse courtesies. I bet Thomas Lynch, the undertaker-poet, has a better word for this but right now, my death lexicon has dried up. I'll have to close their eyelids, or arrange their tails, or whatever it is you do to expired cats to dignify their passing and make them not look grotesque. Even though I know I should check on them, my tongue gets first dibs.

I stand in front of the bathroom mirror and stick out my tongue, but it only gets as far as the back of my teeth. The hydraulic system is malfunctioning. I am an elephant that cannot lift its trunk, an octopus that cannot stretch out its arm in search of a tasty clam. The oblong lump of flesh is too painful to move any further. Except it isn't flesh, it's a matrix of muscles, with no bone supporting it, and the radiotherapy has scarred the muscle tissue. Up until now, my tongue has been able to do the usual gymnastics: twist, move up or down or flop, Einstein-style, over my bottom lip and down to my chin. I've been doing the jaw, tongue and swallowing exercises given to me by UCLH's first-rate team of emotionally supportive, kindly and painstaking speech and language therapists, though admittedly not as often as I have been told to. Now the invisible clamps are squeezing the sides of my tongue and as I try to push it forwards and between my lips, the membrane that anchors the base of the tongue to the mouth, the lingual frenulum, is straining. I am tongue-tied. In the end, ignoring the pain, I force myself to stick the thing out. I see an expanse of sea foam scattered by the wind and washed up on my beached whale of a tongue. Titus's Lavinia had her tongue ripped out, and that was an act of barbarism; I would rip out my own, it hurts so much.

I should be more respectful. My tongue has served me well up until now. Taste, eating, speech, oral hygiene, infection-fighting, romance, it takes care of the lot. Remember that sweet Gilbert O'Sullivan song, 'What's in a kiss? Have you ever wondered just what it is?' The answer is, a tongue – unless your heart's not in it. As organs go, it does not seem fair that the heart alone has been turned into a universal symbol; perhaps, when I'm done with all this, I'll rebrand it, get some iconography going, appropriate the Rolling Stones tongue loll. The trouble is, though, the tongue, unlike the heart, is not a mysterious thing. We see it all the time, use it round the clock, feel it every second, see other people's. The tongue does not have the heart's pleasing shape or good looks, either. I've seen drawings of cross-sections of the papillae, the tiny bumps on the tongue's surface, in *Gray's Anatomy*, and they are quite surreal.

In one drawing, the tongue's surface appears as a collection of button mushrooms with spots, stubby macaroni tubes topped with anal creasing (not a culinary term, admittedly, but visually accurate) and tall macaroni tubes with prongs. The mushroom ones are the fungiform papillae, found mainly on the front of the tongue. They contain taste buds. The macaroni, cylindrical ones – the filiform papillae – don't but, like all the papillae, they help to increase the tongue's surface and provide the friction needed to grip broken-down food as it is turned into the bolus we then swallow. Or don't, in my case. There are two others – foliate papillae and circumvallate papillae. The foliate papillae look like folded leaves. There are only eight of them on either side of the back of the tongue. The circumvallate, of which we only have between six and twelve, are the biggest ones. The next time a rude child sticks her tongue out at you, take a look at the V-shape at the back of it; it comprises the circumvallate, the gag guys. Taste something horrible, and they make you retch.

The word papilla, I discover, comes from the Latin word for nipple, derived from *papula*, or swelling. Which makes me wonder: which came first, the nipple or the tongue? When those medical nomenclaturists were going through the human body, they must have named the nipple first, and then the tongue in order for the latter to be defined by the former. That's not fair. The tongue is more important than the nipple.

You might disagree. I say nipple and you might well say tassel, and more besides. I might say, providing I know you well enough, breastfeeding and tell you about the first time the nipples on my post-partum cannonball breasts turned into high pressure shower heads with holes pointing in all directions, and how the whole room got sprayed with human milk.

I eventually go back to bed and doze off, only to wake a couple of hours later, hungry. I take some more Nurofen and head to the kitchen, but don't know what my tongue will tolerate. I remember the small pot of hazelnut yoghurt I have bought for myself; it's an old favourite. I scoop out half a teaspoon and as I raise it to my mouth, I inhale its rich flavour and creaminess. So far, so normal. My sense of smell is still intact. My lips settle round the tip of the teaspoon and my hesitant tongue moves towards the metal. There's too much yoghurt on the spoon. My lips and tongue, as if wise to what's coming, only want a quarter of what's there, just the tip. If birds ate yoghurt, I would call this feed for a damaged chick. The coldness of the yoghurt makes the nodules of tissue on my tongue scream blue murder. I can't even taste the yoghurt or make my tongue, the gatekeeper, do anything with it. Meanwhile, what feels like a tiny chip of dead tooth is stuck on the front of my tongue. It's a bit of hazelnut. The tip of my tongue has risen to the roof of my mouth. And that's it. There is no next. My tongue is supposed to propel the moistened foodstuff, the bit of nut, backwards and down the hatch. The epiglottis, that gross pendulum at the back of the throat that I remember from Barney's biology lessons as particularly revolting, should be about to flip into place, acting as a barrier so that the food mush, or bolus, doesn't go down my windpipe. But the fleck of hazelnut won't budge so the swallowing mechanism I have been taking for granted does not swing into action. There isn't enough saliva to break down and soften the bit of hazelnut, so my tongue isn't letting it pass. I probe its bumpy surface with my finger, locate the offending nut particle, remove it and swallow some water. I wasn't expecting the eating to become this difficult this soon, and feel defeated. I try to think of something else I can eat. Then I remember. On her note, Vicky said she had left some smoked salmon for Chilli. I nick a minuscule sliver but, in an act of karma, the fish squats on my tongue and then, when I close my mouth, it sticks to the roof of my mouth. There should be movement of jaw, cheek and tongue, a jigging about, mastication. Nothing doing. I open my mouth, the sliver is back on the surface of my tongue. I suppose I should commend the papillae for doing such an excellent job of keeping the sliver in place. I stick my finger in my mouth to unpeel it, then pinch it between index finger and thumb like a worm in a bird's beak and, without looking at it, flick it into the bin.

Then, feeling guilty about the cats, I creep into the study. Chilli, the blind, incontinent one, is in the middle of the carpet, paws curled under her belly, stranded. Basil, the arthritic, deaf one, is asleep on a heated cushion on the sofa. If I were a transcendentalist like Emerson and had commendable views about nature and humanity being part of a whole, I would empathise with these pitiful, dependent creatures of our interconnected, sacred universe. I would prepare their food with love. Instead, I spoon out their gelatinous tinned glop without looking at it and retch. As I put down their bowls I try to feel a modicum of love and light. 'There you are, kittens,' I say, even though they are old hags and I am repulsed by their infirmity. Pot black, clearly. Nevertheless, if Vicky has installed a webcam, I am covered. Basil licks at her food with her tongue. It's all right for some, I think, hurrying across the room and shutting the door behind me.

Back in the kitchen, I decide that the only way I am going to get anything inside me is to use the PEG, which I brought with me to practise shooting up water. I can't say I feel ready. I thought I had way more time before it got to this stage. I feel humiliated and demeaned. Happily it is still dark, everyone is sleeping, no one will chance upon me. I lay out the syringe and warm up some fresh tomato soup. Idiot, I think, taking it off the hob, it's going straight into my stomach and might burn it. Or will it? I don't know, I can't find an answer in my fuzzy head. I do know it doesn't matter whether it is a nice soup, or a disgusting one, since I won't be able to taste it, a fact I find alarming. I am going to bypass the eating process and put food into my stomach. I pour the soup into a bowl and in another I pour some cold water, so I can practise using the syringe. It's fat, like the toy versions toddlers play Doctors and Nurses with. The nozzle has an opening of 3 mm. I practise drawing the water up and pushing it out, one half of a hydraulic system in action. It is child's play; the syringe shoots the water across and over the bananas in the fruit bowl like a water pistol. I try the soup next. In goes the nozzle, up should come the soup-filled syringe. But the soup is too thick. I add some cold water and stir it with the tip of the syringe. I lower the syringe, draw it up. Again, nothing's happening. I can't see why soup won't work. Then I remember the Abbott Nurse telling me about the man who tried to feed himself porridge through his PEG. Well, this isn't porridge. It is liquidised tomato. I am failing to see that, far from being thin and smooth, it has bits of tomato and onion in it. I add more water. It still won't be drawn. Crushed by my own hopelessness and helplessness, I weep. Then I tidy up the paraphernalia and stash the syringe out of sight.

Later that morning I go to the Anglican church while Richard prepares an Easter roast. The Southern American vicar is like something from the QVC channel, only I am not sure what he is selling. He is a Bible man, and I can't get the measure of him, or any sustenance. Back at Vicky's house, Richard is readying the house for our guests. One is a local photographer whom Richard has recently interviewed for a prestigious international photography prize. I've never met him. He brings his wife, and daughter, and then Laurence comes with his son, and another friend arrives. We open wine, pass round smoked salmon blinis (using salmon we bought, not Chilli's), chat. Or rather, they chat. I sit, unable to speak, my mouth an old garage full of sharp tools and dust and stale kerosene, and I float like I did back at that first dinner party a week after the chemotherapy started. I've subjugated my hunger; it is startling how quickly one can do that. I just watch and listen. My eyes switch from Bassy to Reuben and then to everyone chatting away, doing all this living. And then the calm cleaves, cracks, and up comes panic, takes me under in a single tug. I know I need not be pulled down like this, must keep my head above the surface. But down I go, and here, in this moment, there is just me, and there's no light, it's a tight squeeze, the air elsewhere. Minutes pass and then, finally, I'm back up again, back in the room, breathing easy. But I'm exhausted, my mouth too much, not talking too awkward. I slip off to our bedroom, curl up on the bed and hold my knees, regroup. I give myself ten minutes, and then I go and check on the roast and lay out Easter eggs and chocolates on each plate.

Everyone tucks in. I move a roast potato around my plate with my fork, and try to ignore my hunger. We go for a walk after lunch, following Wellow Brook for a little bit before heading up and over hills stretching into a show-off distance I don't care for, the landscape so insensitive and full of itself. It is hard to get my feet to move forward, I feel too tired. I don't know where we are going, and feel the panic rising. I can't walk to nowhere. There's so much grass and mud and trees. Way too many trees, rooted, reaching, doing their own thing. I fall behind. The boys stay at my pace. Then, unable to continue, I say I am going back to the house. Reuben offers to come with me. No need, I say, but he takes my arm and back we go, admitting temporary defeat not so calamitous, pretending everything is normal not necessarily the only way.

On the drive back to London the next day I sit in the back of the car and size up a banana. I can't face eating it, but I'm really ravenous now. I peel it, can't bite into it, ask Richard to stop at a service station and buy me yet another Mars milkshake. Ten minutes later, I ask him to stop the car so I can throw up. You're going to Mordor, the boys' school vicar said when I told her about the side effects ahead. The Easter weekend must be a trial run.

17

RADIO GIRLS

I am back on the radiotherapy couch straight after Easter, but not before my morphine intake is ramped up by the registrar, who assures me that the tongue horror is part of the trajectory of escalating side effects. The speech therapists have also stepped in, giving me more tongue and swallowing exercises. I need to avoid my tongue becoming completely immobilised.

Something has shifted today. As I lie on my back, the tips of my cowboy boots pointing to the ceiling, my naked upper half covered in the giant blue modesty tissue that is not my shroud, a gloom has set in.

The radio girls – not girls of course, but they are so young, so optimistic, their soft hair in ponytails – attend to me as usual, one either side of the treatment couch. They smile, fuss, make reassuring noises. The ink freckle on my chest is checked for positioning, a bare shoulder cupped then nudged, a hip moved, legs tugged, one side pushed a fraction over, my own ponytail rearranged, a question asked: are you cold? and my answer always yes, I am. A blanket is laid over me, though not to cover the whole of me, I am not dead yet, thank you.

Four hands lower the mask, every session the same, the known world gone, this my day job now. I am Cleopatra and the radiographers are my Charmians, my girls, making me feel important and that nothing is too much trouble, everything must be just so. Admittedly I've swapped Cleopatra's bronze and gold for plastic and pale blue, my mask identical to all the others waiting on the stack. Every day now it is tighter on my face; the lowering of it embodies my sense of separation from others. I don't want it near me, want it away from my neck, sore now, raw. It snubs my nose, and there is no making the snapping gentle, however gentle the hands. Snap. Snap. I never get used to the noise, always gasp, don't always feel brave. Snap. Snap. My eyes are long shut, and when the two radiographers leave the room after the 60-second warning, I say thank you. Thank you for this treatment, and then I try to breathe. I have heard that others scream, take tranquillisers first. Into the tube, the tomb, I go, or so it feels; really it is the radiation machine going round my head. What if I have been tricked into lying here? I imagine the radiographers as my torturers pushing freshly cut daisies into the perforations of the mask and watering each one, drop by drop. I imagine them leaving me inside the machine. Then I think about the Ancient Egyptians wearing death masks in their own image so that their soul – or their version of it – could recognise their body and return to it. If I die now, how will my soul find me?

Heal me, Lord. Let me live in your light.

I start the chant, try to calm down.

Heal me, Lord. Let me live.
Heal me, Lord. Let me.
Heal me.
Heal.

I know healing is what's happening, albeit in a roundabout sort of way, and I have a basic understanding of the radiotherapy process. It is not entirely reassuring. When the radioactive beam hits the good squamous cells in my head and neck – the ones making up the surface tissue of my mouth, throat, larynx, oesophagus – the cells that have got to the stage of dividing, as opposed to fulfilling their particular functions, or getting ready to divide, are killed first. When the beam hits the rogue cancer cells, the same thing happens. But neither the good cells nor the cancer cells die instantly. The healthy ones don't grow back as fast as they should but – here's the plus side – the cancer cells don't divide as fast as they would if they were left to their own devices. All the cells take weeks, even months to die; in fact, they will still be in their death throes when the radiotherapy finishes four weeks from now. This should be obvious, and partly explains why I will have to wait four months before the oncologists can tell me whether the treatment has been successful. It may be obvious, but it scares me all the same. I had thought, in my ignorance, that as soon as a cancer cell is hit by a gamma ray, it dies. In fact, a cancer cell is like a cockroach, quick on its feet, determined.

I am not the fragrant sort, yet I really miss wearing perfume. It isn't allowed during radiotherapy. I hadn't realised what a pick-me-up the choosing of a scent is, how a dab on the wrists and spray on the neck first thing is a ritual that sets you up for the day, marks your readiness for it. The Ancient Romans and Greeks used it to ready a dead body for the next life. Not me. As soon as my skin heals post radiotherapy, I shall use it to engage with this life again.

In the meantime, there are other perks to my radio days. After the morning sessions, which at least get me out of bed, I have my Home Girls to look forward to. Fliff, and my girlfriends Kate and Gabsie, have elected to be with me at set times. Three times a week, on my return from radiotherapy, one of my Home

Girls arrives. They bring lunch, at least in the early days when I can eat, they chat, potter about, do the things a wind-up relative would do. They hoover, tidy the kitchen, put on some laundry, make my bed, simply be with me. Sometimes they lie on the bed alongside me, not minding that, as the weeks go on, I begin to fall asleep in front of them. Once, when I wake up, Gabsie is in the same place on the bed.

'I watched you sleep,' she says.

Instead of blanching with embarrassment, I think: this feels like love. Not just BC, but even a few weeks ago, I would have felt compromised to find myself so exposed. Now being vulnerable no longer equates with failure, or giving up. It is just how it is on Planet Cancer.

And here anything can happen. One morning I get a card from Mother Theresa. Not formerly of Calcutta, but of St Helens, near Liverpool. This Mother Theresa is from a Carmelite monastery. Unbeknownst to me, Rota Sue's mother has asked the sisters to pray for me. It is quite a card. Jesus is on the front in a white tunic, his heart exposed and aflame, his raised hands aglow with stigmata. Beneath him there's a gold heart sticker, a mini red envelope, opened and displaying a plastic ruby. A message in gold reads: *With Love & Best Wishes*. It couldn't be more kitsch and yet I take the whole thing at face value, including the Mother Superior's long note inside. When she writes that 'Our Lord never asks of us more than we can bear, although He sometimes takes us to the very edge, He is there and holding us tightly in His arms,' I don't dismiss this as incontinent holiness, as I would have done BC. I think, she's right about being taken to the very edge, and I feel comforted. She signs off, 'With all our love and prayers, Mother Theresa.' I don't even laugh.

Ordinarily, if ever someone says, 'I am praying for you,' I cringe. They sound so credulous, and as if they have access to a VIP hotline to God. In the hierarchy of prayer I realise

I have been operating under, my own occasional praying is quite different. It is knowing, superior. It is private, and considered, not crowd behaviour. Now I put the card down and I think, blimey, are those nuns really praying for me? – that's nice. Positive energy, if that is what prayer amounts to, is not to be sniffed at. If prayer can hold you up, then hold away. Then again, if I knew I would be dead in a matter of months I might well say, sod prayer. But for now, a stranger writes to say she and others are praying for me and I feel less lonely. And I am grateful. Because cancer is very, very lonely.

A week after Easter and the halfway point in my thirty-day radiation programme, I open my mouth to thank the radiographers for the session and hear a sparrow voice. My unsung tongue is a container ship in a dry dock, not going anywhere. I pity it, this fallen hero, my Mr Universe, my boneless hunk of flesh. And yet I've never liked tongues much. Kiss frontman Gene Simmons sticks his out of his black and white demon face and I think, put it away. I'd say the same to Mick Jagger. At university a flatmate once produced a tin of tongue for supper. It was a round economy tin, as big as a Frisbee. He ran a can opener's blade round the lid. We peered over as he peeled it back, revealing the pressed pink flesh covered with suction cups within. A cow's tongue, once. I heaved at the sight of it – unaware that it was my own tongue that enabled me to do so. Cows' tongues are giant things that swoosh about and froth and do a sterling job of digesting grass. And don't forget the jaw. There's no tongue action without a functioning jaw, as I also discover when mine goes into lockdown. Chewing the cud, what a newly lovely thought: down goes the grass in an easy swallow, up comes the cud, down it goes again, using 40,000 jaw movements in a single day. What good is a tongue in a tin?

My own is not much good in its new, seized-up state. Determined to override its malfunctions, I have a routine that enables me to talk and get my jaw moving. If someone telephones, for instance, I ask them to ring back in five minutes. I then dissolve and gargle an aspirin mouthwash, a phial of the liquid anaesthetic lidocaine, and mix up between 20 mg and 60 mg of morphine – I've got a colour-coded selection box, like a box of herbal teas they give you in hotel bedrooms. Then, mouth numbed, I call back, breaking to sip water every few seconds. But it's not my system that needs water; it's my dry mouth and throat. There is no mucous membrane for the water to stick to, so water only relieves the dryness for the second or two it is in my mouth before being swallowed. It is as if water is an illusion, everywhere, and not a drop to drink.

I use the same routine if we go out, which is rare now. It is all about timing the pain relief. We accept an invitation to have supper with local friends. It's a short, fifteen-minute walk, but I'm not up to it so we drive. I down pain relief just before I get in the car, which buys me some conversation on arrival. My capacious Longchamp handbag, rudely commandeered, is jammed with jingling glass phials of lidocaine, sachets of morphine, a plastic cup for the morphine, baby toothbrush and paste for when I throw up, and a couple of cardboard bowls for the it-no-longer-rains-but-it-pours vomiting moments. The bowls don't fit in the handbag and their frayed cardboard rims stick out over the black patent leather.

The host, David, is a very good cook, and ordinarily I would be really looking forward to the meal. We sit in the kitchen. The smell of sautéed fresh tomatoes makes me nervous. Everyone chats, but I am an old person again, planted on a hardback, upright chair, wishing I was in a comfortable armchair with a blanket on my knees and another round my shoulders. Attentive to timings, I leave the moment the pasta is brought to the table, hurrying up to the bathroom with my bulging handbag. I dose up as fast as I can, the lidocaine no longer tasting of anything, the white granules of morphine turning bright red the moment the water is added, me forgetting, as always, to bring something to stir it and using my finger, then it's the aspirin mouthwash, and back downstairs I go. All done in a couple of minutes. My mouth and jaw are ready for action. Just a little, I say as a spaghetti spoon hovers over my plate. Less, I say, when a dozen strands are on my plate. Really? David asks, surprised. I end up with three or four strands of spaghetti and a dollop of Amatriciana. I size up this insurmountable mountain of food, wanting to eat it, but not knowing how I will get through this much. Soon I will lose this desire altogether. Food will be the enemy and being near anything I might be expected to eat or drink will trigger anxiety. I twizzle a strand of spaghetti around my fork, move the forkful around the plate like a metal detector. Eventually, unable to put it off any longer, I open my mouth, drop my jaw, raise the fork half way. But I can't face the food just sitting on my tongue, going nowhere, and lower the fork. At the next attempt I skip the spaghetti and put a bit of sauce on a prong of the fork, try swallowing that, but wince at the spiciness, think I will throw up, decide to wing it, drink some water, force a bit of pasta down. Try again. Give up. I'm a toddler now, wishing this hateful food would be removed.

It's a good evening and worth the effort. I am trying my darndest to follow Blondie's advice that we eat together and keep things normal for as long as possible, plus I feel sure that I have read somewhere that the more active you are and the more positive, the speedier your recovery will be. It's my mind that is the biggest challenge: it doesn't always do my bidding. Getting out of my bedroom and out of the house helps to lift my spirits, and I am trying to keep them buoyant for the sake of the boys. Any socialising or party I can still manage will surely do me good. They certainly did, BC, and so, I tell myself, overlooking my increasing fatigue, self-consciousness and unsociable side effects, they should do so now.

That's why I find myself, a few days after the spaghetti challenge, standing in a marquee and holding a plate of curry at another fiftieth birthday party. Not able to eat the curry, I go into boarding-school mode and push the rice up on one side of the plate, and shore the prawns up against it. This reduces how much it looks as if I am leaving. But it's a steep bank, and the prawns keep tumbling down, willing me to eat them. Enough, I think, suddenly, insanely furious at these un-evolved bottom feeders taunting me. In one bold arm thrust, I chuck the plate, fork and all, past the awning and into the flower bed. Richard, my ally, as ever, does not so much as blink. Together we go into the adjoining room and join the throng of guests. I make myself chat to someone, or rather, I plant myself in front of a woman, kick-start conversation with a question, let her do the talking. Five minutes in, I am looking at her throat as she speaks and thinking about my own. Is it wise to be standing so close to her? I know the answer, leaving her mid-sentence to push my way past the punks and hippies (it's a fancy dress party) to the guest cloakroom. I know this house well and, on this occasion, have judged the distance with precision timing. I get my head down the loo just in time. Then we go home.

Bassy is already in bed. I lean across and give him a kiss. You smell of medicine, he says, moving his head away. Eau de Cancer: I had no idea I smelt of anything at all.

In the Lansdowne pub in Primrose Hill the next day, I am squaring up to a pizza. It is Fliff's fiftieth birthday and she is celebrating with half a dozen friends, all of us seated at a long wooden table. I watch them eat. Jaw, lips, cheeks, everything moves and then, as quickly, all is still again. The chewing happens somewhere along the way. Often, without even letting go of their fork, they prod or scoop, barely glancing at the food, and then they are off again. Gobble, gobble. What tongues they must have, and how much saliva. Saliva, the champagne of bodily fluids, the word no longer slumming it with football hooligans and old people, with spit, drool and dribble. I take my chance, see if I have enough of my own to swallow a morsel of pizza. I pick up a slice of Fliff's mushroom and taleggio pizza and nibble half a centimetre off the tip. The smidgeon of dough gets stuck on the roof of my mouth and my tongue refuses to curl or extend. I cover my mouth with my hand, stick my finger in, and hook out the unsoggy morsel, then swig some water. Attractive.

Vic is sitting diagonally opposite me. I know all about Vic. She had bone cancer and had to lie in a bubble in a sealed-off hospital room for six weeks at a time. Only members of her family were allowed to visit her, and they had to wear special clothing to protect her from germs. Early on she would meet Fliff between treatments for coffee, have a piece of cake, a drink. Chat. Be normal for a few days. And then she would go back into her hermetic chamber. I have made Fliff tell me about Vic and her visits to the café and her subsequent disappearances and her recovery again and again. And here she is now, laughing, chatting, eating, living, a live exhibit, a cancer survivor.

Seeing Vic makes me believe I'll get to the other side, too, and I am inspired by her recovery during the next few weeks. But then I hit an impasse. I turn up for radiotherapy, knowing that I have only two sessions to go after this, and the mask is lowered. It is tight on my red face, too harsh on my raw, blistering neck, the snapping inside my ears and the reverberations suddenly more than I can stand. The warning is sounded, the radiotherapy girls dash off to the control room and I think, don't go, and the machine takes me. A sob wells up, I feel a surge in my chest and my eyes welling, but I can't move my shoulders, they're caged by the mask. I have not said my thank you for my healing, try to, can't, can't breathe. My ribcage is raised and won't flatten. And then, suddenly, the machine stops. *Sorry, Genevieve, we'll need to start again.* It's the radio girls, speaking to me from the control room. It is the only time in twenty-eight sessions that this exemplary team has had to turn the machine off and come back and reposition me, so expert are they. Seconds later they are back in the room, and they're at me. The snaps crack, the mask goes up, my neck gasps. I'm not strapped down but I might as well be; there's no escaping. *We'll just get you in the right position.* There is the prodding and the nudging which usually I don't mind now I say get off me stop touching me keep your fingers to yourself and all the while my radio girls issue instructions to each other and they cross-check and use numbers and now I must interrupt. *So sorry, but I cannot do this. Not any more. I'm afraid you cannot put the mask on again. I can't go into the machine again. I just can't do it.* But it's too late – clingfilm is placed on my neck this time to protect it, the mask is going on. *We're OK now, Genevieve. Here we go.* And down the mask goes. I can't speak let alone shout. Snap snap. Snap snap. Snap snap. Snap snap. Snap snap. *Just a few minutes now.* Then the warning goes off again and out they go and in I go.

I open my eyes and see the blue white light through the mesh and I say sorry thank you heal me whatever get me out of here just hurry the fuck up. But of course the duration is fixed: time does not shift. Four minutes is four minutes, and for ever. And then it's over, and I feel small. I put my top on as fast as I can and leave the big blue tissue on the chair instead of giving it to the radiographer to put in her medical bin. I scuttle out, not even saying thank you, and my red face is redder from fear and the tears and the heaving shoulders.

Two days later, my treatment is complete and never to be repeated, even if it has failed. The head and neck can only take one bout of radiotherapy, and hooray for that. I say my goodbyes to the radiotherapy girls, not so much bounce in my voice now, talking not so easy, and I note that they are talking to me in quieter voices in return. I blanch, embarrassed that my reduced state should be so noticeable.

I should have bought them gifts. I don't know what the etiquette is for one's last day of radiotherapy. I've seen chocolates and cards on some of the reception desks. I've done soap, vouchers, and wine for teachers, but I've no idea what you give people who are trying to save your life. A box of Celebrations? Champagne?

In the end, I fall back on the offering of two humdrum words, never so heartfelt. Thank you, I whisper as they get ready to heal the next patient. Thank you.

18

DISGRACE

When I was thirteen Tamsin put down the telephone to my brother, who had called from New York, and cried, 'It's the last straw!' and this time, it was. Her sobs seeped under her bedroom door, across the landing and down the stairs. I opened my own bedroom door and her sobs were on me like leeches, sucking away my defiance. The air held its breath and so did I, that evening and in the angry weeks that followed until – poof! Tamsin was gone. She wasn't coming back.

Everything went AWOL after that. The cigar chair. Her wardrobe. The small tables for putting drinks on. Her tapestry zigzag cushions. Her wool. The unfinished tapestries. Paintings. Ornaments. Her double bed. Her bedroom chair. Her bedside table. The curtains. The chicken brick. The sofa and the armchairs in the living room went, too. It turned out they had been a grapevine loan. The TV went. A metal hospital bed, like the one I had in my first dormitory that night I peed in the bin at school, appeared in Tamsin's bedroom. It had a thin, pinstriped mattress.

The Fox orphans were officially in disgrace. It was my fault. Weeks earlier I had told my brother, in my excitement to be talking to him when he called long-distance, how horrible it was living with Tamsin. He was working in New York, between his Oxbridge exams and going up to Cambridge. I, the uncomplaining one, complained. It was thrilling, being listened to, feeling important. There was so much he did not know, this big brother with his questions, so grown-up-sounding, and attentive. Having been at boarding school himself, he never spent much time at Lewes Crescent during vacations. I have no idea where or how he spent his time. Even so, I was surprised at his reaction to my litany of grievances; this was my life. It was hardly news. But it was to him.

My brother wrote Tamsin a long letter from America and swore. Or perhaps that's not what happened. My brother wrote Tamsin a long letter from America when he was stoned, and said hateful things. Or, my brother wrote Tamsin a long letter from America, and asked if she might look out for his younger sisters, who he understood were unhappy. My brother wrote Tamsin a letter from America, and said things we shall never know. And then he followed up the letter with a phone call. It was in the phone call that he swore. 'Bloody something,' he said. Or perhaps he didn't. At the time I didn't know exactly what happened, and since then the facts have been passed around like Chinese Whispers, but I know what happened next. Three years after she moved in, Tamsin moved out in the half-term of the summer term, the furniture went with her and my brother was summoned back from New York. He was living in our Uncle George's downtown brownstone at the time, working on a local newspaper called the *Village Voice*. His punishment, for that is how it felt, was to be summoned back by our half-brother and to look after us. Look after. It's an approximate term. He was eighteen years old.

At the end of term, we returned to the virtually empty house, Tamsin's flight and our failings the dead albatross around our necks thereafter. The three of us spent the summer being grown-ups. My brother bought an orange Saab 96 V4. It was low-slung and curvy. It had seats in the boot and you could watch the oncoming traffic and wonder about the normal families coming at you or fold the seats down and load the very foreign car with groceries. One day my sister and I made shepherd's pie. We boiled the potatoes and mashed them with milk, then butter. We put the mince in a dish and laid out the mash across the top like a duvet. We brought the shepherd's pie out of the oven. I sank in the spoon, brought up the mixture. The mince was pink. You were supposed to cook the mince first. There were angry voices then. The sea air swirled in the empty house, pushing its weight around now that there was no adult and no furnishings to keep it out. Each morning, I pulled up a black metal upright dining chair and sat at the end of the glass dining table, both of which Mother had shipped over from America. I had a school reading list and I systematically worked my way through all thirty-two books, like a lawyer reading her briefs. I put the book in front of me on the otherwise empty table, and read it from beginning to end. When I got to the end I ticked it off the list and started on the next one.

When there were no books left on the reading list and still weeks to go before the autumn term began, I rode my bicycle up and down the seafront. There was something about that bicycle that wasn't right. It was mail order, for a start, and had arrived in a large flat rectangular cardboard box. I put the thing together myself, using the spanner that came with it. It was a dud, the Clothkit of bicycles, and I wished I had got a normal one from a shop. I wrote to my Uncle George in New York and told him about my new bike. George was a Trotskyite, which made him sound mysterious and important, and he had been married, until her death, to Aunt Connie, one of Father's three sisters. I always knew, and I suppose Mother must have been the first person to tell me, that during the McCarthy era of the early 1950s Father was blacklisted for various legal positions he applied for because George, also one of the founder members of America's Socialist Workers Party, was his brother-in-law. He was the perfect uncle. Packages from RadioShack, the American store that attended to every electronic leisure requirement, started arriving, following the announcement of the new bike. First, there was the indicator belt. The strip of white plastic had yellow arrows on the back, operated by corresponding buttons on the front. Instead of sticking your hand out and balancing at the same time, you just hit the indicator button. After that he sent a handlebar-mounted radio, red to match my bike, with a speaker and dials that faced inwards. To round off my mobile leisure zone, he sent me a drinks helmet. This comprised a holder for a can or a bottle in a mount just near my sticking-out left ear, which meant I could drink Coke while I cycled along the promenade. But by the time of this *Cement Garden* summer, the blankness and the baffling abandonment captured in the eponymous Ian McEwan novel that came out a year after our own bleak summer, I had grown out of my bike.

I resorted to my skateboard, which I could not ride. I would take it to the top of one of the hilly streets in Kemptown, stand on it and let it do its thing. Down the sidewalk it went, racing to the seafront, me wobbling on top of it. I jumped off before it hit the coast road, retrieved it from wherever it had continued on to, walked back up the hill, and did the whole thing all over again. I didn't do any jumps or twists. I couldn't do a darn thing with it on the flat. Going out with it filled me with ennui; I wasn't doing it right. I wasn't a proper teenager.

The girl who lived a few doors down was. She had surly legs that oozed over her living-room floor. She would never be seen dead on a skateboard or a sofa, even though there was one, and armchairs, too, in her living room. In our new and urgent bid to be like everybody else and have days marked by human connections, the necessity to be so hung in our air like yet another reproach. Socialising is what people did, what we should do. People functioned in units; families functioned as units. I could see that. I knew of the girl with the legs because of Tamsin. Perhaps there had been drinks with the parents, or something similar and awkward, such as tea by the fire with Tamsin's octagonal teacups with handles bent like a spider's legs. Somehow, the three of us knew the girl rode and so, reluctantly and only because one of us had come up with the idea and thought it might do the trick, that is to say, give us the sense that something normal was happening when it wasn't normal to knock on the door of an unfamiliar house and ask a child you did not know to do something with you, I knocked on the door. The girl answered and I said: do you want to go riding with me, up at the stables on the racecourse? When she did not answer immediately and her dark eyebrows moved closer together, I said: I'll pay – money the orphan's reach, the adult gesture in lieu of the adult. All right, she said. When?

After the ride, she asked me back to her house and that's when she sat on the floor so I had to as well and she rolled a joint and passed it to me and I thought, no, I don't like your raven hair, your cheekbones and your lambent skin, all so knowing and confident. You make me feel lonely.

I went home and my siblings were pleased, for all of us: I had pulled off an outing and a connection. I hid my failure and our empty house that reeked of abandonment swallowed me whole. Our half-sister came to stay, the only adult who did, and we knew it was not to look after us because she was not that sort of adult. She needed looking after herself. She arrived with thirty-two pork sausages in her handbag and eyes that looked lost and I thought, things must be bad for her if she is reduced to staying with us. She must have been sent; we were a purpose, again, a means of keeping my half-sister occupied. She slept in my brother's bedroom. He had gone somewhere. His bedroom was big and had dark brown cork tiles on the walls covered in posters and Polaroid photographs and badges. Some of the posters were layered on top of each other, their sides seeping out, which felt rebellious and cool. One evening, when the sun had packed up and there was more sea air than usual in the *Cement Garden* house, I walked past the open door and felt a whoosh of cold air. The light was off. In I went. My half-sister was sitting on a chair, spine like a ruler on parade.

'What are you doing?'

The window was wide open.

'I am piercing my ears, but I can't get the needle in.'

'Shall I turn on the light?'

I was afraid of her dark. Without waiting for her answer, I turned on the light. She opened her palm and the fat pearl stud was just lying there, its silver pinhead playing the innocent.

'Shall I shut the window?'

She put her finger to her earlobe.

'They used to be pierced. I thought I could push the pearl through.'

I saw the blood and looked at the blunt pinhead and felt frightened and repulsed and I thought, poor her, let loose with the orphans. We deserved each other, the broken, the lowest of the low.

Afterwards, my half-sister gone, my brother back again and the three of us alone, our voices flew at each other, swooped out of sight, came back for the kill, except mine, not so loud. Then one day, when voices weren't enough and hard objects flew through our cold air and not for the first time, there was ducking and dodging. I picked up the phone and dialled the first nine. Round went the dial, back it came, my index finger in the hole all the while, determined, and then all the way round again, and me sobbing *police! I need the police!* and the other voices my brother and sister saying *no, don't, they will take us away, they will give us to social services.* I put down the receiver at that, our voices all three of them hushed in the gloating air. From that moment, we were one, joined together then, baptised into the communion of orphans by our own fire, fire we had lit ourselves, and Mother, who had been alive and living less than a mile away, was a no-show at this, her children's second baptisms, our first by holy water, Mother and Father holding us at the font – and now this. I could not reach her and she did not come and oh, I wanted her then. It was as if we did not have a mother at all, and never had had one, for all it counted for now. She did not put out the fire. What on earth does a soul do all day, day in, day out? Does it only connect with fellow disembodied souls? Is that why the rest of us have to wait for death to be reunited?

Later that summer we went on holiday to Italy to stay with our half-brother and his second wife in a palazzo outside Florence. Before we went, I shopped for holiday clothes in Churchill Square and the Lanes and bought a new suitcase, a small taupe holdall with blue trimmings. My last holiday had been aboard the SS *Uganda* in the Easter holidays, before Tamsin left. It was a school trip and my sister and I both went, along with teems of children, the whole ship wriggling, all of us sleeping in bunks below deck, pipes everywhere and portholes for peering through and shouting *Land!* We ate pizza in Naples and bought evil-eye beads in Bodrum. Men in a market offered us a camel for our blonde friend Janie, or so we told our friends, and during a lecture one evening a boy I didn't like sat next to me and put his fingers between my legs and I squeezed his hand to trap it and kill it, I didn't say anything to him, just glared, and he didn't say anything either, the lustful little twelve-year-old.

In the disco on the ship we danced to 'Fernando' and 'Don't Go Breaking My Heart' and had snogging competitions. I did the timings on my Timex watch. Tongues weren't a must but if the lips separated, it was game over. A boy from Eastbourne College took me up on deck one night and he went to kiss me and I, fearing his tongue, said, look at the moon, which he did. Then he asked me to look at the moon with him the next night, and I said yes and the moon didn't get a look-in. When I got back to Lewes Crescent we wrote to each other by return and I kept his blue denim cap that smelt of him under my pillow, counting the days til we could meet up again, and we did, every Saturday afternoon in the Wimpy in Eastbourne. We sat opposite each other at the Formica table, drank milkshakes, and butterflies looped the loop inside me.

The leaves on the trees in the garden in the house outside Florence were pale and coated in icing sugar, the air smelt like burnt perfume, and the ground was dry. Our half-brother showed us how to make pasta sauce with garlic, olive oil and blood-red tomato paste you squeezed out of a long tube and into a solid black frying pan where it sat, a giant sandworm, until the heat came through and you squashed it with a wooden spoon. We cooked the pasta and we swam in the swimming pool and listened to the dryness and the heat. The three of us slept in the studio flat on the ground floor, where we were left to our own devices. There were two beds and a hammock. I, the smallest, got the hammock; the first night, and every night, it sucked me up like a Venus flytrap, the string wrapping itself around me and digging into my skin. Turning on my side was out of the question. On the third or fourth night, the three of us cooked more pasta and tried to make it *al dente* whilst still not entirely certain what that meant, and definitely not knowing how to spell it, just knowing that it was sophisticated and Italian. Then I got in the hammock. It was way too early for bed. As I hung there, between two pillars in the middle of that stone room, tears spouted, and wouldn't stop.

Mother used to kiss my eyes with her eyelashes. A butterfly kiss, she called it. Lean in, sweetheart. Closer. Be still, and then, eye socket to eye socket, noses touching, her breath so pure you didn't know there was any other kind. Breath of life not God's, my own mother's, all I needed then, and after. Love incarnate.

'Ready, darling?'

'Ready.' Then the brush of lashes locking, the body shiver.

Stop, my siblings said, stop crying, their voices insistent, perhaps afraid. What's the matter? Then new days came and off we went, sightseeing, the three of us, further afield this time, Florence's sights exhausted, the tension growing. We took the train to Siena and walked across that horrible shell-shaped piazza and our voices took flight again, bashing into each other, and then there was the pushing and shoving between us that had no malicious intent but was hurtful and hurt and was frightening, too. We ran out of money. We made a plan. We bought a big bag of soft Italian cakes for rations and nursed our hunger and got ourselves to Pisa to take the aeroplane back to England. The Tower leaned over us much more than I ever expected and we went inside it and up to the top and looked at the traffic. That evening we walked amongst the streets looking for a *pensione* we could afford; in and out of old houses we went, asking the price, realising we did not have enough money, walking away and after the last one, me thinking, I should go back, I should ask the old lady in black with the droopy, dimpled belly and the grey-wire hair if I could please use her bathroom, but I didn't have the gumption. We walked some more and our voices came out again, scratching, clawing. Needing somewhere to stay for the night, we climbed over the wire fence at Pisa airport, a high fence that ripped my trousers. It was hard getting over it and there was impatience; it felt like every man for himself, hurry up, and over on the other side we walked past the empty terminal building and across the tarmac and found a hangar looming in the dark. We lay down to sleep by big cement bags, my sister and I next to each other, my brother on the other side. I still had the upset stomach. I waited and waited until I thought my brother and sister were asleep and then I had to get up, and go, but where? I couldn't squat on the runway. Or I could, but it was dark, and I didn't fancy my bottom out there, in the Italian dark. Suddenly there was no time and I hurried to the other side of a sandbag and pulled down my trousers and even though nothing could have gone any faster, I willed it to in case someone came. Then I crept back to the other side of the sandbag.

At first light there was an apocalyptic roar and then lights. It was a plane, hurtling down the runway, brakes on, but coming straight for our hangar, and I thought, it's close. Then I saw men in overalls and uniforms, hurrying about, and I knew it was time to slip off to the terminal before they found me out. We were too slow. The men in uniforms came and got us. They were very cross. I was very relieved when they marched us back across the tarmac, me off the hook, my misdemeanour undetected. There were people in the airport now and men took our brother into a room and left us outside, sitting on plastic chairs. He came back out, phoned our half-brother, something must have been agreed with the police or the airport officials, and I wondered how the Fox orphans had messed everything up, again.

When we got back to England, we took out the orange car and went house-hunting. We were leaving Lewes Crescent and buying somewhere else, maybe in Brighton, maybe somewhere else in Sussex. We went to all sorts of places, like we did when Mother was looking for a new house with Richard Williams. We looked at a house in Peacehaven, a desolate post-war linear settlement with ticky-tacky houses and no signs of life. Our great-aunt and great-uncle had lived there. We used to visit them in their bungalow with Grandma, who didn't drive, so we took a taxi and it floated down the dead roads. It was hard to feel alive in Peacehaven, even then. Our great-aunt had a cosy husband with a concertina chin and a fondness for boiled sweets. He was always on the sofa in his slippers, sucking on the sweets shaped like rugby balls. Peacehaven was a halfway house, not really a place for unattached children. We looked at a terraced house on a hill near Brighton railway station next. A man, the owner, showed us around. He had a look on his long face that said: are you children for real, coming to look at my house like this, and I could see we were an odd proposition, but I did like his banister that curved like a woodlouse at the top and the bottom. We looked at another house in a boring part of Brighton that was nowhere near Churchill Square or the shops and could have been in Peacehaven and was nowhere near a bus stop or the sea either. And we looked at a house on Sussex Square, at the other end of Lewes Crescent, but that was too close to home, if you could call Lewes Crescent home. After that, the house-hunting in Sussex petered out. It was felt London would be a better option, and talk turned to us moving to the capital when the right place could be found for us.

When it came to the first exeat weekend of the autumn term, I invited my friend Louise to come and stay with me at Lewes Crescent because it was definitely my turn to invite her. I had stayed at her house so many times. She said yes, which didn't seem odd to me then, but it does now, how a mother would let her thirteen-year-old daughter stay in a house without adults. But things were different then. People made less of a fuss. Louise's mother, being Swedish, was perhaps more open-minded than many British mothers might be, and open-hearted too: she was always so welcoming and generous. Louise and I slept in Tamsin's old room. The hospital bed was in there, and there was a second bed now too, and the stars and the black night hung outside the curtainless windows. It was freezing cold. It rained and stormed. We shivered, both of us hit with a flu we didn't see coming. I thought, I shouldn't have brought her here. By day, we did our favourite things: Louis Tussaud's waxworks museum to see the man with the entrails being prodded with a hot poker and the ribby man in the creepy dark vault being stretched on a rack, a red light bulb behind him and a plastic rat on the floor, the pier, the tunnel down to the beach, and then we got the train back to school.

19

CAPITAL LIVING

Halfway through the autumn term, we moved to Little Venice. The garden flat had been advertised in the rental section of *The Times* and was 'north of the river', but nowhere near it. It formed the bottom of a fat, four-storey stucco house the colour of buttermilk that sat on a wide road with a canal – the Regent's Canal – running through it. Otherwise, the area wasn't particularly watery or Venetian. A tower block overlooked our back garden. Coloured barges called *Siberia* and *Mayflower* lined the canal, periscope chimneys sticking out of their roofs and geraniums in pots marking out their patch on the towpath. If you followed the canal from our house down to the bridge at the end of the road, it opened into a desolate basin, overlooked by tiered, low-rise apartment blocks that had once been modern and now looked fierce. If you took a right past the Puppet Theatre, which wasn't a theatre at all but another barge with a painted sign on it saying LITTLE VENICE PUPPET THEATRE, you went under another road, or bridge, and you could keep going, by barge at least, all the way to Birmingham. Alternatively, you could take a set of steps up to a small municipal garden and walk under the flyover to Paddington, one of the four railway stations on the Monopoly board and the one my sister used to get to her alternative, rules-free boarding school in Totnes, Devon where she was studying for A levels.

Back at the house, half a dozen broad stone steps led up to the main-event front door. To the right, six steep, narrow steps led down to our half-glass, half-wooden front door. The overhang from the main steps hid it from view and blanked out the daylight. My brother took the bedroom with the bay window to the left of the long hall. We left the bedroom to the right empty for the mystery woman who was coming to live with us in a few weeks' time and my sister and I took the biggest bedroom, next to the kitchen. It had French doors opening on to a small courtyard, off which a narrow opening led past the back of the kitchen and into the 100-foot garden that had a rope swing at the end of it like the one from the Pears' soap advert. There was a bathroom off our bedroom with no windows and when you switched on the light a whirr went up like a tractor on the home run.

My sister and I had gone back to Lewes Crescent earlier in the term to pack up our belongings. My brother organised the move. He got hold of lots of tea chests – high boxes made of thin, blond wood with no lids and metal around the rims – and we packed everything up in newspaper he had also got from somewhere and he said, do you want to keep this, do you want to keep that, and I threw away my Mrs Pepperpot books and kept *Jaws*, which had that sex scene in it, and the *Lord of the Rings* set my brother had bought me and my Superman duvet cover, and the teddy bear and knitted rabbit I still kept on my pillow.

We unpacked the tea chests, discarding the sheets of scrunched-up newspaper on the modish pine floorboards in the living room. There was a mantelpiece and a plug socket inside the hearth. We installed the fake fire with spindly silver legs we had brought with us from Lewes Crescent and arranged on the mantel the fox ornaments that had been part of Father's Vulpine Society collection. Mother, who must have packed them up herself when she left America, had done the same on the mantelpiece in Marine Gate. My favourites were the pair of dancing foxes, paws on each other's shoulders, bushy tails ahoy, and the smaller fox in coat-tails, playing the violin. There was a conductor, too, with his own music stand, and he held one paw aloft, a miniature baton keeping his musicians in time. There was a hunting cup in the shape of a fox's head, and, standing next to it, a tall, elegant vixen with cheeky eyes and a wide grin. The painting of a fox running through a wood that had hung above the mantelpiece in Marine Gate we put on the opposite wall, next to the abstract splodge print my brother had bought in Brighton post-Disgrace when we had needed a few things to put on the newly empty walls. Hanging the running fox was the finishing touch in the rehabilitation of the Vulpine Society which Father had founded and made official with a crest, imprinted on his signet ring and on a rubber stamp, bearing a fox's head and the Latin inscription *Cave Vulpem*, or Beware of the Fox. Little Venice was the Vulpine Society's new headquarters. To the mantelpiece we added a photograph of a young Granny Fox striding across a golf course in plus fours, African-American caddies walking on either side of her. My hold on my American heritage was already tenuous. This photograph added to the sense of unreality. It was hard enough to believe an era like this had ever existed, let alone that my family was part of it.

A large black and white photographic portrait of Granny Fox with Father and his three sisters, Genevieve, Cathleen and Constance (at the time of being propped on the mantelpiece: alive, dead, dead respectively) had a similar distancing effect.

The family poses against a studio backdrop of blurred trees. Granny Fox is seated in the middle, her hand angled a jot to the left, her dreamy eyes staring at the camera, her heart-shaped lips pouting. One fat pearl pops out from her short, wispy hair and there's a dark, dead animal around her neck, resting on her white blouse and a long string of pearls. Her left hand rests on top of Genevieve's, seated to her left, her right sits demurely on her lap. All three girls are solemn and bright-eyed and have their mother's classical lips. They are wearing ornate lace blouses under dark pinafores. Cathleen and Constance are standing behind their mother and Lyttleton, my father, is standing behind her right shoulder, sporting a tie and a belted and pleated woollen jacket and matching trousers – plus fours, presumably – with one hand sitting jauntily in a sizeable crisp bag of a pocket. His white starched collar is almost as wide as his face, which is soft and round and has a look of Bassy.

We didn't have many other photographs, even though I periodically stole one or two back from the photograph albums Mother had compiled and which my grandma and aunt kept for themselves. We did have one, a colour one, small, square, with curly white edges, that depicts a family scene as homely as anything from *The Waltons*, only with better-dressed children. Granny Fox is in the middle of this one too. She threw a Christmas party for her family and grandchildren every year and this photograph is taken the year before we left for England. She's older by now, of course, in her late eighties. Because Father was fifty-four when I was born, our first cousins were the same age as Mother and their children were our age. There are ten of us, sitting cross-legged in a row in front of a seated Granny Fox. She's got set, silver gelatin hair, red lips and high cheekbones still showing through her chalky face and we've got happy ones, all of us at ease, everything familiar, dressing up for Christmas and being lined up for a family photograph nothing out of the ordinary. The girls are wearing party dresses and white tights and black patent Mary Janes and the boys are looking round and smiling and are smartly turned out. My sister and I are wearing matching velvet dresses.

The vulpine artefacts constituted a sort of shrine to where we had come from, representing a past the three of us, in our own ways, tried to revisit and even resurrect. Foxes are bewitching creatures, but the vulpine mementoes made it harder for us to let go of a past that became increasingly mythologised as time went on. Nor did they help us find our place in the present.

When my sister and I had looked around the Little Venice flat with our half-brother, before we took on the lease, we chatted to the nice woman who was moving out. As we stood in the kitchen, she said we could buy her furniture if we wanted to – the wooden table, a church pew, three hard-backed dark brown dining chairs with tanned fake leather seating, and a pine dresser – and we did. The pew was exotic and thrillingly, blasphemously out of place, the dresser was homely, and therefore also out of place. We bought her old brown hessian curtains that hung over the French doors in the living room, her hall mirror, a pine chest of drawers with amber handles, and a low double bed with a stained mattress that rested on coiled springs within a square wooden frame. I wondered what this woman with the long blonde braids thought of us, buying the furniture she and her family no longer wanted. I thought: it is a wonder what adults will buy and sell.

We supplemented this job lot with a few purchases of our own, including a shocking pink silk two-seater sofa. Everything else – the pair of chinoiserie lamp bases with their white silk shades, the calico three-seater sofa covered in acorns, the console table in the hall – aped an English country house

aesthetic. We had a lot of books – our own, and Father's – and
agreed we needed bookshelves, with deeper shelves at the
bottom for the turntable and the amp and all our records. We
arranged for someone to come and build them. All three of us
were governed, in our own ways, by a desire to do things in
the way they were supposed to be done. We took playing house
very seriously.

And then the woman our half-brother found to live with us
unravelled all of that. Danielle, his inspired choice, was small,
passionate, full of zest and, almost best of all, half-French, half-
Spanish – an outsider, in other words, a fearless foreigner who
followed her instincts and had no knowledge of British mores.
She had short black hair, wore thick blue eyeshadow and she
had verve and passion. She felt much older than us but much,
much younger than Tamsin. She lived in Paris but had grown
up in Madrid and was coming to London to study Fine Art at
Christie's for a year. She too had been found on the grapevine,
but of a very different sort: a north London social network,
one branch of which was connected to a bohemian sub-network
which had at its epicentre a formidable and, we would
later discover, legendary half-Russian, half-German former
Communist, wartime resistance fighter and Chelsea restaurateur
called Elisabeth Furse. By the time the orphan Foxes came into
her orbit, Mrs Furse, as we always called her, had long made
it her business to do things for people, especially younger
generations. She knew of us and she knew of Danielle, and the
match was made. Danielle arrived just in the nick of time. We
were in the throes of a domestic drama hinging on interior
decoration. A trip to the Sanderson headquarters near Oxford
Circus had been lively. Rattled by the fear that we might not
do the right thing and that our choices might not meet with
approval – albeit of absent, unspecified forces – my brother,
sister and I yelled and cried our way through the two floors of
fabric swatches, paints and wallpaper displayed on banners

befitting a medieval jousting arena. Divided, we left with no
decisions made. In due course, my sister and I settled on Laura
Ashley, a safe bet. We already wore their smock dresses, and
chose a fawn and terracotta acorn print for our bedroom walls,
and matching curtains. For our bathroom, we chose a green
and white leaf motif because it was similar to one in a country
house we often visited. That still left the hall bathroom with
no wallpaper. Danielle joined in the debate, and back we all
went to Sanderson together. She suggested a William Morris
print for this bathroom, which she was sharing with my brother,
and we all agreed. My brother chose blood red for his bedroom.
Even the ceilings. To me, it was an unusual, and therefore
alarming, choice. Danielle simply found it amusing. She made
doing up the flat fun. She made everything fun. She cooked
chicken, but not in a brick. First, she whisked my sister and
me off to Church Street market to buy the chicken along with
the vegetables to go with it. It was an outing. When we got
back to the flat, she showed us how to roast it with garlic,
rosemary and lemon.

A few years ago, reminiscing with Danielle in New York –
where she has lived and worked as a gallerist and curator for
many years – she revealed two things: that she was twenty-six
when she came to live with us, so hardly ancient, and that she
had never cooked a chicken before. I was learning too, she
laughed. She had angel's wings, and under them we went. She
took my sister and me to Paris to stay in her tiny flat near Gare
du Nord and when I asked where the shower was she took me
into the kitchen, produced a square plastic tray, put it on the
kitchen floor and pointed to a shower head coming out of the
ceiling and the sheet of plastic you could pull round on a runner
to shield you. She took us to the movies, only letting us watch
French films, and to art galleries, too. When we changed Metro
stations at Place d'Italie she always stopped and gave money to
the beggar with no legs who played an accordion and tapped

her feet and jigged her shoulders. She inhabited the moment, she connected and was so quick to laugh and loved to talk, even to the formidable Mrs Furse who lived in a dark basement in Belgravia and fired questions at my sister and me as if we were target practice. Danielle fielded the worst of them, batting them off with an easy comment, in the process opening our eyes to the harmlessness of our interlocutor. Mrs Furse could make me feel inadequate, grown-up and worth bothering with in a single dragon's breath. Danielle was our firefighter; she had our backs.

One day she found a pigeon with a broken leg in the garden so she brought it into the kitchen and made it a bed. During its recuperation it strutted across the wooden floor and shat everywhere. Once it had recovered, she released it into the neglected garden, so it could do the same out there. Danielle was there when we went home for exeat weekends and she was always pleased to see us, seemed to look forward to seeing us, and wanted to know all our news from school. And she was there as dynamics shifted once again between the three of us. Tensions intensified, emotional distances grew. Our shared loss made itself manifest in unique ways, and each of these marked us out as the outsiders we did not want to be. We covered a range of tendencies between us: social awkwardness, an excess of independence, an excess of vulnerability, a bent towards brittleness, depression, eccentricity.

Danielle was the buffer between the *Cement Garden* summer and the desolation that set in for good after her tenure ended and she moved out. But she was there to see my sister and me off to Victoria station, where we camped out all night to be the first in the queue to buy tickets on the pioneering 'no frills', low-cost airline Laker Airways to New York. Eight years after leaving, we were going back to America. My half-brother had arranged the trip, writing to relatives and making all the arrangements. The drawbridge was down.

We made makeshift camp beds on the pavement in front of the Laker Airways kiosk using cushions our half-brother had pulled off his sofa for us. The kiosk was opposite the bus terminus at Victoria station. The police erected a pen around us and all the other Laker hopefuls, using metal barriers. When the tickets went on sale in the morning, they pulled the barriers back and out we all spilled, running with our suitcases and our bags to get the one-way tickets. They were £45 each.

20

AMERICA REVISITED

The British nuns may have slapped the Americanisms out of me, but I loved America from the moment I was back. I showed the man at the airport my new passport, the photograph inside just of me now, no Mother with bouffant hair and me and my sister positioned around her any more. He looked at me, then back at the passport and said, have a great stay, and I did. Time of my life more like, life-changing.

Cousin Jim was waiting for us at JFK, the first in a line-up of hosts signed up by our half-brother to the Orphaned Cousins Exchange Programme. Jim drove us in his VW van from the City to the expanse of blue sky that sat above his Long Island summer house like a Welcome banner. What a wonder it all was: the sky and the hot air and Jim, my first cousin, old enough to be my father. James, his son – Sweet Coz as he became known to me, and I to him, it just happening to be that we both loved *As You Like It* – is exactly my age, and his daughter, Catherine, only a few years older. Jim's wife, Biche, was a revelation, her attentiveness felt day after day, and each day with these friendly strangers even easier than the one before. Mornings kicked off with home-made pancakes small and round like coasters, followed by sailing in a boat that was barely a boat at all, more like a slab of white plastic with a sail in it. The dinghy sometimes jived and sometimes sulked, depending. Jim with his strip of white sunblock on his nose shouting 'Ready about' and us shouting 'Ready' as he taught us to do our first time out with him. Me being whacked on the head by the boom all the same and not minding one bit, though it hurt like hell. It was fishing for snapper with nothing but a thin pole for a rod and jumping off the dock and Sweet Coz saying, just lie on your back, see, the current will carry you, and landing on the small horseshoe beach, dodging the poison ivy that was waiting to turn you into something bumpy and hot, and doing the whole thing over the next day. There were excursions, for Baskin Robbins ice cream in a store that sold nothing else, for giant pizza we ate straight from the cardboard box sitting right there in the restaurant, and for clamming on Fire Island. There was no fire when we got there, just a long sandy beach, the water warm, no need to count to ten like we did at the sea in Brighton and Eastbourne. In we went together, all of us in a row, just up to our calves. We dug our heels into the sand and felt for the ridge of the shells. Sweet Coz made a fire right there on the beach and I said, I can't eat the clams, I'm allergic to shellfish but not even trying to conjure up Mother like a genie from a bottle, no need of her just then. It was tuna fish sandwiches and iced tea on the deck and in the evenings sitting around the table, all of us together, talking about our day, and so much laughter.

When the visit came to an end and we stood on the sandy driveway, it was hard to say goodbye.

Jim handed us over to Uncle George. It turned out that his brownstone on the Lower East Side, the one my brother was staying in before he was hauled back for the *Cement Garden* summer, was round the corner from RadioShack. I couldn't believe my luck, to be near that great store, and to meet George, with his whiskery beard that tickled when we kissed each other on the cheek and his plump lips pursed into a perpetual smile. He produced an inflatable canoe from the roof of his car and set it on the shore of a lake in the White Mountains, though how we got up north in the first place I don't know. We set off for the lake from the big old house in Concord, New Hampshire that was home to his second wife, Muriel, who sometimes wore her long grey hair done up like a Danish pastry. Here, take a paddle, he said, there's one each, and we did, the three of us on the water, everything effortless, George's belly sticking out like a crescent moon in broad daylight.

Biche was thoughtful and now here was Muriel, more of the same, though quieter, and she was ready with pitchers of home-made lemonade and let's-see-what-can-we-do-to-make-this-stay-sing. Her million-year-old father had invented a board game, a variation on Checkers he called Geese and Ducks and he taught us how to play it. His gentleness was something you could wrap around yourself. We sat with him in his conservatory in the old house on the wide street and he watched while we played. The house held back, and so did Muriel, but only when it came to words, and it was hushed, as if closed up for the summer, dust sheets out, blinds drawn. And it smelt of something, the old days and ways, perhaps. We had supper in the dining room at five o'clock, so early my sister and I collapsed with giggles in the upright chairs, being served something called meat loaf, and Muriel slicing it as if readying it for the toaster just about finishing us off.

There was no hokey meat loaf with Uncle Chauncey, whom we stayed with next, and supper was dinner and served at seven. Chauncey wasn't our uncle but Father's best friend and our brother's godfather. To get up to his country estate, we took a train from Grand Central Station to Amenia, which is in

Dutchess County in upstate New York. The carriage was way up on giant wheels and it had steep metal steps going up and a door at the back of it that led out on to a viewing platform. There we stood, only a railing keeping us from tracks which cut through countryside not much different to English countryside, everywhere we had been giving way to the next unknown newness that lay ahead.

When we climbed down off the high train a man in a blue suit was waiting by a blue Mercedes saloon. This was Eddie, Chauncey's butler. We knew all about him from Mother, and from our brother, who had been back to America and stayed with Chauncey many times and we knew that they were inseparable. Eddie was angular, neat and quietly spoken. He was also Polish and Catholic and when he and Chauncey went to Mass in the local town, they sat together in the family pew. Chauncey was also impeccably turned out, and he had pizzazz. I'd seen him in photographs, smiling away in a three-piece suit and a boater by his front door and, in another, at the reins of a horse and carriage, a whip in his hand like a shepherd's crook. He and the lady sitting alongside him had checked blankets across their knees. Mother had told me that the lady was a princess from Portugal's deposed royalty and that she was my godmother. She was poor and never sent me any cheques or invitations to the castle in which I presumed her to live, and then she died. When we got to the house that was supposed to be a farm, there was Chauncey, standing on his stoop, frozen in celluloid in his signature three-piece, his hands clasped in front of him. His house was called Wethersfield Farm but we hadn't seen so much as a cow, let alone a gated yard with rolls of hay piled high and a rusting car by a manure-filled cowshed. The estate sat amidst lazy hills and on the way up to the main house we passed a building painted red and white with an arch and a clock tower and horses' heads peering over stable doors. Chauncey walked down the flagstone path to greet us, then we followed him into the marble-floored hall and a man appeared from nowhere. Chauncey said to him, the Fox girls are in the goldfish room, won't you show them up. And up a sweeping staircase we went and there were goldfish all over the walls. The man put the hard blue Globe-Trotter suitcase our half-brother had bought specially for the trip on one of those stools with straps we'd seen in English country houses. We went downstairs and when we went back up to change for dinner, the suitcase was empty and the chest of drawers was full.

At dinner Chauncey sat me to his left and my sister to his right. We kept those places around the walnut table for the rest of our visit. When we had finished a course Chauncey would either pick up the gold bell beside him and ring it or slip his hand under the table and ring the hidden bell instead. Then Eddie, or another man, called Francesco, would appear through the green baize door and take away the plates. There was a porthole in the door. Whoever was serving would look through it first, then float in with the next course. Francesco never seemed sure about timings. He spent longer and longer looking through the porthole, sometimes not even bringing in any food, just staring. I began to wish I could swap places with my sister.

The days had a routine; timings were precise. Breakfast, served at 8.30 a.m., was always the same: farm fresh melon, the orange flesh sliced away from the bright green rind, chopped into bitesize pieces and put back into position. A tiny glass of freshly squeezed orange juice, served at stomach-turning room temperature. Scrambled eggs, runnier than the ones in the Sussex house. Warm bread rolls. Butter in individual silver pots. Strawberry jam in a glass bowl. Halfway through the visit Chauncey announced breakfast wasn't working out. We were always late coming down. From now on, it would be served in our bedroom. At 10 a.m. each morning Chauncey and I rode.

On the morning of our first ride, I went out to the driveway to meet him, as instructed. Four horses and two grooms in jackets and riding hats – sadly not a Stetson between them – were already in position. I was hoping for cowboys. My charger was as spectacular and poised as any that Stubbs glorified. It held its head high, too high; it was preposterously tall. When I bent my knee and stretched my foot up to reach the stirrup, I very nearly did a back flip. Take her to the mounting block, Chauncey said over his shoulder, which sounded a bit medieval. The block was a cube with three steps carved into one side. One of the grooms led my horse parallel to it. I nipped up the steps, the well-brought-up horse stood stone still, I swung one leg over the English saddle and I was on top of the world. Chauncey, then aged sixty-nine, led the ride. He didn't wear a hat, and he rode fast. His horses were thoroughbreds and hunters, not the riding-school refuseniks I was used to, and we cantered much more than we walked or trotted. The moment we hit the open spaces of his estate, the Berkshires and the Catskills all around us, we galloped abreast. Chauncey's long legs lolled about in his stirrups and my feet came out of mine. I slid in the slippery saddle as my horse-god flew, the double-reins spaghetti in my hands. I clung to the horse's mane and whooped inside.

Instead of finishing the ride at the stables, we rode past it and up the long drive all the way to the house. I thought the horses were coming in for lunch. But we dismounted, the sensation of my feet hitting the ground a long time coming, and then the grooms led the horses away. I wanted to go with them and help out. But that was not the done thing, no catching me out there. So I went inside, got changed and spent the rest of the morning in the demure swimming pool that looked like a pond. It was a large oval with lawn growing right up to its edges. Frogs lived on the inner edge and rode the waves my tentative strokes made. This was not a pool for splashing. Sculptured horse heads positioned either side of broad steps kept watch over it. The neat lawns and yew trees fashioned into lollipop heads and candy cones kept order, and every vista trained the eye to a view of rolling hills.

I don't know what I was expecting from that first trip back to America. But I liked the sweetness of the just-picked corn and the mentions of Mother or Father, softer than first rain. They had lived in a cottage on the Wethersfield estate at some point before I was born. I wish, even now, that I had asked to see it. I have a photograph of Mother sticking her head out of a car window, one elbow resting on the door, behind her a white picket fence and a clapboard house. That's the one they stayed in. Mother used to talk about Chauncey, and spoke fondly of his two daughters, who were her age. They each came to lunch during my first visit back and I was riveted to be in their company. Nonsensically I thought, would Mother be like each of you, is this how she would be? Would she be quiet, or would she be talkative? It was her voice I wanted to hear; for years and years I listened out for it. I think the voice of someone you love and who loves you back is a tender touch. The local schoolteacher came to lunch on another day, and so did a young priest. He was a house guest, and he stayed for three days.

We always took lunch on a terrace under some vines. The table was laden with cutlery, even scissors for cutting the home-grown grapes. Once, a guest ripped a few off with his fingers and I thought, oh dear, there are special grape scissors for that, didn't you know? I had seen someone using a pair at the chateau in France our half-brother had taken us to for a holiday soon after Mother died. That house even had scissors whose blades were forged into hoops; you put one hoop over the top of a soft boiled egg and squeezed the other to meet it, and off came the egg's head.

After lunch, Chauncey napped and my sister and I swam. Then, at 4 p.m. and not a minute later we stood in front of the house that was covered in ivy and joined Chauncey, who was starting to cover us in his own kind of old-fashioned love. Not love. Affection, perhaps. Whatever it was he was putting our way, I lapped it up. Within seconds there was the pounding of hooves on gravel, two horses' heads appearing first, then both grooms at the reins of a carriage. Chauncey always took the reins and off we went through twenty miles of trails that wove through his 1,200-acre estate, dust flying against the gleaming wheels, the horses so lively, the smell of them like musky pine in the sweet, wooded air, the happiness making me feel I was on to something. Sometimes we went for an afternoon walk instead of going out for a drive in one of the two dozen nineteenth-century carriages housed down at the stables. Chauncey called these afternoon walks his constitutional, and he had an outfit for walking, too, which he finished off with a cane. We fed the peacocks that strolled about the gardens like Elizabethan courtiers, Chauncey calling to his treasures in his high-pitched peacock voice that belied a tenderness that surprised. Then we would leave the formal gardens for the Wilderness. The carriage trails marked its circumference. Inside this magical woodland a path awaited and it was covered with a hint of grass so that, each time, you felt you were the first to walk on its downy spine. In we went, and there were statues of classical figures like the ones on the carriage trails, but these took their place amongst the trees, discreet. Some not discreet enough, the naked man with his penis hanging down and a gown on his arm making it hard to know where to look.

In the quiet between the return from the afternoon carriage drive or constitutional and evening drinks at six, I sometimes got a poetry book from the panelled library, pulled down the flap of the prim desk in the drawing room, and read. I would spend hours like that, lost in whatever new world the poem offered but also in the expansiveness of Wethersfield. Even when indoors, you could feel the rolling greenness outside, the cushioning air. Time tiptoed. If my boys found themselves in a similar situation now, filling the hours like the Brontë sisters, they would suffocate from boredom or, in what was a pre-computer age, play hunt-the-television. There wasn't one.

I can't see how any child would feel comfortable going to Mass in the Wethersfield chapel. It was a room off the hall, just a crucifix on the wall and a thing you could kneel on, not enough otherness about it to set you off into suspended disbelief. We went on our first Sunday, perching on upright chairs, arranged in a row, no pews to hide in. Mother and Father might have sat on them, but that was no help now. The priest, the one who was staying for a few days, stood a metre in front of me, all done up in his priest robes. On went the Mass, all the usual words, and then, in his low, holy voice, from nowhere came a question, addressed to us, the mini congregation: who amongst us would like to offer up a prayer? I squirmed in the silence. Yes please, I'd like to say a prayer for my dead mother and my dead father in heaven. That's what was expected. That's what I should have said. Instead I rode the silence out, singed by my own sinful silence. The priest got Holy Communion going next, and there was no getting out of that one, not in this small room. I didn't want to go near him but I didn't want Chauncey to disapprove of me either. Suddenly I was up and stepping forward, my shoulders shaking with nervous, stifled giggles. Out went my tongue to receive the nasty little wafer that sticks like a suction cup to the roof of your mouth, the intimacy mortifying, the obligatory meeting of eyes as you say 'Amen' lasting for ever.

That afternoon, with everyone retired behind closed doors, I met the priest on the staircase. I was coming down from my bedroom; he was going up. The whole house was still. He reached out and took my hands.

'You know something, Genevieve?' He cupped his hot hands around mine.

'What?'

'I really like you.'

The stair beneath me needed to disappear, and me with it. But it didn't, so I held his gaze, smiled, withdrew my hands, got down the stairs and walked, very slowly, down the hall to the Flower Room, where the vases were kept and all the floral arrangements prepared. It led on to the terrace. Once outside, I ran.

After dinner we sometimes took tea in the Gloriette, a sort of gallery-cum-Sistine Chapel manqué. It had wild frescoes on the walls and when Chauncey said they were by Annigoni, we made ooh noises. We knew the artist's name by then as he was one of Chauncey's favourites. Chauncey's head was on a plinth in the middle of the stony room and Cupid was in a fountain at the far end. We sat around a small, low table on gilded chairs. The first time Eddie asked me what *digestif* I would like, a fortuitous bout of shyness prevented me from replying, a chocolate one, please. Chauncey stepped in and suggested we all have peppermint tea. We sat and chatted, Chauncey gracious, our company never seeming to bore or vex him.

On another evening we went to the drawing room after dinner instead and Chauncey asked my sister to play something on the grand piano. It sat, black, shiny, imperious, amidst the wooden panels, unfurling blue sofas and gold in unexpected places. She declined. What about poetry? he asked. We seemed to be playing a parlour game in which you rewind the clock a couple of centuries and see what you come up with for entertainment.

Sensing, with alarm, that we were in danger of failing to rise to the occasion, I made willing noises. I may have had no musical accomplishments – I played the triangle in the school orchestra – but I could read aloud, entered competitions for it. All you had to do was stand on the edge of a bare stage, three judges lined up in the front row of an empty auditorium, and read out a few paragraphs, smiling or frowning and looking up whenever you could. Easy. Perhaps 'Kubla Khan', Chauncey said, passing me a cross old hardback with four ridges placed in intervals on its curved spine. I'd never seen the poem before, never even heard of it. I got off to a bad start with 'Xanadu', sounding the X as in X-ray. Chauncey and my sister stiffened, I lost my nerve, stumbled, stuttered through the rest of the poem in a monotone.

I've thought this opium-induced fantasia overrated ever since, overlooking the fact that the humiliation it occasioned is what turned me against the poem rather than its content. I've also thought about Chauncey's love of ritual, how nerve-racking it felt, but how, when you knew what to expect, how reassuring and pleasurable it was. Chauncey immersed us in his rarefied world as if he expected nothing less of us than to fit right in. And I did, 'Kubla Khan' and the fact that I kissed Eddie goodbye when we left notwithstanding. I was a fast learner, and Wethersfield honed the chameleon-like social adaptability that is another orphan hallmark. Or so I erroneously believed. Chameleons don't change colour to blend into alien environments. They make sure they are never in them in the first place, putting themselves in environments where they blend in. The veiled chameleon is green and lives in trees, the dusty grey and brown Namaqua chameleon lives in the desert, and so on. Chameleons only change colour to send out a message, such as sexual readiness, or impending danger. The difference between orphans and chameleons is that a chameleon's survival skills are innate; it never even meets its parents. Chameleons, unlike human orphans, are born survivors.

We only put one foot wrong during that first Wethersfield trip. We referred to our stay with Uncle George. Chauncey was a cat with his hackles up at the very mention of him. Chauncey Stillman was a Catholic with three papal blessings under his belt, and the grandson of the founder of Citibank. Like his forebears, he was good with money and he gave a good deal of it away, through philanthropic channels. George Weissman was a Jew and, as a Marxist, more taken up with redistributing money than with making it. Chauncey had the Wethersfield Estate. George had Trotsky's literary estate, which had been left to him and of which he was the executor. So, they had nothing in common, except our father (mine, not the divine) and the belief that we are all created equal. Which they came at in different ways. Forewarned, in later visits we defused any potential Chauncey–George clash through a cocktail of precision planning and subterfuge. If, for instance, we were going to stay with George straight from Wethersfield and we hadn't been able to wriggle out of Eddie driving us into the City, my sister would get him to drop us at Cousin Jim's on the Upper West Side. Eddie and the doorman would help us with our bags, a tense moment as the doorman was not expecting us and we would have to stall his enquiries, making sure he did not buzz up to Cousin Jim to announce our arrival. Once Eddie had driven off, we would tell the doorman we had changed our plans, grab our suitcases and take a yellow cab down to George's brownstone on East 17th Street.

Until that first summer back, my knowledge of internecine animosities was limited to Grandma referring to Protestants as Prodidogs. As for Jews and socialists, I had never met any – until George. I couldn't see what all the fuss was about, blacklistings notwithstanding. George was a humdinger of a man.

We went to stay with my godfather Freddie next on Long Island Sound. His wife collected us from somewhere, the train station probably, and she pressed a button from her car seat and the garage door opened and I said 'Wow!' Later my sister said I shouldn't do that; it showed I wasn't used to it. Well, I wasn't. To this day I find my ready enthusiasm regrettable. It is akin to what my brother calls an orphan's gratitude. I've never successfully suppressed that either. My godfather was Father's first cousin and another Catholic of Jesuit persuasion. They had been close. He sent me cartoons he had drawn, and cheques for Christmas and my birthday, too. I had been looking forward to meeting him, fancied we might strike up a relationship. He made an appearance on the first evening, frail, unable to speak, none of the stories I was hoping for about Father forthcoming. He was dead within a year of the visit, which made me feel cheated. Adults had no staying power.

Back in the City my sister and I shopped for homewares. My godfather's New York apartment was on Park Avenue, Chauncey's was too and we had already stayed in that, so we knew where to shop. If you took a right once you had said good morning to the liveried doorman you pretty much walked into the Helmsley Building, after which we would make for Bloomingdale's and Barneys and the stores on Madison back on the Upper East Side. We bought white guest towels embroidered with WELCOME and napkins with ivy on and anything else that would lend our home adult touches. We did the sights, too, and these included a ghoulish visit to St Patrick's Cathedral. Mother and Father had got married there. Not married. Blessed, as I found out later. Catholic divorcees couldn't remarry in a church, which explained the photograph of Mother and Father on the cathedral steps on their wedding day. She's in a day dress with one of those hats perching on the side of her head like a cabbage leaf; no white dress and veil.

The cathedral was less a trip down memory lane, more a back alley with a dead end. I wasn't reliving memories, I was constructing them using fragments, photographs and hearsay, affording myself a Saturday matinee glimpse of what our lives might have looked like had Father not dropped dead following a heart attack and we had stayed in America. What might have been is another way of describing loss. It is what, in different ways and to different degrees, my brother, sister and I have been defined by all our lives. What might have been is a curse, or can be, if you fall under its spell. It is a trap, like nostalgia. But it can help you keep going, too. That first trip back, seeing how well our lives had started off and how full of connections it had been, was a shot in the arm: an orphans' reprieve, a taste of belonging.

There is a black and white photograph on my American moodboard of Chauncey and me sitting in the Gloriette, having cocktails. There's a neo-baroque Annigoni fresco behind me and, just visible in the left of the frame, the edge of an Old Master painting behind Chauncey. On the table in front of us are two bottles of champagne and a bowl of camellias. I am sixteen by now. Chauncey is dapper in white suit and tie, I'm in a high-necked blouse with sleeves as puffy as the halberdier in the Old Master painting, later sold to the Getty Museum for $35 million. It's not the ubiquity of priceless artworks that holds the secret to the magic of those Wethersfield visits; most of the artworks felt odd or boring. It's the fresh camellias floating in the silver bowl. Every evening, before dinner, Chauncey would cut two stems, one for me, one for my sister, lowering his head into their rose-like petals, burying his nose deep. He would inhale, look up, and smile, and then he would present each of us with a flower. Petals are soft, but these petals had a softness you would never expect from looking at them; it was a wonder how they kept their curve. And then there was Chauncey's gesture, the delicacy of it. I was enchanted. I can step right back into the feeling, can remember the ease of inhabiting it, and how it was over in an instant.

Happiness isn't a one-off, it isn't contained in a single moment, though we experience the sensation of happiness time and again. It is a feeling, and the feeling of happiness must accrue, if it is to provide ballast. It will be embedded in memories, and these will accrue also, and alter over time. Happiness is learned, it seems to me, and is cumulative. It is also in one's own gift; one can choose it; it is not only conferred. But it helps if it is expected; to be able to default to a state of happiness is a question of entitlement and habit, as is love.

I see with my own children how emotionally entitled they are; what love does for them, what it gives them, how they expect it. They default to a state of happiness whose roots reach deep, down into the constancy of love. There is no question of where the love came from, or if it will end. The question simply does not come up.

Of all the experiences during my first trip back, Wethersfield gets the gong for having the most dreamlike qualities, outstripping any in Coleridge's 'Kubla Khan'. But they were all surreal, in their own ways. None had any context to speak of, and I took each at face value, which is the child's way.

That included learning to shake lime daiquiris with cousins in Darien, Connecticut. They had a sunken caviar pit in their living room, seven children, televisions in every bathroom and a driver who deposited my sister and me into the city for a show and then picked us up and deposited us at an upscale steak house for dinner, then drove us back up to Connecticut again. One day we flew in a plane with ten seats to an island called Nantucket. Some of the children were teenagers or at college and everybody talked and made plans, the energy of their gilded, go-getting lives electrifying. Into these lives we swooped, and then off we went to LA and Cousin Dorothea, sister of Jim. She had a crisp white house and a kidney-shaped swimming pool beneath a bright sky. It was a pool for splashing in, and this time we were overlooked by HOLLYWOOD spelt out in giant letters on the hill opposite. It was like stepping into a David Hockney painting. Cousin Tim lived nearby and he was a professor of Latin American studies and was quietly spoken. But when he and his late-teenage children reached for their guitars and played their South American music and sang and caught each other's eyes, there was an instant fiesta. Every family we met was entirely different to the one before; it was something, trying to join the dots. My sister and I took walks in the Hollywood Hills and one day a man drew up in a convertible Cadillac and asked us to jump in and we felt like we were in a movie.

We flew from LA to New York and then back to London. Uncle George took us to the airport in a cab. He sat in the front, which passengers don't usually do in yellow cabs, and chatted to the driver. It was very early in the morning and George asked the driver to pull up at Dunkin' Donuts. He got out and bought a big bag of donuts, which he offered around, first to the driver, then to us. I didn't even know adults ate donuts. But what really struck me was how George treated the taxi driver as though he was part of our unit when our unit was the three of us. The taxi driver was, well, he was the taxi driver. It was a respectful way for George to behave, an egalitarian one, and it stuck with me. I've often replayed that scene. As with happiness, behaviour is learned. Children copy adults. They watch, and they learn, and it's usually their parents that lay down the templates for living. I see that now. It took the threat of being lost to the boys and rumination on what makes a family something to cling to before I worked out the personal significance of George's comradely behaviour.

I went back to America every summer for the next four or five years, and pretty often after that. The visits provided me with a handy narrative that I have called upon ever since.

Before, if an adult said: 'Is your mother collecting you today?' I would have to reply, 'Er, no, she isn't.' Then the adult would ask another question, such as: 'Oh, why not? Is she away?' Well, they asked for it: 'Because she's dead,' I would reply, though only occasionally. Usually, I put my interlocutor at ease by adding something disingenuous and reassuring like, 'Both my parents are dead, but I have lots of brothers and sisters.' After the first American trip, I was able to say, 'My parents are dead but I've got lots of family in America.' The responses suggested a cohesive family network; they took away the sting of orphanhood. I particularly liked using the American family line to friends. It made me sound not only normal by virtue of having family to speak of, but glamorous too. I left out the fact that we had parachuted into the lives of near strangers and that, understandably, not all the connections held. The people we foisted ourselves on both during that first trip and in the ensuing years were doing us a good turn, a favour. The Orphaned Cousins Exchange Programme was a one-off, not a lifelong commitment. I actually did rather well out of that first visit: four adults became key figures in my life, and their fondness has been a life raft. Which isn't to say the water wasn't sometimes a little chilly.

Another occupational orphan hazard is the propensity to latch on to anyone who takes an interest in you. There is an inbuilt imbalance; the orphan wants more than is on offer, takes a mile when given an inch. It's a problem of containment, I see that now too. Parental love is a citadel: its walls protect a place of safety and of abundance. The impulse to peer over the walls and look for more on the other side is not felt; there is no need to look for more because the child has everything he or she needs. But when there are no walls, and only an expanse, the child keeps looking, near at hand and into the distance. She moves on, and she keeps looking, and when she finds a bit of what she is looking for, she takes it. Grabs it, even. Think of the camellia. And of the chameleon, and its darting tongue that, in a flash, can extend the length of its body, twice the length of it in some species, to catch its prey. Back comes the prey, down goes dinner. And then the chameleon wants more. The child wants more, and on she goes.

During the first few years of going back to America, my sister and I unearthed more unsuspecting distant relatives; complete strangers, in effect. We would initiate contact, with the hope of being significant to them. I want doesn't get. On one trip back, we looked up two more of Father's first cousins, the Preston brothers. John was my sister's godfather and the unassuming younger brother to his socialite older sibling Stuart, who I remember for wearing a good suit and speaking with a long jaw. He was the *New York Times* art critic and, having turned down a commission in the US Army, his numerous society friends called him 'the Sergeant'. Evelyn Waugh fictionalised him as 'the Loot', as in lieutenant, in his Second World War trilogy, *Dark Sword*. Years later I discovered the writer James Lees-Milne and his diaries, and saw that he was the one who had come up with 'the Sergeant' and that Stuart Preston had been offended by the nickname. And I thought, look what offends people. I also thought, James Lees-Milne is from a bygone age, along with Evelyn Waugh. How could I have a first-cousin-once-removed from the same era? And then I had to look up Father's dates, again, working out that he would be 107 when my friends' parents were in their late seventies or early eighties. Such comparisons were a bit childish. The orphan thing can do that to you, too: make you compare notes, stop you moving on. It doesn't always. But it can. It drove our forays into the past, each a quest for connection and belonging.

John Preston, Father's other first cousin, lived in an apartment block on the Upper East Side. He was a quiet, blinds-kept-down man. We spent an hour with him in his dark apartment, conversation something for which we waited, and eventually he said, 'Oh my dears, I have an appointment, I really must get going.' We left, he left and, smelling a rat, we secreted ourselves in a neighbouring doorway as he set off round the block. He was back five minutes later. That an adult would lie about having somewhere to go to get out of where they found themselves felt injurious. Now, of course, it seems entirely reasonable.

Back then, wanting a part of what might have been, we moved through a shadow world of our own creating, never much substance to be got at. It was years before I admitted as much, though I knew it in my heart; the knowing undercut those camellia moments. I knew, deep down, each sensation of happiness wasn't for keeps, it wasn't part of something bigger. I took the attention when it came my way, no questions asked, and, like all children, when I caused offence or was found wanting, I smarted. Chauncey made avuncular observations from time to time, and some were chastening. During dinner once he pointed out that I mumbled, which I did; that I did not sit up straight, which I did not, and still don't. We wrote to each other when I was back in England. 'Return soon,' he wrote, and 'gladden the heart of your fond "Uncle" Chauncey S.,' once signing off with two hearts, drawn in thick red ink, and a PS updating me on his new pair of big carriage horses, the hackney foal in the offing and the wellbeing of the riding horses.

One day an envelope arrived, his italic hand in blue ink and the American stamps on the long white envelope immediately identifying the sender. I eagerly opened it, but found only my previous letter. There was no letter from Chauncey. I unfolded my own, written on stubby Basildon Bond paper. It had been marked up with circles of red ink. My handwriting, he wrote at the foot of the letter, was florid and immature. Indeed it was.

The y's and g's dangled and curled like trapeze artists. But I could not see as much at the time, and couldn't see that his was an exacting, Edwardian mindset that kept a tally of a child's accomplishments; instead I felt hurt. I took it personally; but it wasn't meant that way. Nothing that offended in those years was meant that way, but my sister and I, my brother too, took much of what came our way personally. It goes back to the yearning, and the expanse of need. Narcissism and need; it is a pernicious combination.

I now chortle at the escapee cousin and see that Chauncey was only trying to help, but I would like to warn my boys about perceived slights nonetheless. They spawn misunderstandings, which can last entire lives; the trick, as adults, is to unlock the cage of resentment and unfulfilled needs that often engenders the misunderstandings in the first place. Release them, I'll tell my boys, because once you get trapped inside with them, it's hard to get out alive.

One of the most frightening things I can think of now is to ask for love, and then not get it: there's a darkness in that. It's the child in the night, spooked, wanting her mother to come and give her a hug, and waiting and waiting.

I think, perhaps, that being an orphan is frightening because you never dare ask for what you want. You don't have the right to. And besides, who would you ask?

When I got into my mid-twenties, I tried not to think about my childhood. Adulthood was much more fun and, like boarding school, a great leveller. All my friends were living on their own now, rather than at home. I came to realise that while my friends had mothers and fathers, some were the cause of all manner of disappointments and resentments. I began to see not only the ties of love that bound the parents to their children, but the adult flaws that pushed the children away. Family, I told myself, is not all it's cracked up to be. I was off the hook.

Until that realisation, there was making do, which is what we did in Little Venice on our return from New York. Danielle was gone, as planned, and a very nice replacement moved in. It was business as usual: a default to a state of abandonment and to emotionally fending for ourselves. The old bleakness rolled back in. Mirabelle was also half-French, half-Spanish and another contact of Mrs Furse. She, too, was in London for the Christie's art course. She was quiet and affable and no Danielle. She needed somewhere to live and didn't connect with us, as most students in their early twenties wouldn't. Looking back, I think I had a subconscious desire for her to be another latter-day Mary Poppins in disguise, one with a practical, domestic streak. One day, during the holidays, I asked her if she could take the bin out, and she left, even though her study-year was not over yet. I don't know how I asked her, but it was the wrong way and I offended her, burned with shame, wanted to make amends, didn't know how. She left, and it was my fault. I thought, since she was a grown-up, she might help us on the domestic front, keep some kind of order. There was a gap of several months after that, then a woman whose name I don't remember moved in. I came home one weekend and in the night I went into the kitchen to get a glass of water and a man in a pair of pants and a landfall belly slipped into the hall bathroom. The woman kept her clothes in the hall closet. She would walk up to it in her underwear and stand there, flicking through the shirts and skirts, deciding what to wear for work. I was still changing in the wardrobe at school. She didn't stay long. She sort of fizzled out, and that was the end of our carers.

I had a time of it with my own underwear the night I woke up with daggers digging into my ribs. I had my nightdress on but no pants and the doctor was on his way to see me. My brother, who was down from Cambridge, had called him out. Manoeuvring into a pair of knickers required breathing, so I had to endure the shooting pains for reasons of decency. If I had heeded my housemistresses and kept pants on at all hours, including a spare on the chair, I would have been saved the discomfort. I was sixteen and we had been living on our own for over a year by now, and when the doctor came into my bedroom my brother, trying – as he had done so many times – to morph into a multi-purpose, hermaphrodite parental figure, remained in the corner of the room as the doctor asked me questions. He asked me about 'passing water' and the pattern of my periods. For this last word to be uttered in front of my brother was all wrong and he, alert to the fact, hurried out of the room. The doctor put the stethoscope on my stomach and said, it is renal colic and I said, OK, and he said, that's a stone in your kidney, which is the sort of thing Roald Dahl would say. How did I swallow it? I dared not ask. We'll know in the morning if it's that or something else, he said, you can see the day doctor and he'll be able to confirm it.

The following morning, my brother brought Doctor Tate to my bedroom door and left us to it. I knew Doctor Tate. I had been to see him before in his practice on the ground floor of an apartment block on Sloane Street in Knightsbridge. He arrived in a dark suit and I had my best knickers on, big pink flowery ones that went up to my waist. He put his stethoscope on my ribs and said, breathe in, and did the same when the stethoscope was on my back, and then he said, you've got pleurisy. He also said something about my lungs having membranes and sacs of fluid and I paid little attention until he said, you can't wash your hair, you'll have to use dry shampoo for two weeks. That didn't feel right, and neither did being ill. We weren't really set up for it.

Mrs Furse kept up our relationship for years after Danielle left for New York. She invited us to visit her during the Christmas season, giving us re-gifted gifts, and she diligently invited us to her curious dinner parties. We piled in with other strays, intellectuals and artists as if we were as worthy of a place around her table as they were. The fact that we were children didn't matter to her; she looked out for us. Never in my life, save on a visit to Myanmar, have I had to negotiate such disgusting food as the unidentifiable offerings she served up. At least I could barely see what was on my plate. Electricity didn't seem to be a feature in her Belgravia basement home. The long wooden table was lit with candles, stuck into wine bottles. As for enjoyment, there was little of it: in her presence I regressed to rabbity shyness. I willed her, and the rest of the adults, not to address their conversation to me, but I was not always spared. On one occasion Mrs Furse addressed me directly and declared in her Middle-European accent that the time had come for my brother to visit a brothel. Coming from a Resistance fighter who, as her autobiography later revealed, had hidden British servicemen in a French brothel, and secret messages and a million dollars in condoms stashed in her vagina, it was an innocent enough suggestion. But I was shocked. Even now I wonder what a witty retort might have been.

On home territory, I was bolder. Thanks to our US caviar cousins, we imported the art of cocktails back to London and I mixed a fine lime daiquiri. I liked playing the hostess, and so did my sister. We threw regular soirées for our teenage friends, and did most of the shaking and less of the drinking. I invited my school room-mate, Mary, to come and stay for an exeat weekend and her father said no, because there were no adults in the house. Mary had never been to London before, and to do so in the company of a minor seemed perilous to her protective father. In the end, our housemaster served as my advocate, assuring Mary's father that I was quite responsible and that her daughter would be well looked after. And so she was. I took her to Camden Market and we had dinner in the King's Road Jam, a trendy restaurant in World's End in Chelsea. The tables were stacked on top of each other like bunk beds and you had to climb up a ladder to get to the top booths. Once installed, there was a dial to control your own music and floor-to-ceiling mirrors so that you could check yourself out and, in my case, pimp my spiky gelled hair and admire my leopard print jeans and mohair sweater. And that was as wild as the weekend got. We took the train back to school on the Sunday night and, as ever, it was a relief to get back. Not only did someone else empty the bins, I knew where I was at school. As my sister and I got older, with our brother living elsewhere, first in Alaska, then Saudi Arabia, New York and West Virginia, my Little Venice existence became increasingly unpredictable.

21

FOOD WARS

Everything is going as expected post-radiotherapy. I can't open my mouth, swallow or talk without morphine, which I no longer bother to measure. I swig it straight from the bottle. I've got three on the go, one in my handbag, one on my bedside table, one in the bathroom. My neck is oozing honey diluted with paint thinner. I dab it with radiation gel bought on the Internet to avoid scarring, and shoot up my shakes through my PEG, two or three times a day. Not enough, the speech and language therapists tell me, and I promise to take more. But they make me throw up. Water makes me throw up. Nothing makes me throw up. One morning, getting my timings wrong, I shower the bathroom wall with vomit. I lie to the speech and language therapists and say I've got up to four milkshakes a day. It is not a complete lie, because I mean to take them.

Ten days before Bassy's thirteenth birthday at the end of June, I take myself off to stay with my friend Sally in her house in the Dordogne to practise eating; I have promised Bassy I will be eating normally by his birthday. I think the jaunt will do me good; they have always done so in the past, Easter notwithstanding, and I've always liked to get away. My present is rather different to my past, but I don't let that stop me. It's the recovery period now and I must focus. I am determined to eat. It's just a question of mind over matter. Or rather, of denial. I have barely any saliva, my jaw hurts, and there's the constant vomiting. I press on and, insanely, kick off the first eating trial with a baguette. I pull out some fluffy inside, add some butter, put it in my mouth, chew. It sits like woodchip on my plank of tongue. How foolish I am. I fill my mouth with water, wait for the bread blob to soak it up, swallow. The next morning we go to a local café, a simple pleasure never before deconstructed because never denied. Sally orders a pastry and a coffee. I look at both, feel no longing, feel perplexed. The emotional links with food and drink are hanging by a thread, the pleasures, rewards and nutritional benefits they afford very nearly cancelled out. Sitting on the terrace overlooking Sally's garden in the evening, I force myself to sip red wine. I want to be who I was before. It sears the sides of my mouth. It's not the liquor I crave. It's the companionship and sharing that I hanker after, the life-affirming food that accompanies a drink, the talking, the engagement with life, the sheer energy of it all. This is what I am trying to reclaim, and it's taking its toll.

We set off for a mini local excursion on the second morning. As I approach the car, I don't feel up to getting in it, let alone going somewhere. Gingerly, I climb in. Sally starts the engine and I pluck up the courage to admit defeat. Can't do it, I say, and ask her to turn the car around. I sleep for the rest of the day. The next day I have some success with a savoury crêpe in Bordeaux but then have an unsavoury time on the return drive, constantly out of the car and throwing up.

So that's it. I return to London, my mind having recalibrated itself so that I am dimly aware that food and I are over. I am not resigned to the fact; I am too weak and, quite simply, too hungry for that level of awareness. I don't even pay the hunger any attention; I am used to it now. The illness has set in motion an incremental shift of consciousness, an erosion of self; I can see how it is possible to give up on it altogether, too much fight required to get back to your old self. For now, I cannot imagine being able to taste, let alone enjoy food, ever again. As for wine, I want it far less than I want to be able to glug down a glass of cold water without giving it a second's thought. I fantasise about that, picture myself lifting the full glass, bringing it to my lips, letting the cold water into my mouth and then my throat, the whole glass downed in seconds.

Bassy's thirteenth birthday arrives. We shower him with presents, and then we take a dozen of his friends bowling in Shoreditch. The boys stand in huddles by the lanes, laugh, joke, give each other high fives. I am watching them from one of the booths in the adjoining bar area. I only really see Bassy. He picks up a ball, lunges haphazardly, hurls the ball down the alley, turns to look at his friends and his brother. Then his head goes back and he does his laugh, deep now, his voice long broken, his long legs everywhere, his smile so quick and bright, the brightest. I can feel my own smile mirroring his and then I suddenly remember all those evenings I worked late on newspapers when the boys were younger. I flash back to Bassy, nine years old. It is his bedtime. I call him from the *Daily Telegraph* to say goodnight.

'Are you ready?' I say. 'My arms are getting ready for the hug.'

'Ready,' he says, and I can hear the excitement in his voice.

'I am putting my hands through the phone now, pushing them through. Can you feel them?'

'Yes, I can feel them.'

'And now my arms are through, they are all the way through and they are wrapping themselves around you and I am hugging you tight. Squeezing you like toothpaste. Can you feel my arms around you?'

'Yes,' he says. And then it's goodnight and I love you and I love you, too, and God bless and I will kiss you when I am back and you are sleeping and I will see you in the morning.

If I don't make it, and the results in September are negative, and the cancer has spread, I don't want anyone to say what they have said already, that whatever happens the boys will be all right. They may well be. If it comes to it, I hope they are, obviously. But I want them to have a mother. I want them to have me. I don't care if they've had more of me than I had of my own mother, or father, or more of me than other children have of their mothers. I want them to have more of me. And I want more of them.

If I didn't have cancer everything would look different. I would not be looking back. Why would I, and break the habit of a lifetime? Now I look at my thirteen-year-old self and I look at Bassy on his thirteenth birthday and am pleased they are worlds apart. But the contrast is not stark enough for my liking. What I would like is that his world, and Reuben's, had not been redrawn by my illness. I am back to where I was in the library in Babington House on New Year's Day with my friend Vicky, making deals again. This time I want more than extra time, I want the future, and I'm done with compromises. The boys have endured my being ill, I've done my bit, done the treatment, and that's enough. Don't ask any more of me; or rather, please don't put them through anything else. Bassy's got the bowling ball again, his smile so big and no, I cannot countenance any further redefinitions of their lives. Sorry. I know they could take it. I know children are resilient, but resilience can come at a price. Now that a mirror has been brought up to my childhood self, I've seen sufficient. I've seen with my adult, mother-love eyes what grows, or does not grow and flourish, in dry soil in a dry river bed. I see who is affected by loss, and how. I don't want my boys to get anywhere near that kind of landscape.

People say: the boys will be fine, you've set them up. I say: I know my circumstances were unusual. Things were different then, for sure. People also say, and they better not say it again:

the boys will always have Richard. They might not. If Father had been given advance warning of his imminent death, as opposed to dropping dead from a second heart attack, he too might have said: at least the children will have their mother after I am gone. And look how wrong he would have been. Yes, we did have Mother, for 1,146 days after he died, in response to which I would ask: Is that (a) sufficient? (b) insufficient?

Please do not answer. It is not that it is a rhetorical question. I just don't want anyone to answer (a).

Bassy and his friends pile into the diner for lunch and sit at a long table and have burgers, the lot of them chatting or playing on their wretched phones, or staring about them in a contented, teenage fashion. Richard, Reuben and I sit at a small table nearby. To celebrate Bassy's birthday, I order myself a chocolate, caramel, peanut butter and banana milkshake and set my morphine on the table. It takes its place like a bottle of bourbon in a speakeasy. I take a swig, then grab a straw and get sucking and swallowing. Milkshakes and morphine, Reuben says, it's a good title for a book. I hold up the shake and the morphine and he takes a photograph and I think, maybe he's all right with this cancer thing. I look across at Bassy and I think, what about you Bassy? I hope you are too.

A week later, I step into a houseboat in Amsterdam and ask myself why, exactly, I am having a mini break and, worse, staying in a budget caravan-on-water. I hate caravans on land. The grotty houseboat bobs on the water like an apology. There is only a layer of wood and a slab of concrete between it and a canal which, for decades, received human waste. Not any more, obviously, but a provocative thought all the same, especially on the lavatory, from which vantage point the inky canal water is at eye level. On the other side of the canal, on lovely dry ground, is a row of solid, five-storey houses. Staring at me from beneath the bathroom sink is a pair of Sliders – the rubber slip-ons men wear as slippers-cum-sandals. The Airbnb owner may have just taken them off. The rubber, I think, is probably still warm.

There are two other rooms – a bedroom, and a bedsit. Small and bare save for two single beds, the bedroom looks like a holding room for young offenders. Come and look at your room, boys, I say. Great view. Richard and the boys are on our bed or rather, two beds pushed together, in the 'living zone'. It takes up most of the floor space. There is a kitchenette on one wall, wardrobes on the other, those elegant houses lording it over us through the narrow rectangle of window. I open a wardrobe door and the owner's Y-fronts tumble out and hit me on the head. It's one thing choosing to put a man's underwear on your head; it's another when it catches you unawares. Disgruntled, I turf the boys off the bed and curl up, wishing I was on my own bed back home. I don't like using strangers' sheets, and the ones on this bed are flannelette verging on nylon. I can't see why we didn't stay in a hotel. Really, I can't quite see why we are here at all. You need energy for a weekend break, focus, verve. All I want to do is sleep.

Two hours later we go and explore. We're here as a late birthday present to Richard. Amsterdam is orange. Holland is playing Costa Rica in the World Cup and every bar and café is full of football fans and big screens. The city is buzzing, music everywhere, a street party round every corner. I am a fly on the bunting, wings wilting, wondering how I alighted here. The feeling intensifies the following morning when Richard takes us off in search of a café sequestered within a Viennese-inspired riding stable. We walk and walk, first through a park, then in the same park but in a different direction, then into a police station to ask for directions, then back through the park and up and down various streets. I haven't upped my Ensure shake intake and I am down to two a day, with the occasional banana milkshake thrown in. So I am on 600 calories, which is not tourist fuel. I lag behind, long to hail a taxi, hate being unable to keep up in front of the boys. We eventually turn into a courtyard, a row of horses' bottoms and twitching tails indicating we have arrived. Never has horse dung smelt so sweet. Our destination turns out to be part riding school, part museum, and no part café. Refreshments, for want of any word that might suffice, are upstairs in a long room that may once have been a ballroom, though it's an odd ballroom that gives on to a gallery overlooking an indoor riding school. At one end of the room is a makeshift bar and there is a teenage girl wearing jodhpurs behind it. We order what is on offer, and it's clearly only ever ordered by the children who take lessons here: fruit squash and dry biscuits. The girl serves us at a table long enough to entertain an Austrian empress and fifty guests to a banquet.

It was a relief to get here, and a greater one to get out of it and visit the Van Gogh Museum, a mercifully short walk away. In my own altered state, I feel a new affinity for the Dutchman's. Maybe it's the lack of calories, or the fact that I have not read for so long now, let alone been to an exhibition, but I suddenly see why Van Gogh painted, have an insight into the process. This famous artist for whom I have never particularly cared feels suddenly real to me. I see his humanity, his bafflement, how he is driven to make sense of things. I am alert to his sense of urgency and, moreover, to the process of making sense of things through painting. I stand in front of *The Garden of Saint Paul's Hospital* (1889), which Van Gogh painted during a year's voluntary incarceration in the asylum in Saint-Rémy-de-Provence, and I am riveted by the duality he conjures. There are easy yellows and ochre, a golden sky daubed with blues and purples and speckled with white, and there's a flower bed of white roses. Trees – I think they are pines – take up most of the canvas, and they are anguished; there is nothing relaxed about them. They look like they want to be on the move. The leaves are frantic, swirling, thrusting. They are nothing like the vibrant trees outside my friend Tim's apartment window back in London. There is too much movement, and so much grey. Even the trunks are partly grey, one of them sawn-off. I spot a lone figure, so small beside a single tree, and two others in conversation by the high golden wall on the right. Are they trapped, or do they want to be there? I can't tell, but seeing the two men makes me feel much better, takes my mind off the lone figure.

When we go to a café that night, the four of us together, Richard telling us stories about university and all his pranks and making us shake with laughter, I know this is my world, whole and everything I need. It's the best moment of the trip. Then I blow it by feeling overwhelmed. I have to get away, just for a moment, and retreat to the Ladies' Room. I stand by the sink, Van Gogh's yellows and greys clashing in my head, the yellows my absolute happiness, the greys my own piercing anguish. I feel and see the colours, but I can't deploy them to make sense of my own feelings as Van Gogh did; I can't make anything out of them, have nothing to show for myself except these sudden tears. A moment ago I was part of my family. Now I feel like a ghost, looking at what I love the most, unable to connect with the three people in the world I love the most. I splash my face with cold water, then go back and join them.

There's none of this at the Anne Frank Museum the next day, and quite right too. It is impossible to be even slightly self-referential here, which is refreshing. To see the young Jewish girl's family house, so ordinary, and a monument to such bravery, is profoundly moving. I leave, reminded of how lucky I am, which I then realise is self-referential, and feel confused and harried. Is it inappropriate to feel lucky after being reminded of such suffering? I don't know. My head is no longer up for the job. By the time we get back to London, it seems to have short-circuited altogether. A switch has gone off. There are no yellows or greys. It's as if someone has unplugged me and the battery has drained to zero. Everything goes blank. I am all out of drive, and I'm stuck with the realisation that the trip to Amsterdam was a mistake. Yes, there was the night laughing in the café, the delight in looking at the Van Goghs with the boys by my side and the moment of illumination about the mind's relation to creativity, and a catch-up with old friends, too. All rich and good, and more so in retrospect. But at the time I kept watching myself and thinking, is this it, is this the best you can do? Can't you *buck up*? I regret that I let the boys see me struggling. I had wanted it to be a perfect weekend break. And it's left me exhausted and quite unable to reboot.

For days on end, I lie in bed holding my legs as I try to warm them up. I curl up tighter and tighter, not a second thought for Van Gogh now or Anne Frank or the millions and millions of people who are suffering far, far more than me, or who have properly suffered and endured in the past. One morning I give up halfway through sending a text; it is too much effort to depress the keys. I stop texting after that. I stop sending emails, too, because I am low on mind-over-matter. I'm all out of topspin. I wake in the mornings, my mouth stuck together as usual, and think only about how I must move in order to go to the lavatory. Two hours later, I am in the same position, still trying to make myself move. In the end the only way I can get out of bed is by manhandling my legs to get my feet on the floor and force myself to get up. Then I come back to my island-bed, curl up again, my spine a child's jointed plastic toy snake, my knees an anatomical diagram, all bits and hard bone. Still cold, always cold now, I ask Richard to check that every window in the house is closed. It's boiling in here, he says, and I think I hear irritation in his voice. Time has him on the rack, pulling him this way and that. When will he say: enough? Is he coping? I have not even asked. He never complains, keeps the house running, wraps the boys in his indefatigable cheer and his love. But what is he doing with his grief, and his worry? Who does he talk to? Who is holding him up? Is he holding up?

Pepper lies alongside me. Bassy sometimes comes in and does the same, and that just about breaks my heart. Within days it's not just my spine and my knees that ache, it's my whole legs. It must be the tumour; some of the cancer cells must have got away and formed new tumours. They are in my legs now. What would that be? Leg cancer? Bone marrow cancer? Is there such a thing? I can't think, I don't know. Then there's my breathing, suddenly shallow. We go somewhere in the car. It's parked near the house, just a few metres away, and by the time I get down the five front door steps I realise I can't make it on my own. I am too short of breath. I take Reuben's arm and he slows down for me. I need his support, ask for it, get it. He readily offers his arm, and that's a nice feeling, but it irks all the same. I remember a friend being in hospital last year for a straightforward but painful condition and not letting her children come and see her. I don't want to be vulnerable in front of them, she told me, I don't want them to see me like this. Only now do I fully understand what she meant.

I don't like being out of the house. I only want to be on my island-bed, even though the walls of my bedroom have pulled back, leaving me in a blankness that has risen from some old, dark place. It's the same dread blankness as the *Cement Garden* summer, the same sense of being uncontained, abandoned, cut off. More than ever then it felt shameful to be an orphan; the shame I feel at being helpless and ill takes me back to that childhood state for the first time, only now my shame holds a mother's anguish. I cannot be dependent on anyone, or anything. I must be dependable. The boys depend on me, yet here I am, ineffective, helpless. Is this how Mother felt when she was dying? I hate to think of her, out here. I'm sorry, I whisper, I never knew.

But I thought I knew. I thought I had an inkling of what Ruth Picardie must have felt, and Cassandra Jardine, too, in the face of their own dying. But I think now that it was the child in me that was grieving for them, as well as the adult me. I felt for both brave women, with a full heart, but I felt for their children, for the pain that lay ahead, more keenly. I lived it, or relived it, wanted so badly to keep them from it. Now the mother in me lies curled up on the edge of my bed and I say to all three mothers, how did you endure your imminent passing? How does any mother endure the prospect of being lost to her children?

The boys' first nanny, the one everyone lovingly called a white witch, was called Rachel. She enchanted every child she looked after, and she had two sons of her own, the same age as Reuben and Bassy. When her boys were two and five, by which stage she was no longer working for us, she became pregnant with her third child. One evening, she collapsed and died. We'd been on the phone three days earlier, arranging to meet up. When I got the phone call telling me she was dead I could not stop screaming. *No.* That is what I screamed, nothing else. It was partly for myself, for the pain I felt, but mainly it was for her boys. I saw the years ahead without knowing their mother's love, and what I saw was desolation and longing.

I come across a letter from Mother to one of Father's relatives, thanking her for taking my sister and me out for the day. 'Being ill is terribly boring,' she wrote. She comes alive with the sentence, and it made me think that if I had only known she had been strung out on the plains of boredom and could wind back the clock, I would sit with her, read to her, draw her pictures, prattle on. My nine-year-old self might tire her. So what? Maybe the mother who considered that sending her daughters to boarding school was the done thing also thought children did not belong in sickrooms with their dying mother. Maybe she was in too much pain to have us near her. I don't know. But oh, to have been with her.

The white days pass inside my white bedroom, and outside the sky could be any colour and I think, so, this is what happens when you are dying. I don't know if I am allowed to think this, fear censure from the terminally ill, but this is what I think. Did Mother start slipping away, and did she care a great deal that she was doing so, and then care only a bit, and then perhaps not at all? How I've got to this point where I am thinking about those who make the transition – Peggy the guru's word, resonant now – I don't know. I have no right to be here, on the edge. I know that. But my mind keeps coming back to the physical sensation of slipping out of consciousness and into oblivion. I slide over it, trying to pinpoint what it is that I am feeling. I need something to focus on. Perhaps Ezra Pound, confined like an animal in his cage as a POW, became fixated by those ants on the floor for the same reason. Perhaps he shut everything out except what it was to be the ants at his feet in order to feel something himself. Van Gogh may equally have believed that by embodying his anguish in those dead-head rose bushes in that painting in the asylum he would alleviate his own anguish. At least he could paint. Being able to paint, or write, talk or, if all else fails, think coherently is a lifeline; it connects self with others. I see that now. Otherwise you are stuck in a void, outside of time; you inhabit a space where self – or soul – is suspended, where time taunts because you are out of time. You can't measure it because you aren't doing anything; you may as well be dead. This siding with the dying and the mentally anguished is wrong and distasteful, but I am too tired to work out why and maybe I am putting the wrong words together in my head anyway. The usual distance that keeps us safe and sane and not mindful of our mortality is reduced. Shame at my weakness starts to dissolve; I feel far less distaste for my deterioration now. Perhaps this is acceptance, finally. Yes, all right, I accept my cancer club membership. And all the while the boys are on the periphery; I can't bring them back to the centre. I cannot reach them.

Peggy said that Buddhists say: The body does the suffering, you do not.

I go to the cancer, I go away from it, I come back to it and I say: cancer, you do not define me.

But this is not true. These are just words. The cancer is me. I have cancer.

The fear is back, and my throat is slacked. There's no wind. When will I ever get away from here?

Yeats said: 'The centre cannot hold.'

Now that is true.

These are my days. Is this Mordor? Everything is white. Where are the flames? Where is the enemy? There is no end in sight, and nothing to aim for. It's two months since the radiotherapy finished, and whilst Caroline, with her palliative care expertise, and Blondie, with all her experience, have both warned me that the psychological aspects of cancer can be the worst, knowing as much doesn't enable me to shake out of my desolation. I can't get out of bed, don't care that I can't get out of bed, I cry at random, have no sense of connection and no agency. The sun shines. Let it shine. The boys come in and out. Whatever. Whiteness closes in on me, and so does a new thought I have tried to fend off. Perhaps when you are very ill you want to be held, as you would hold your own children. The thought comes at me, at full force, winds me. And then I ponder what it would be like to be looked after by a mother, a preposterous, childish thought in every sense. Some of my contemporaries do not have extant mothers of their own, and of those that are alive, some are in key ways, lacking. It is just a thought. But the thought, emboldened, repeats itself until suddenly, there I am, sitting on the edge of the bed, and I allow four words that have been waiting in the wings to step forward. I say them out loud. I don't say them, I howl them. *I want my mother.*

Appalled, I sip some water, move across the room, away from the moment. I pretend it has not happened.

22

HOME ALONE

When the woman whose name I can't remember left our Little
Venice flat, I moved into her bedroom. I was fifteen by then.
The huge, low-slung bed had a whiff of the bohemian about it,
which I mistrusted. A saffron chest of drawers painted with
flowers and featuring a matching triptych vanity mirror stood
beside it. The chest of drawers had been bought for my sister
with great care and fanfare from Tamsin's parents' antique shop
in Lewes. It had little drawers beneath the mirror that didn't
quite open, the wood was warpèd and the splintered wood inside
the big drawers was musty. I kept my own triptych, a folkloric
wooden icon of the Virgin Mary, on the top of it. Tamsin's
father, a landscape painter and a warm man, had given me the
icon after I had admired it in the studio of his Sussex home.
You can fold the side wings in like shutters over the Mother and
Child and open them when you feel like seeing them again.
I usually kept them closed. Marian iconography made me uneasy.

I had my bedroom walls painted a rose pink, and covered
the main wall with the same dark brown cork tiles my brother
had had on his bedroom wall in Lewes Crescent. He'd worked
a teenage vibe in his room. I tried to do the same.

We spent a lot of time inside the flat I won't call home, now that I know what home is, the family outings or dutiful visits other children went on no longer part of the patchwork of our lives. If you were in the big bedroom with the French doors of an evening, about six or seven o'clock, Arthur Lowe, the actor from *Dad's Army*, and his wife would start arguing in the room above. He barked like a Basset Hound, low and deep. Whatever sounds his wife made didn't make it through the floorboards. The furniture would start crashing its way across the ceiling. Five or ten minutes later, the piano music would start up, Mrs Lowe on the keys.

I spent the best part of my Easter holiday before taking my A levels lying on my bed and learning my lines for the school production of *Antony and Cleopatra*. I was Cleopatra. I practised my lines as a trainspotter would a train timetable: mechanically, and with a deficiency of passion. I summoned up the courage to ask Arthur Lowe to give me some coaching, only to discover he had died the week before. When it came to the performance, I failed to capture the sexual appetite that ate up the Egyptian firebrand, even though her longing for her beloved Antony, and the fact that she wasn't as strong as she seemed, completely cut me up. Otherwise, the production went well. I managed to get a wiggle into the tail of the plastic toyshop snake I clutched to my breast in the suicide scene and, after my death, Enobarbus dignified my passing by recalling how I had sat on, rather than shat on, my lovely golden barge.

Unless I had lines to learn, I was rarely in my bedroom, or in the living room for that matter. It wasn't a place where you hung out, or watched TV. I think you need atmosphere for that, and the right kind. I went out whenever I could, my door left open.

My brother kept his bedroom door shut when he was back from university in the holidays. He had a bay window mirroring mine, but the outside wall was only a few feet away, which made his room darker than mine, even before the scarlet paint. He kept the curtains shut. One afternoon, sensing he was inside, I pushed open the door as quietly as I could and laid my duvet over him while he slept.

My sister also kept her bedroom door shut. She made herself a No Entry sign using red felt tip and pinned that up on it. Increasingly, as the years went by, there were yellow Post-It notes on her door and, on the inside, words written in a private code of her own devising. They were messages to herself, mantras perhaps. I don't know. I never deciphered the code; never wanted to.

When friends came over, my bedroom door would often be the only one left open.

We played a lot of records and tried out a lot of cookbooks. *Cuisine Minceur*, Sophie Grigson, *The New York Times Cook Book*, Mrs Beeton, *Darling, You Shouldn't Have Gone to So Much Trouble*. My brother was forever cooking up new dishes for us all, everything measured, precise, a mark of something, something that wasn't failure, something that people everywhere were doing in just this same way, cooking all the rage. An alternative health movement had sprung up too, its disciples living off raw juices and nuts. My sister was way ahead of the curve, a pioneer. She meditated and levitated and boiled chickpeas to make hummus. She held a coin dangling from a chain near my head and watched to see which way it would swing, and she gave me regular updates on my aura. She made us fresh carrot juice and consumed so much of it her skin went orange, and that was funny and alarming and another way of being. We played opera and *lieder*; sometimes I thought all this classical music was only to bring Mother back from the dead and wanted less of it. We had hundreds of records, the sleeves strewn across the wooden floorboards. Talking Heads, the

Ramones, Philip Glass, Erik Satie, Schubert, Barbara Streisand and David Essex. The Streisand and David Essex albums were mine, my singalongs my dark secret when my musically sophisticated siblings were elsewhere. Between us, we had eclectic tastes, and we had a very good sound system. When the ghetto blaster flew across the hall at head height, you couldn't hear it coming.

There was screaming, and there were tears; need rubbing need raw.

Sometimes Grandma and my aunt, temporarily detached from her husband, came to stay in the flat for Christmas. We cooked turkey and all the trimmings. One year, at Midnight Mass, my aunt stood up in the pew, teetered backwards and forwards and, before she could involuntarily prostrate herself, we manhandled her home. She slept in my bed, not with me in it, and she took a tumbler with her in case she got thirsty in the night. I rinsed the last few drops of whisky out in the morning.

She had form. I remember, with Mother, how she once slept in my bed at Marine Gate, and I squashed up with my sister in her bed. In the night her snores let loose like a hippo in a tizz and then there was a thud. She was on the floor. I tried to roll her up the side of the bed. When she was nearly over the edge and on the mattress, gravity got her and she fell back on to the floor.

I always thought it was strange to have a close relative, your mother's twin, no less, who had not only managed to stay alive but was everything you did not want or need.

Grandma was always very game. We sometimes took her to Camden Market where she admired all the punk rockers and their imaginative clothing. As she got older, she got smaller and smaller, and the dignity that had defined her ebbed away. She seemed to throw in her lot, including her money, with her daughter. It happened without me noticing, and then it was too late. We lived in different worlds by then, and, from my vantage point, I was ashamed of the straitened circumstances to which she and my aunt had been reduced.

My aunt had resumed her relationship with her estranged husband so any visit to see Grandma meant seeing him too. On one visit, my aunt served an obscure brown fowl for lunch because, as she saw fit to explain, it was cheaper than chicken. I noticed that she and her husband had switched to supermarket brand cigarettes, and shuddered. Need, like weakness, ferments fear; I think there is a risk of contagion.

About seven years later, my aunt's husband wrote to me at university. His handwriting on the envelope triggered the old revulsion; his request for money fuelled it further. How much could I give them, he asked, and how was my studying going? I did not reply, and that's something else I am ashamed of.

The fuse box was in the cupboard on the left as you opened the front door into the hallway. The black switch in the middle of the fuse box was the one you flicked up when you wanted to make sure all the electricity was off, to clear the waste disposal unit without chopping your fingers off, say, or to prise the piece of fat, burnt toast out of the toaster without getting electrocuted. Flick it, and OFF appeared in red letters against a white backdrop.

The hall bathroom had no windows, just a ceiling light and a noisy internal fan. One night, I was in the bathroom, sitting on the floor with my back against the door, hiding. Suddenly, everything went dark, and silent. Someone had flicked the switch.

Occasionally we went to see my half-brother or my father's first wife, and it would be like going out into the real world. There was a yearning for that. Then we would go back to our hollow home and each continue to try out our different ways of being, some more successful than others. We became the orphan's dread: difficult, different, bad in company. We were too thin, too odd, we had the Ancient Mariner's eyes, we hovered in doorways, unable to step inside, retreat preferred, solitude the safe place. We stood out. Look at us, look away. We grew angular, jagged, the shoulders hunched, the breath arrested.

When I came back to the flat at the start of each school holiday, and university holidays too, it was the stillness that made me wobble, did something to my gut. It wasn't the stillness after everybody has packed up and left, or the stillness just before the rest of the family comes home – I know both now. The Little Venice stillness was a flattened thing, and it hung in the air. Some things you never get used to. I had to adjust to it every time.

In my first year at St Andrews University I took a psychology module. I didn't enjoy the graphs or the time spent in the lab, or not spent, as was more often the case. But I was grimly gripped by the psychologist John Bowlby and his evolutionary attachment theory, first published in 1969. I set out to disprove it.

Bowlby's work was informed by that of fellow psychologist Harry Harlow who, in 1958, subjected eight rhesus monkeys to an unconscionable experiment on maternal deprivation. Each was separated from its mother after birth and then caged up with two surrogates, one fashioned from wire mesh, the other also made of bare wire but covered in tactile fabric. The wire surrogate was a source of milk, provided in a bottle, but only some of the time. When given a choice, the monkeys spent more time with the cloth monkey, embracing it, especially if they were scared; they only chose the wire monkey when they were hungry and it had a supply of milk. There are photographs of monkeys clinging to the cloth surrogate.

The results underpinned Bowlby's evolutionary attachment theory, which holds that early attachments are emotional rather than physiological: an infant attaches to a nurturing, emotionally responsive figure, rather than, as the learned or behaviourist theory of attachment held, to the provider of food.

In my essay on maternal deprivation I set out to prove, in the manner of a tabloid journalist who writes the headline first and then the story to go with it, that both theories were wrong: neither infants nor children need an attachment figure in the first place. I worked hard to make my essay watertight, twisting the data and finding some of my own to demonstrate that maternal deprivation, including continuity of care, was not a factor in an infant's emotional development and was not a root cause of emotional damage in later life.

I had wanted a high mark. Instead, I was commended for my tenacious reasoning, but marked down for my conclusions. I minded, very much. Even though maternal deprivation did not pertain to me – I had had a mother of my own during the formative period from zero to five months stipulated by Bowlby and, by all accounts, formed a healthy attachment – its findings felt personal. I did not want a mother to matter, at any stage of a child's development.

Years later, when I was in my thirties, I met a contemporary of my brother's at a party and she said: Oh, I always felt so sorry for you. I used to come to your house for parties and everyone was taking cocaine in your garden and you were so young. I don't know what it was she found upsetting. I've always liked a party. Drugs, not a bit. I occasionally came across people in their twenties, not friends but people I knew from my childhood, who had turned stick-insect-thin. The adults connected to them would say, 'She's got anorexia' because they didn't want to admit that whoever it was used heroin. One particular casualty came from a fully fledged, signed-up, cosy family and I thought: you've got everything and look how you've messed up. I couldn't fathom it. My friend Louise ate some magic mushrooms once and she told me how creatures tunnelled through her eyeballs and into her brain. I couldn't see the appeal.

I think, living home alone, you veer towards the self-protective side. I remember one party which Louise and I co-hosted in the Little Venice flat. My bedroom door was shut. When I opened it to get something, five strangers were sitting on the floor, cross-legged, spaced out and looking very bored. I left them to it, and hit the dance floor.

That was my childhood. We all tell stories about our lives, and everybody has a story. But to tell a story, you have to be selective, which is why parents cherry-pick what they tell their children about their pasts. We protect them, or try to, by withholding information, saving some of it up for when the time is right, keeping other stuff under lock and key. With my children, I've done midnight feasts, running away from school, sleeping on Pisa's airport runway, my ice-cream-loving, pint-sized grandmother, key people in America, a dead mother, dead father and Danielle, and that's about it.

23

MIND GAMES

Lesley, one of the Meals on Heels posse, calls to see how I am two weeks after the Amsterdam weekend. My conversational skills are down to sounds: splutter, snort, warble. She clocks the extent to which I am reduced and that there is not much eating going on and quite a lot of not much else.

'We need to sort you out,' she says in her Glaswegian lilt. 'What we need to work out is, who will be your mummy?'

The question sends me reeling, though it is straightforward enough and one she might have put to any one of our friends who, with a mother either living far away or no longer alive, is in need of practical, as well as emotional, love. She won't know, of course, that only days earlier I had called out for my own mother. With the extraordinary timing that seems to come with the cancer territory, she was invoking Mummy, or Mother, as a metaphor for loving care.

The following afternoon, not yet dressed, I will myself to get out of bed. It is my friend Julia's fiftieth birthday party tonight, but mind-over-matter is not working and I remain curled up in a ball. The party had seemed so far off; it has been a goal for weeks. I have nothing to draw on to get me there. If I do go, what will I talk about? I can't do a Ruth Picardie and bring the house down with gallows humour. Some of my oldest, dearest friends will be there, but many others, too. I draw the shawl of shame tight around me. I don't want to be seen like this, diminished.

I keep thinking about Lesley's question. It has got right under my skin. To her, it was a practical question, yet its effects are wonderful and far-reaching. It has made me see that I need some reinforcements. First I call Mary, my beloved school friend who stayed with me all those years ago for that unwild weekend in Little Venice. She is a consultant psychiatrist and, throughout my illness, she's made my fears feel legitimate and normal – again, that word, normal. Then I call Caroline. I explain that I seem to have turned into a static jellyfish, and a miserable, insane one at that. I need to know where this depression has come from. I add that something has happened to my tear ducts. The valves, or whatever ducts have, are permanently open. Each woman says: you feel like you are going mad, and that's normal, in the circumstances. Get antidepressants. Can't, I say, I don't do antidepressants, never have done. They both insist, saying: stuff is happening in your brain, neural pathways are rerouting. You *need* antidepressants. So, I go and see the GP, snort, blubber, explain that I am not depressed. Or rather, that I might be, but it is circumstantial. I ask for drugs to get me back on my feet, literally.

I need to get a grip for two reasons: one, I can't go on like this and two, after we broke the news of my illness to the boys I promised that we would go to America in the summer, stay on our favourite lake in Maine, go to New York, do all the things we love. Also, when I emailed friends about my treatment plan (worse than a Christmas round robin, I know), I assured them that we would be eating lobster rolls in Maine in August. 'Sunny uplands' was the subject header of the email. OK, so Maine is too much energy. And the lobster rolls are looking unlikely. But we can at least get to America, or try to. The GP gives me sleeping tablets as well as antidepressants. Mary tells me to double the dose on the antidepressants. When I tell Caroline that I've got them, she screams 'Attagirl!' down the phone. She's like that.

Technically, the antidepressants need two weeks before they kick in, but they have an instant placebo effect. I have fresh wells of resolve to draw on, feel like an agent of my own well-being. I address my leg cancer fixation, asking Khalda, my specialist nurse, if she can squeeze me in to see one of the oncologists. It's my legs, I explain, could the cancer have spread to my legs? I shouldn't even be calling her. I am supposed to be seeing my GP from now on and not bothering the hospital. Khalda sorts it, as always, and I feel better the moment I walk into UCLH. I've missed the place. Blondie had warned me that the no man's land after treatment finishes is a hard place to be, the radiotherapy routine gone, other hospital contact reduced. Left to my own devices, I don't know how to get better. I can't make my one surviving salivary gland grow new cells, or whatever it needs to do to start producing saliva. I can't think my body back to being strong, can't just will it back to life. Who said body and mind are linked? I am powerless. And what if there is something going on in my legs? I feel fantastically stupid even asking the question, but I force myself to ask it of the registrar anyway: could the cancer have bypassed various vital organs and somehow shown up in my legs? No, he replies, explaining with his usual patience that it's not cancer in my legs, but the fact that I am not eating and not moving much and my system is battered. It's obvious when he says it; I wish I had asked him before.

I do get to Caroline's fiftieth birthday a week later. This is a black tie, swish affair at Senate House. Sue and I get dolled up in my house, take loads of photographs, and I swoon at

Richard, so handsome in his black tie which he bought from Marks & Spencer half an hour before the party is due to start. We arrive to find most of our male friends are also in brand new Marks & Spencer dinner jackets, Caroline looks like a movie star in a designer ballgown, and I take more photographs. I feel so much love and light I should be certified. I even engage in cancer banter with one of Caroline's colleagues.

'Oh, hello,' she beams. 'The last time I saw you, you were naked. You look great.'

She is referring to the night she came to see me, despite not being my doctor and being off-duty. I had telephoned Caroline when I was convulsing in agony and about to give birth to Ridley Scott's alien, aka the night of the dreaded PEG fitting. Caroline, off duty and out of range, had enlisted her colleague to check on me.

'You look good in a dress yourself,' I say.

She then asks me how I am, and boy do I want to tell her, could bang on about it for hours. My Cancer Etiquette rules hold me back. She's off duty tonight. I would happily not talk to anyone else tonight, except the medics; the room is full of them, but it wouldn't be fair to talk shop. I can't think of a single interesting or funny thing to say to anyone else. What do people find to talk about on Planet Earth? I keep sneaking off for a snooze on the squidgy chairs in the hall. But when the disco starts, Richard, Sue and I get straight on to the dance floor. It's huge, and it's just the three of us, and we use up all the space, working it like Mick Jagger, arms doing anthemic swaying and crazy hands. At least I've got an excuse, unlike Richard and Sue. When my legs protest, I ignore them and when I can't, I sit down. And then I get up again. Richard later tells Sue that this is the first time he has forgotten I am ill.

Usually the last to leave, we slink off early and in the morning all four of us go to church, which shows what a strange old time of it we are having. This never happens; not even on

Christmas Day. I'm on a roll with the taking-help-wherever-I-can-get-it and have accepted the school vicar's offer of a laying on of hands ceremony. Julia, and Sue and her family are here too. We gather in a side chapel after the main church service. Reuben puts his hand on my head, Bassy's hand is on one shoulder, Richard's on the other. Everybody puts a hand on me. It's like a scene from a Louis Theroux documentary on bonkers believers, and the joke's on me. I am so up for it. I close my eyes and as the vicar prays for me, I say: Let it work.

When Reuben was a baby and, unlike Bassy, used to scream his head off, I sometimes placed the palm of my hand on his head and let it rest there. It was an instinctual thing to do. Touch, I think, is a salve. There have been occasions when I have wanted to hold someone, someone brittle and lonely, and to take their hand. My half-sister was one of these people. I wanted to take her hand and hold it in mine when she was in the hospice. Always I am repelled by the thought of doing so, convinced my instinct is misjudged, have never had the confidence that it would be the right thing to do – except with my own children. I am glad that others feel able to touch me now. Glad, too, that I have had the confidence to involve my children in an ancient ritual that makes public my vulnerability, and my submission to it. By formally asking for healing, I am also acknowledging to them, for the one and only time, my fears about making a full recovery. It is a risk; I fear doing so may upset them.

We read the passage in Psalm 23 next, the one about being protected by God in the valley of the shadow of death. The boys' school vicar quoted it when I told her how terrified I was shortly after receiving my diagnosis. I felt, then, that I was hearing the passage for the first time. It was so kind and reassuring, and it reassures me now, no longer feels like more hackneyed, hollow words ignored. I recall how I told the vicar about my dream back then, too, and how she had said, Why don't you trust it? But I was in the shadows then, couldn't see my way through.

The laying on of hands is mumbo-jumbo, I suppose, no different to seeing a white witch or a witch doctor. But that's not how it feels to me. I've stuck my neck out, asked for healing, asked my husband and sons to stand in a church and join me in this ceremony. I've also exposed my hotchpotch, half-formed, work-in-progress faith, inviting them to take the leap with me or, failing that, to witness my own willingness to do so. Though I am a mother and my role is to protect my children and be strong for them, I am putting myself in their hands. What was it the priest said in hospital seven months earlier? 'Your boys can help you.' Perhaps this ritual can help them, too.

Afterwards we go to a café. The boys have burgers, I have a vanilla milkshake. Julia is with us, and she comes over to the house the next day, too. She is full of reasons why I must not go to America. You are not strong enough. You can't even eat. Look at you yesterday. You didn't eat – you had a milkshake. You're underweight. How much do you even weigh? There are medical risks. What if you can't get health insurance and can't pay for an American hospital? What about the plane journey and the long drive from JFK to the Hamptons? It's too much for you, too exhausting. Look at you. She works up to a climactic I don't want you to die.

La-la-la-la. Won't die, won't listen, refuse to be moved. It's a bit like Blondie giving me the treatment options back in January. What Julia says makes sense, and there are indeed health risks, but my fingers are in my ears. You're right, I say, I'll think about it.

Which I won't. I want to go to America in mid August. It is nearly four whole weeks away, for heaven's sake. Plenty of time to put on weight and build up my strength. But Julia has put the wind up me. Is it foolhardy to go? There is only one person who can answer that question. I make an appointment to see Dr Suleman.

I ask him if it is selfish to be taking the boys to America in the state I'm in, tell him about Amsterdam, how I thought it would be good to get away and how difficult I found it. Richard and I had discussed him taking the boys to Amsterdam without me, I continue, and that's what we should have done. But I vetoed it. Now I worry that the so-called jaunt did them more harm than good.

'And what was the harm?' Dr Suleman asks.

I was a ghost, I say, a shadow of my usual self.

'But how was it for the boys?'

They had fun, it was amazing to be together, hanging out in the houseboat, going to museums, having a laugh.

'So what was the problem?'

Me: I was bad company, I rubbed my recovery status in their faces, I was weak and cold. I want America to be different, I tell Dr Suleman. I want to use the trip to wipe the slate clean, prove to the boys that everything is all right, move on. But what if I can't? And what if everything isn't all right? Now that the end is in sight, I gnaw on the prognosis statistics – a 75 to 80 per cent chance of the treatment being successful – and the 25 per cent chance of its failure bites back. I've ignored it until now, or rather, reduced it to 10 per cent in my head after various people assured me that oncologists play down positive outcomes. They dare not offer false hope, they say, but how can you get through the treatment without hope? I've been so intent on getting through, I now don't know what I'll do if it has failed. My brain isn't wired up for it. What if I have to have surgery, and then more chemotherapy after that? How will the boys cope with a round two? How will Richard cope? I am telling Dr Suleman everything in a splurge. The results will come through at the beginning of September, I explain, when we would still be in America. Waiting for them could sabotage the trip and my ability to be present in it. One of the oncologists has said he can give me my results over the phone, but if the results are negative, our Big Holiday will be tainted by the disease from which I am trying to give us all a break. It could be the stuff of nightmares, not golden memories. Would I withhold the outcome from the boys until we got home? And, if I don't take the phone call, what if I can't manage the anxiety caused by not knowing?

Dr Suleman treats my what ifs with gravity. He does not say: well, the chances are you will be fine. He says: these what ifs, these fears, are very real. He acknowledges how debilitating they are, how overwhelming and frightening; hearing this from him sloughs off my anxieties like dead skin. He says: give all these legitimate fears due respect. But consider this: There is nothing you can do about the outcome. You cannot control it. It might be helpful to park these fears. To put it another way, he continues, imagine this consulting room is full of balloons. They are everywhere, he says, and he points all around him. They are on the ceiling, lining the walls, floating amongst the furniture. One of them could burst at any moment. But there's no knowing when, or even if, any of them ever will burst. And there is no way of stopping them from doing so either, so accept that you have to live amongst them, and get on with living. Do the same with your fears. They are all around you. Acknowledge them. As I say, they are very real. And then try to turn your thoughts away from them. When they return, as they will, acknowledge them once more and then, once again, try to carry on.

He then returns to the question of the American trip.

'What are you most frightened of?'

'That aside from the tumour having survived and the cancer spread, the trip will be a re-run of Amsterdam.'

'Amsterdam need not be the same as America. You have had Amsterdam, seen what was difficult. You can learn from it.'

And then he asks: 'Do you think it will do the boys good to go to America?'

'Yes.'

'Will they be disappointed if you don't go?'

'Yes.'

'Do you want to go?'

'Yes. It will be good for us. It will mark the next phase. We'll have fun.'

'Do you know what you need to do to go to America?'

'Yes.'

'What?'

'Get strong.'

'Then do it.'

I love this man. He speaks my language, a positive, proactive, pre-cancer me language. He helps me reconnect my mind to my body, makes me feel it is possible for my mind to drag the latter, kicking and screaming, back into action; the old governance is restored. In a single session, he has given me strategies to manage the anxiety that has exploited my physical weakness and gained the upperhand. Where there is a will, there is surely a way: I'd forgotten how good that feels. Suddenly hopeful, I go and see Steven Hannah, UCLH's senior specialist dietician. I always feel better after seeing him, and today is no different. I outline the America plan. In that case, he says, you need to get up to six milkshakes a day and you need to start eating again; I can't get you off the feeding tube until you are. It's a deal, I say.

The following day, Caroline drops round to the house. I am in position on the sofa in the living room and she fusses over me, asks if she can get me anything. Yes please, I say, a glass of water. Down to the kitchen she goes, back up she comes. She leans in as I ramble on about America and my physical state and then, wham, she swings into action. In that case, girl, you start right now. No more asking people to get you a glass of water. Get it yourself. Get up and down those stairs. Get to the local shops. Get moving. I am taken aback, but after she has gone, I walk up one flight of stairs, then down again, and make myself do it again. The next day, I do the same thing, with more repetitions. I also walk to the dry cleaner's five minutes away, and feel triumphant. I go to the GP and ask him to write me a letter saying I am fit to travel, for purposes of insurance, and to throw in a request for a golf buggy at the airport. 'A golf buggy?' he replies. 'It would be preferable if you didn't need one.' What you do need, he adds, is stamina, and no, he can't sort out the golf buggy. It seems the NHS does not stretch to concierge services, which is a shame. I'd have liked an upgrade to First Class, too.

I sort the stamina next, excavating a phone number for Amy, my personal trainer from a million years ago. I spit out my ill-health bulletin but, even so, when she comes to the house a few days later I am embarrassed for her to see the broken me. I used to be like her. Not in so far as she is as tall as a gazelle, has visible muscles, and looks like Christy Turlington; I just mean out there, full of zest, or so I like to think. She's a Pilates instructor now and sets me on the path to strength and well-being that began when I asked the GP for antidepressants. I stopped taking them after two weeks, so they never did get beyond the placebo stage but, like Dr Suleman's toolkit for managing anxiety, they put me back in the driving seat.

Amy and I start with the basics, boomerangs and body rolls not for me just yet. I have to be reminded what my core is, can barely get my leg in the air when she asks me to lie on one side and lift one leg, and have to break off every twenty seconds to sip water. Amy waits for me to sip, takes the bottle from me, places it within reach, and continues. When I do the exercise where you lie on your back and bend your knees and raise your head to meet them, my body remembers what stretching is like. I love hugging my knees, could stay there for ever. Best of all is the feeling I get when I reach my arms skywards or spread them wide and open up my shoulders. I open my arms and it's no longer just a body stretch, it's a gesture of both strength and vulnerability, signifying my open heart. It takes me back to the beginning, to Babington House and the deal I struck: I will open my own heart to God in return for getting time with the boys. Open my heart: I'm not there yet but, without even being conscious of the fact, I am getting there.

I move straight up to four milkshakes a day and start weaning myself off the system-blocking morphine intake, swapping glugs for the measured sachets I started out with. And then I embark on an eating rehabilitation programme, for which I call in the Meals on Heels posse, plus extra friends and family. I not only ask them to cook for me – strictly no culinary flourishes; hideous soft foods only – but to sit with me while I learn to eat. This entails swallowing again and, crucially, ending my face-off with the food I have come to mistrust and dread. They rally, delivering a new round of fresh dishes, from dahl to fishcakes, and they sit with me and watch me eat, as if I were a political prisoner, or a baby. One evening Estelle brings thick home-made soup, and two cartons of cream cheese, which she dollops into it as she heats it up. The sight of the white mass makes my insides constrict. Cream cheese is what her father added to his soups when he was weaning himself off his feeding tube, apparently. She pulls up a stool and sits next to me at the kitchen island, and then she waits. I pick up the spoon, lower it, raise it, leave it there in mid-air and start chatting. Estelle, wise to my distraction tactics, raises her groomed eyebrows. She looks at the soup, at me, tells me what's in it, how much good it will do me, and then she points at the spoon again. She may as well say, Open the tunnel, Thomas the Tank Engine is coming. I bring the tip of the spoon to my mouth, close my lips around it, suck the gloop on to my tongue. It lands bang in the middle, spreads out to the sides. I can feel it at the back of my teeth. Then nothing happens. I can't give the command to swallow, and so what feels like liquidised cardboard stays put. It is not accurate to say I have lost my sense of taste. I can't differentiate between sweet, sour, salty, bitter and umami, but the soup tastes of something, I'm just not sure what. Something pasty and unwanted. All food is unwanted. It is the enemy now. It causes me discomfort. It makes me throw up. I don't care if it has positive properties. I can live without it. However, with Estelle perched next to me, I have no choice but to attempt to swallow. I must shift the soup puddle on my tongue. The swallow hurts; the mechanism is inflamed. One of my strengthening exercises is to bite the tip of my tongue and to swallow at the same time. It feels like I am biting my tongue now, deliberately thwarting the act of swallowing. But I am not. I just can't make myself swallow. I keep trying, a tyrannised toddler. I prevail. Down goes the gloop. And so it is with each half-spoonful. I manage half a dozen.

In the days ahead, one egg, scrambled, takes me half an hour to get down, watched over by my sister-in law. Julia makes me a two-egg omelette, a woeful thing, dry and flat. I give up halfway through. When presented with a chickpea stew by my brother, I say I feel nauseous and will eat it later. The truth is, I know the pulses will be too dry and that the fresh lemon juice he has just added will sting. But little by little, the effort of sitting in front of food breaks down my learned habit of repulsion; the prospect of eating becomes less distasteful and by the time a friend brings over a fish stew baked with soft orzo in a clear broth, I get two spoonfuls down in less than five minutes. This is a breakthrough. Another friend brings Jewish chicken soup for the boys and I try it, breaking my no-meat regime in the name of protein. It goes down faster. I put in a request for another delivery. Then the fresh-prod-squad turns up: Lesley, her husband and army supplies of fresh fruit and vegetables, plus a Nutribullet. They've come to teach Richard and the boys how to make me smoothies and juices. I admire their optimism. Getting in the mood, I dig out the unused wheatgrass powder and turmeric Tim the Buddhist gave me months earlier. We try different variations and I drink a whole glass of apple and kale juice. Kale has finally slipped under the radar, like the Nutribullet. Lesley makes another smoothie, fortified with oats and honey this time, and leaves it in the fridge so I can have it after she and her husband have gone.

And there it languishes. Alone, I don't put anything in my mouth. I have zero interest, maximum resistance to a nutritious regime. Left with bags of po-faced fruit and veg and that self-righteous Nutribullet, all I do is snarl. I bet I'm not alone; the pressure to 'beat' cancer with food and supplements is surely felt by most cancer patients, even those who are able to eat and drink. Being reduced to baby food, or old people's food, is way too Seven Ages of Man for my liking. Then, when I do eventually try to have one more bowl of super-food soup, I look for the cream cheese to add to it, but both packets have disappeared. Richard has had the munchies. It's the excuse I need. I skip the gloop.

Orthorexics would be horrified. Health yob! I hear them cry. Cancer troglodyte! They would be purging their bodies of all the toxic drugs by now. Well, I can't be bothered. Nutrition and no life to go with it is gruelling and grim. Food with no social context is bleak, functional, and since that's what food now means to me, I remain out of love with it. The life-enhancing kind is out of my reach. I won't be able to eat full meals in America or even in the foreseeable future, so what's the point in force-feeding myself? In the short term, it's calories I need so I keep my pledge to my nutritionist and, finally, ramp up my Ensure milkshake intake to six a day and eat the odd token bowl of Shreddies, soaked in milk for twenty minutes until they turn to mush. I also shoot up more water. I measure out my days in bathroom dashes.

Which is where Amy the personal trainer comes in. She turns out to be exactly what I need, but not for the reasons I had identified. I wanted someone who could train me back to something approximating functional physical strength. My spine felt rigid, even when I curled up in my tight ball, my knees right into my chest. I did not stretch out my legs on the bed because that made me feel exposed and colder than I did already. My fingers ached. Instinct told me I needed to stretch, but I didn't have the energy either; my mind couldn't stretch to a stretch, couldn't even get to a place where I could contemplate it. I did do stretching, earlier in my treatment, in a yoga class at Healing HQ. I only went three times. It broke my heart, just four or five of us in the class, some women without hair, a man in ordinary trousers and a shirt, sportswear never part of his wardrobe or his world, this new cancer one leading him to a place where the damaged go. The instructor's thoughtfulness was bruising. Was it warm enough? Too hot? Would we like a blanket? If anything is too hard, just stop, she said. I had never been to an exercise class where you're not expected to be hitting targets, pushing yourself. The class reminded me of what you never forget, never for a single moment, but would like to, even at this stage: that you are in a different club now, the cancer club.

Amy is a full-octane force of a woman who knows how to dial down, revealing a generous spirit I didn't even know was there. Why would I? I never looked for it, was never open to it, never needed it. She does frailty, doesn't seem to mind it at all. Using what I suppose is the power of suggestion, she takes me forward. As we stand and breathe and stretch, she surprises me by saying things like: let your body be whole, let your body be free of cancer, let your body heal. And I surprise myself. Instead of doing a quackery audit, the old barriers lift: I hear her words and I let them in. And I think they function at the level of prayer: they are her offering and, by accepting them, I have made an offering to myself.

The boys' Turkish foodie nanny Elif, now an actress, makes an offering herself in the form of her Taiwanese Qi Gong master, Ching-Wen Yang. She recommended him once before, during my chemotherapy, but I forgot about him, didn't know what Qi Gong was, didn't care. It turns out it's another way of moving energy around and, I think, can't do any harm. She tells Mr Yang about me. 'I can help patients with cancer,' he tells her, in an email. At least he doesn't say cure. He checks with Elif that I have finished my chemotherapy. The Qi Gong healing can't have any effect if I haven't, he says; Cindy the healer had said the same thing. Book him, I say. I trust Elif.

I like Mr Yang the moment I meet him. He puts the palms of his hands together and nods and says thank you over and over as he takes his shoes off in the hall. His deference does wonders for the ego; I feel like the Dalai Lama, again. I sit on the sofa. He sits on the other one, in the window, and Elif, who has accompanied him, sits on an armchair. In my pre-cancer life, the calmness he embodies would have made me self-conscious, but I'm better at calm now. I ask him what he's going to do. Heart attack exchange, he says, which sounds a bit Hannibal Lecter. His Taiwanese accent is light on English consonants. I scan you, he continues. I use chi to check your body situation. You say the cancer is here. He points to his neck. I nod. I scan your neck, he continues, then whole body. I do the healing to here. He's got his hand on his neck again. Then disperse, disperse the articles and become healthy cells. Articles. Oh, he means particles, as in particle exchange, not heart attack exchange. That's a relief. We're all particles, apparently; the idea is to get rid of bad ones in exchange for good ones. This treatment might be better suited to quantum physicists, I think. Then relax relax relax internal organs. Internal organs, relaxing. I may have moved quite some way along the we-are-flesh-and-blood front, but relaxing my organs I cannot do. The very idea is repellent.

You lie down now, he says. I lie down on the sofa, everything suddenly tensing tensing tensing. Mr Yang perches by my bare feet. My head is on a cushion. I shut my eyes, and chant like mad in my head. Heal me, heal me, heal me. I need to disperse my scepticism before Mr Yang gets wind of it. I take a peek at him. His own eyes are shut. He is peaceful, rooted. One hand rests on his knee, the other hovers over me, palm down. Presumably it has been moving up and down the length of my body, the stagnant pond. I shut my eyes again and try to give off more flowy, let-the-right-one-in vibes. The minutes pass. Eventually Mr Yang speaks. *Cancer gone.* Two words, no preliminaries. Kapow! My eyes ping open. I don't believe him, obviously. I'll only believe these two words, if and when I hear them, from Blondie or Dr Dish. Still, if Mr Yang's only got two words to say, I'd rather they were 'cancer gone' than, say, 'cancer big'. No problem there, he continues. No stagnation. But I still did some chi particle healing to you. I did healing to you and to your chest. Stagnation there. Breathe more. Chi particle to make your body become healthy cells. In the end I give you some energy. Empowerment, that is term used in Tibetan religion. I disperse energy from your head to your toes to me, and the energy go through your whole body.

Mr Yang stands up and offers to check the energy of the house before he goes. Be my guest. Hand-of-God Howard and his wife sent me some information about how you can get cancer because your bed is in a place of geopathic stress or, if you are already ill, how you can improve your condition by moving your bed to a stress-free position. A practitioner friend of theirs had generously offered to check out my bed by distance dowsing, for free; you might think it's bonkers, Howard said, and I did, especially when I read one of the dowser's case histories, published in an alternative health newsletter. There's only so much end-of-the-pier someone with cancer can take.

John P. was diagnosed with terminal lung cancer and was only given a few weeks to live, so the hospital did not offer him any treatment.

I found that John's bed was on a very strong Geopathically Stressed line. He immediately moved his bed from A to B on my advice. Next morning, he slept from 10 p.m. to 11 a.m., which he had never done before and from then on slept so much better. After dealing with his very high micro parasites, low blood pH, low Q10 levels and using two MagneTechs on his lungs, John soon felt so much better. So when John went back to his hospital, about three weeks later, seeing that he looked so much better, the doctors agreed to treat him.

I mentally filed GS under More Stressful Cancer Quackery; it was the notion of causality that spooked me, and still does. Now, post-treatment, the pressure's off. If Mr Yang wants to chase off any negative energy it's fine by me, though I don't suppose he'll find any. I leave him to it.

I find snake, he says, returning to the living room some minutes later, in your bedroom. Goodness. I can't do snakes. I'd have preferred a rat. I survived one jumping up to bite my bare bottom and felt its nose where it shouldn't be; I was lowering myself on to the lavatory in Uncle George's brownstone in Manhattan when I inadvertently disturbed the helpless rodent. 'That'll teach you to look in the can next time,' Uncle George later quipped.

Elif follows in behind Mr Yang, dangling a metal and copper cobra by the tail. Bad energy, says Mr Yang. Get rid of it. He also recommends putting some amber in the house for its healing properties and I think, how can a stone heal you? I slip him the fee he is too polite to ask for and promise to buy some amber forthwith.

24

LOBSTER ROLLS AHOY

I get my golf buggy at the airport after all. I ordered it myself.
Thank you, cancer. I read in a touchy-feely, hug-your-cancer book
I was given as a gift that it is empowering to say thank you to
your cancer. Well, now I've said it. But only because I frequently
eye up the infirm and overweight whizzing past on mobility
scooters while I, late and laden with hand luggage bulging with
the books, boots and other lead weights offloaded from my
overweight suitcase, stagger to the airport gate.

First, I have to get through security and thence to the invalid
zone where we can pick up the buggy. My medical letters work
like a dream. Three security officers huddle together over them
and my liquid contraband: a litre of water and four Ensure
shakes. The liquids go into a mystery tin box to be scanned.
Then one of the security officers approaches.

'You're all right. Here we are,' she says, returning my precious
stash. 'I know what it's like, needing your liquids like that.'

'Oh, well, yes, it's my salivary gland. I . . .'

'Throat cancer, was it? I had it, a few years back now.
Couldn't swallow for months . . .'

'Really? I'm so sorry.'

'I'm fine now. You pop those back in your bag. And take care.'

Has everyone got cancer? When the writer Michel Faber and I exchanged cancer notes by email, he remarked that the disease is an epidemic. His beloved wife Eva, a gentle spirit whom I had met when I once interviewed Faber, died from myeloma during my own treatment after several years of illness and suffering. Is cancer an epidemic? The answer is yes: as I write, approximately eight million people die from it worldwide every year, though many will survive for more years than ever before. Many recover well, I think, looking at the security officer. I give her a big smile, which is akin to high-fiving a traffic warden. Oh, the paths cancer leads you down. I follow a new one to the invalid desk, as I do like to call it since I am not, let's be honest, an invalid. It is a ringed-off area, bang in the middle of the departure lounge. As I approach the registration desk, alone – Richard and the boys won't cross the threshold – I wobble my head and stick my feet out like a penguin in an affectation of frailty. The Pilates and stair workouts have left me feeling considerably fitter than I had anticipated.

As penance, I have to sit amidst the incapacitated for half an hour before the 'ground transport' officer arrives. He rounds up a gaggle of us and we trip merrily after him, everyone quite mobile. Down a short escalator we go, me barking over my shoulder at Richard and the boys to follow me. But there isn't a single golf buggy to be seen, and much huffing and tutting. Waiting at a bus stop during a London Underground strike would be jollier. One buggy arrives, and is immediately filled – by other people. If I were on my own I would stick my elbows out and get straight in there but Richard and the boys are keeping their distance. Then along comes another buggy, already carrying four passengers. Only the back seat is free, the one where you travel backwards and look out, like we did in my brother's orange Saab as children. Two seats for the four of us, three if we squash up. What to do? Request another buggy, obviously. Richard, however, isn't playing. He is already walking the long walk down to the gate, followed by the boys. They'll regret that when the gate closes on them.

'I am not going on my own,' I call. 'Someone come with me.'

Bassy obliges and we jump on the back.

'We're off!' I say, nudging him. His bowed head is turned away from me. 'What fun.'

The boys hate it when I sound like Miranda Hart but moments like this are made for her. The seat is a lovely cream banquette cushion. I nestle in and happy memories of being shuttled all of 100 metres from luxury villa to luxury sun lounger during an upscale press trip to Parrot Cay in the Turks & Caicos come flooding back. I don't get long to enjoy them, though. We've only just passed the first human conveyor belt of foot passengers when the buggy stops. We're already at our gate, Gate 10. I did clock the gate number back at check-in, and with some disappointment. Ten sounded close, it being so much closer to one than say, 140, which is the high gate number I usually get. But my heart is set on my golf buggy moment, and I stick to the plan.

Richard and Reuben are already at the gate.

When boarding is announced, the queue instantly trebles in size. I toy with the idea of requesting priority boarding, but the boys can only take so much mortification. I make them queue instead, then slink in in front of them at the last minute. Once on board, I hitch up my skirt and pull on my flesh-coloured, elasticated support socks. Forget 1661 and young from the front, old from the back. I'm middle-aged from the waist up, an octogenarian from the thighs down. Half an hour into the seven-hour flight, I am hungry. This provokes a fresh cancer etiquette conundrum. Is tube-feeding in public akin to yanking out your bursting breast and feeding your slurping baby in front of your Edwardian grandfather, which is what I did with my late father-in-law? Taking no chances, I gather up my gear – syringe, Ensure shake, bottle of water and plastic cup – and hog the lavatory for ten minutes as I shoot up. I repeat this three times during the flight; I needn't have bothered with the granny socks. They're for fat people who barely move and order transporter carts at Disneyland or request golf buggies at the airport.

We land at JFK at ten in the evening. Our friend Ford's house in Quogue, somewhere on the South Shore of Long Island, is about sixty miles away. We've been there before and know there's a highway in the middle of the island. Route 27. We decide to head for that, then hang a right. The roads at this time of night will be empty and I'll have a snooze, so Julia needn't have made such a fuss about me getting tired by a long drive. We get on Route 27 without ado, but then come off it inadvertently, and get lost. In the absence of a map, or a satnav, or a phone with Google maps, we're thrown back on our intuition.

'I feel like we are going parallel to the highway we need,' Richard says.

'I know what you mean.'

The skies are wide and the sea feels close.

'If we keep going, we can just cross over and go north.'

'That sounds good.'

It is midnight. I doze off, mouth open and dry, and the dryness keeps waking me up. Famished, I try to have an Ensure shake but I can't get the syringe into the bottle and I've left all my plastic cups in the boot. I nod off again. When I next open my eyes, I spot a sign saying Babylon, which cheers me up because it's near Oak Beach where my cousin Jim has his summer house, only it's on the North Shore, and Quogue is on the South shore. Babylon is west – so far west, in fact, that it's only thirty miles from JFK. We drive over a bridge. There is a lot of water. Great expanses of it, shimmering. Another sign says Robert Moses Causeway. I remember that from my Oak Beach vacations too. Then there is some land, which is hopeful, then some more water, which is less so. We hit a T-junction. Our options are: turn right, into a car park. Turn left, down a sliver of road to Fire Island Lighthouse Visitor Center. Straight on: into the Atlantic Ocean. I don't know what to advise, so shut my eyes. I wake up to the sight of our friend Ford's white clapboard house. Miraculously, Richard has got us to Quogue. I am so pleased to have arrived, I don't notice Ford carrying my holdall inside.

'Wow, that's heavy,' he says, the back door swinging shut behind him.

'Sorry, yes. It's full of milkshakes.'

'Right. I'll leave it in the kitchen then.'

He thinks they are normal milkshakes. I know Richard has explained that I am on medical milkshakes and a feeding tube, but what if he has forgotten?

I wake jet-lag early to soft light and a fix of morning sun. I feel it before I even open the shutters and peer through the mosquito screening. The mesh reminds me of my mask, now face-up on the floor in my study like a *Dr Who* prop no one knows what to do with. I have lofty plans to turn it into an artwork. Richard is fast asleep. I look in on the boys, also fast asleep, as is Truman, Ford's son. Ford is nobly sleeping in the guest cottage in the garden. With the coast clear, I tiptoe down the staircase, turn into the kitchen and, after checking I am still alone, grab the holdall and lug it back upstairs. There is no way I am going to pull up a stool and shoot up while Richard and Ford shoot the breeze over a coffee or a beer, or let Truman or any other child see me with a metre of tubing coming out of my two-belly-button belly.

With the holdall safely stashed away, I come back down, leave a bowl of Shreddies I have brought with me to soak and make myself a cup of Earl Grey tea. My mouth must feel up to it, otherwise it would not have occurred to me to have a cup. I haven't drunk tea, or anything hot, for five months. I take it out on to the deck and settle into a rattan lounger and then feel another urge, this time to read a book. I fetch the one and only novel I have brought for the entire three-week trip and suddenly here I am, sitting beneath a yawning blue sky, the sun hotting up, reading in my PJs, a cup of tea to hand, in our friend's garden in Long Island, America. What a moment.

A few hours later we're on Quogue beach, multi-million dollar celebrity summer houses either side of us, the ocean breaking on the shoreline in lively, lifestyle waves. The boys swim, bodysurf, crash on the caster-sugar sand. Ordinarily I'd be straight in the water. Today I am plonked on a towel, another one covering the bulge underneath my one-piece swimsuit. Richard, Ford and the boys start a game of beach volleyball and after a few minutes a sculpted couple in bikini and Bermuda shorts runs over and joins in. They reach, cheer, lunge, laugh. I film them, zoom out to the grey, shingle-clad gables of Quogue Beach Club up on the dunes behind them, pan across from Bassy jumping blue-skywards to Reuben diving across the sand. But then I feel the call of the milkshake. Not wanting to put a dampener on the Condé Nast scenario, I leg it across the sand and up the boardwalk steps to the restroom. I peel off my one-piece, rolling it down my stomach as fast as I dare without dislodging the two 10 cm^2 waterproof adhesive dressings spread over my feeding tube. I snarl at the dressings. I know I need them; they protect a mutilation, albeit a very minor one, from seawater, should I swim. But a mannequin would feel more sexually attractive than I do now. Ever since

I've had it, I've kept the PEG out of sight. I turn from Richard when I undress, obscuring the 6 cm rubber tube that dangles over my abdomen. I suppose I should swing it about or shake it like a belly dancer, throw in the Dance of the Seven Veils for good measure.

Back on the beach, I clock everybody's tubeless bellies, then turn to the ocean and search for the impulse to run into the waves. More than anything, much more than being active, I would like to have the energy and wherewithal to chat. I miss it. I am with people, but I'm not making connections; it is a particular strain of loneliness. In the evening we pile round Ford's big kitchen table, joined for supper by two more teenage boys. Everyone talks about their day as they tuck into corn on the cob, fries, burgers, salad. I eye up the corn someone's put on my plate, and don't say anything. The kids who've joined us must think I'm a bit creepy. I think I'm a bit creepy, just sitting here like this.

I'm sitting on the floor in our bedroom the next day, surrounded by syringe, glass of water, empty glass, loo roll, adhesive tape and an Ensure shake.

'Are you taking your milkshake?'

It's Bassy, standing in the doorway; I didn't hear him come in.

'I am,' I reply, tugging my T-shirt down over my belly and sweeping the milkshake paraphernalia to one side.

'You don't need to hide in here. There's nothing to be ashamed of.'

I look at him, horribly self-conscious and overwhelmed by his sensitivity all at once.

'You're right,' I say. 'Thanks.'

And he is, sort of. This morning, forgetting to put the bung back after a 'feed', a warm, brown liquid oozed down my belly. I am a sewer, after all. Still, I've got this far without the boys seeing me shooting up, so I'm not changing now. The PEG is disgusting. End of.

Richard makes a reservation to visit Jackson Pollock's house and studio near East Hampton on Long Island's South Fork. I think about dropping in on the cemetery where Father and Granny Fox are buried. I could show the boys the tombstone with my name on it, and no dates, if it's still there, picture myself lying on the grave, trying it for size, the four of us having a laugh. Seeing the family graves might bolster the boys' dubious grasp of their own American heritage and remind them that I had a father, once. But is it normal behaviour to take your children to see the grave of the grandfather they have never known and have barely even heard mention of? Or to take them to see their great-grandmother's grave, given that she's got the same name as their mother, who's got cancer? Worried I might spook them, I bottle out and don't even suggest the visit.

That night, Reuben plays his guitar as we lounge about on the sofas and we sabotage his tunes and make him play rock classics we can sing along to. Truman, who has known Reuben since they were babes-in-arms, takes the lead on 'Hotel California', followed by 'I Would Walk 500 Miles' and then, song of songs, Johnny Cash's 'Ring of Fire'. We belt them out like we're holding Wembley Arena. Karaoke dreaming: it is worth flying over to America for this evening alone. It's a liberating, inhabiting-the-moment high, a life-fix that won't let me countenance letting life go.

For the next leg of our trip, we have to get from Quogue up to Lakeville, Connecticut. Once again, it's not far. As the crow flies, it's a straight north across the Long Island Sound, and then a left after 100 miles or so. Ford takes a less ornithological approach and produces a road map. He spreads it out on the table and explains the route as one might to an extraterrestrial on his first road trip. Taking no chances, I have already asked our hosts, Andrea and David, to email directions. They'll sympathise. Once, leaving their summer rental house in Millerton, New York for the City, we dropped the directions in their driveway and the Royal We did not want to lose face by going back to ask for some more. It took us four hours to make the two-hour journey back to the City.

Thanks to the Ford–Andrea power axis, we pitch up at the picket-fence strip of a village in the foothills of the Berkshires on schedule. Andrea gives me a hug and I think, careful girl, you don't know what you're hugging. I'm different, damaged, not the cheery thing you're used to. We met when we were on our honeymoons in Costa Rica and over the years we've only ever done good times together, with just a sprinkle of life-is-hard. David is a cross between Larry David and Woody Allen, with a sideline in self-deprecation so deep it hurts. We laugh together, we lament the glory days that have not come, we look back at the days when David had an abundance of hair. He carries a photograph in his wallet of himself with a head of curls as proof. And now this.

I needn't have worried. From the moment I walk across their porch everything feels all right. Come, be poorly, Andrea says, do what you need to do. We're here. We'll look after you. She opens the fridge. See, I've bought you yoghurts and soups. We'll get you anything you need. Just ask. Take naps whenever you feel like it. And over the next few days I do, on the sofa, on the deck in the balmy sunshine, up in our cosy guest bedroom under fresh, white, crisp sheets that the Dutch Airbnb barge owner could only dream of. He'd like the walk-in wardrobe, too; there's room for a year's supply of old Y-fronts and rubber slippers in there.

One morning we are down at Lake Wononscopomuc by the water's edge, with Andrea and David's two boys and our own, just back from basketball and about to go swimming. Suddenly Andrea jumps up.

'Oh, look,' she says, 'they are going to do the ice bucket challenge!'

A young woman is standing on the jetty in a bikini. A man is standing next to her with a bucket.

'Henry! Lucas! Quick. It's the ice bucket!'

'Really? The ice bucket challenge?'

Andrea's boys hurry over to their mother and stand alongside her. Richard and I look on as the man raises the bucket. Shrieks go up, the bucket goes down over the young woman's head and drenches her. She shakes herself down like a wet Labrador, lets out a triumphant 'I did it!' The handful of onlookers cheers. The public soaking turns out to be part of a phenomenally successful fundraising stint for the progressive neurodegenerative disease ALS (Amyotrophic lateral sclerosis). We see buckets and drenched heads again and again during the trip. It's the charity sensation *du jour*. I am stupefied. When did fundraising for a chronic disease become such a hoot? I hate the community spirit of it all, the knee-jerk jolliness – a fact I tell no one, except Richard. He knows what I'm like.

When the community spirit is focused on me a week later, I find it altogether more endearing. In Princeton, where we are staying with our old friends Vivian and Frank and their two teenage daughters, Oona and Maisie, we're sitting round the firepit one night in their garden overlooking Lake Carnegie. After a day of untaxing kayaking and very slow cycling through poised, picture-perfect Princeton, we're toasting s'mores and playing campfire games. After a while Reuben and Maisie bring out their guitars. In a lull between songs, Maisie says she has written me a song.

'I could sing it, if you like.'

I am amazed and of course I say yes. Her voice is deep and soulful, the song is jazzy and rises into a four-line refrain:

Well some day can't you tell
You'll be singing along as well
Oh Genevieve
Just trust me, Genevieve.

Maisie the fourteen-year-old jazz singer, embodiment of youth and tomorrows and a self-righting universe, invokes a time when I am no longer tongue-tied and I'm singing as well, back in the gang, joining in. It's just a matter of trust. *Trust me.* What a song. What a girl. What fine community spirit.

Philadelphia is the next pit stop. We'll be staying with Richard's old friend Darryl, a man with a smile like the Grand Canyon, and a deep, infectious laugh. He's more feelgood than Dolly Parton. Despite how much I look forward to seeing him, I get old-person agitated at the thought of getting there, me the planner and logistics queen. I worry about the train ride up, about walking around in a city I don't know, about taking my milkshakes, finding public restrooms when I need them, not being able to make conversation, or eat. I worry about all sorts of things I didn't know it was possible to worry about. In the end I become so anxious, I hide in bed in the middle of a sunny afternoon and curl up, tight. It's a relapse: I can't cope. I want everything to go away, and for me not to have to do or be anything. But a few days later we get there, of course we do, and everything is an effort and the effort is worthwhile and we have fun.

We run up the Rocky Steps, every last one, at the Philadelphia Museum of Art. Then we do a marathon of a walk down horribly long South Street to get to Jim's, home of the ultimate Philly cheesesteak sandwich. I've peaked. The walk is too long and I am so tired and I don't have it in me to say, sorry guys, I can't do this. Jim's is an art deco dream, all black shiny tiles and chrome. It's got a walk-up counter and serves quite the most alarming sandwiches I have ever seen. Bits of shredded brown meat in a hot dog roll with cheese whizz down one side. Bet you wish you had a PEG, I nearly say to the boys when they get their order. We walk the 75 million miles back to Darryl's house and everyone, including Richard and Darryl, take a nap. This chuffs me to bits. It's not just me who is tired by tourist traipsing about.

Darryl and his partner, Coy, are foodies, which would be a happy chance for me, the former foodie, but obviously isn't. They take us to a British gastropub inspired by 'London's culinary revolution'. I sulk on the way, wishing I could tuck in when we get there. Then I see the menu. Highlights include rabbit pie and duck bolognese. It's a farmyard massacre, a pescatarian's bad dream. I order soup. Walking home, Coy, an oncology nurse, talks about getting over cancer himself the year before. How is it that even an oncology nurse can get cancer? That really does not seem fair. He tells me how excellent his treatment was but how profoundly lonely he found the experience, talking with an openness and clarity that amazes me. He is not at all self-conscious about it, does not even lower his voice or steer us out of earshot of the others. He then asks me questions that only another cancer sufferer can ask. We talk about the side effects and how you try to carry on and get back to normal, even as the demons of fear play havoc with your mind. The conversation injects me with a shot of something I didn't know I needed; it boosts me for the rest of the trip. He's made me see how detachment and loneliness gets under your skin, it's what you take with you when you slope off for your nap, what you contend with when you are sitting with friends and not talking; and what a lifeline it is to talk to people who know what you are going through, not just during the treatment, but now, in this far more nebulous, hard-to-navigate recovery period.

On the news that evening an American doctor cured of Ebola in an Atlanta hospital makes the headlines. In his survivor interview, standing beside the doctors who have treated him and whom he thanks, he says that God saved his life.

'It's not God that has cured him,' I say. 'It's the doctors.'

'You've changed your tune,' Richard says. The boys weigh in on a similar vein.

But I haven't changed my tune. Disease is not God's department. God is not a person. I am not an idiot.

Back in Princeton, with a week to go before we fly home, I start fixating on the results of my treatment, running through the probabilities of success over and over. I'll get the results three days after we get back. I keep returning to that phrase from Maisie's song: trust me. I want it to be a new mantra, but the 'what if' balloons are closing in. It's all I can do to ignore them. Part of me wants to be back in England now, so I can get this stage over and done with, whatever the outcome. I've been sleeping well. Now I am not sleeping.

We finish our trip in New York and do all our favourite things, and our favourite thing first. We have breakfast in 3 Guys on Madison, the Upper East Side classic diner a poodle's throw from the Carlyle hotel, otherwise known as heaven on earth. My sister and I used to stay at the Carlyle when Chauncey had an apartment on one of the top floors. If the cook had not come down with us from Wethersfield, we'd order room service. Burgers would arrive inside big silver domes wheeled in on a trolley that turned into a dining table, duly dressed in white linen and silver cutlery. After 3 Guys we hire radio-controlled sail boats on Conservatory Water, the boating pond in Central Park, just a block away from Granny Fox's last home in the

Volney hotel, now an apartment block. We first hired the model sail boats with the boys when they were seven and nine. It is a simple and timeless pastime and the most enchanting thing you can do in the City. The day we go, a quartet is playing jazz in the Kerbs Boathouse café behind us. It doesn't get much better than this.

We've done all the big sights with the boys in the past so we go to the Whitney next, walk the High Line, get upscale take-out at the foodie mecca, Chelsea Market. Reuben gets the obligatory lobster roll from the heaving, buzzing Lobster Place and I look on approvingly – and, joy of joys, longingly – as he tucks into our favourite fast food.

'Want a bite?' he says. 'You said you would be eating lobster rolls by the time we got to America.'

'I won't, thanks. But I will. Soon.' I want to sing Maisie's 'Trust me!' but don't, because we're in public and it would embarrass him. There's also the fact that I might not be eating again soon. I've already broken one promise, to be eating by Bassy's birthday, and now I've broken another by not eating lobster rolls on this vacation.

That night, I make a decision. I'm not doing the feeding tube for a day longer. I've got to get back to eating normally. I can't bear the thought of a life without food at the centre of it. In the morning, I chuck out my syringes. From now on, I will only take my six medical milkshakes a day with a straw and I will also try to get fresh nutrients into my system. A body-as-temple zeal seizes me, at last, and I become perilously obsessed by fresh smoothies and super-juices. I stock up the refrigerator with them and then, when I go out shopping for last-minute gifts with the boys, I buy one from any juice bar I pass. There are a lot of juice bars in Manhattan. The increase in medical shakes, smoothies and juices and my reduction in morphine join forces, making for a memorable few days. One unholy tidal wave after another follows me up and down the streets. I don't get much shopping done, but I could write a guidebook on crashable restrooms in Lower Manhattan.

On our last day Richard goes to The Frick and the boys and I take the aerial tram to Roosevelt Island. They're not very enthusiastic about going. 'It used to be called Welfare Island,' I chirp, 'and it had an asylum!' They are strangely unmoved. I have to cluck and cajole them into coming, which goes to show another thing: you can have cancer, but your teenage children still moan. For my part, I am simply trying to think of something else to do. If it were just me, I would go back to the apartment on the Upper East Side, treat myself to a glass of cold milk, and take a nap. Still, I am looking forward to seeing the views of east Manhattan from the vantage point of the island. We're about twenty blocks away. Two blocks in, what I suddenly look forward to way more is the use of the restroom facilities at the tram terminus on East 66th Street. I lead the charge like a power walker on steroids. But the terminus turns out to be just a booth with a man in it, no nice restroom to be seen. I stick my face up to the glass and mouth the million-dollar question I don't want the boys to hear.

'Pardon me, ma'am?' The man is speaking into a microphone; his voice booms through the bulletproof glass.

I repeat myself, whispering this time, 'Are there restrooms? You know. On the other side?' My phrasing is off; I sound like I am speaking to the Ferryman of the Dead. The boys, nosey as ever, come over to see what's going on.

'Restrooms, ma'am? On the island? Oh, yes ma'am. Plenty of restrooms.'

There's no dignity in cancer, and no secrets. The tram crosses the East River parallel to the Queensboro Bridge. We're so close to it you can almost see the brush strokes on the creamy apricot steel beams. I spot the cheery finials atop the cheery stone towers and feel sudden fury. It's just a bridge. Why all the attention to detail? I bet whoever designed it wanted to go down in history, that's why, and good for them but bad for me, because it makes me think of time and what if, when we get home, I find out the treatment has failed and my time is up and, more critically, what if I don't get to the public convenience in time?

We finally arrive on the other side and step out into what feels like Canary Wharf before they imported human beings, not a recognisable building in sight. I run this way and that, more frantic than a dog on the scent of a fresh, fleshy bone. Finally I identify a modern bunker of a public convenience and make an emergency dash. When I emerge the world looks rosy again; apricot, even. It's Peggy's B-functions that have made me feel mortal and cantankerous, not the poor Queensboro Bridge. I must try to get some perspective.

We walk past the ruins of the old Smallpox Hospital, a dour nineteenth-century Gothic Revival that sits like a Romantic folly near the southernmost tip of the narrow, two-mile-long island. But it's no folly. Both the poor and the wealthy came here to be treated and, mostly, to die. In 1869, the hospital's first unclaimed cadaver, that of a twenty-four-year-old orphan called Louisa Van Slyke, was transported downriver to a potter's field on Hart Island, New York's public cemetery off the Bronx coastline. Today about a million more deceased wards of the City, as those without attachments are known, are buried along with Louisa Van Slyke in unmarked trenches. How wretched. I've always thought that families were the building block of society, and orphans the rubble in the pile. But look what can be built from rubble. Roosevelt Island is part landfill, part original land. Here it is now, home to Freedom Park and a six-foot bronze statue of President Franklin D. Roosevelt. The egalitarian visionary redefined the American Dream, a phrase coined by the historian James Truslow Adams in his 1931 bestseller *The Epic of America*, the very book whose spine Father had daubed in Tipp-Ex and which I had noticed after swiping a cobweb and nearly falling through my study window.

I didn't know then that this history of the American people contained the famous phrase, its evocation of the ideals of economic equality and meritocracy re-appropriated many times since. But I do by the time I am standing on the edge of Roosevelt Island, the boys beside me, the muscular East River racing around us and beneath us. I think to myself, this is my American dream, right here, with the boys, Richard nearby, my family.

Where we are standing, the diamond-shaped island is just twenty feet wide. The plaza's low outer walls are monumental slabs of white granite. They are beautiful and a feat of the imagination, and they are here to protect us. Without them, our position would be precarious.

25

RESULTS DAY

Everything is normal, everything hangs in the air. Reuben went back to school yesterday, Bassy the day before. I get my results at 3.20 p.m. Richard is coming from work and meeting me at Healing HQ; the casual hook-up is our ploy to downplay the appointment. At 1 p.m. I am still in bed, not from jet lag or fatigue but because Dr Dish might pull up his chair close to mine, look solemnly into my eyes and ask me how I am before saying 'sorry but' and then 'the treatment hasn't worked.' I can cope if he tells me I have to have neck surgery, followed by more chemotherapy. Anything worse, and I can't promise much. It is hard to see how a mother given a terminal diagnosis can function. How does she even get to a place in her head that enables her to live for each minute and each day, and how does she love her children enough as the minutes tick by? She must agonise about the quality of the love, the density of it, its durability, whether it is bankable. She must question whether she has given her children enough love to last them after she has gone.

At 1.30 p.m. I drag myself out of bed, shower, put on my favourite top Richard gave me – flouncy, sleeveless, covered in tiny purple, pink and yellow flowers – and blue jeans, and make-up, too. I haven't worn make-up for a hospital visit since Diagnosis Day. Today I want me back, the superficial one who minds about appearances, not the one forever looking inwards, circling her interior world. I take Pepper for a walk and before I know it, I am rushing. I am often late, but to be so today feels wrong, disrespectful, like being late for a funeral.

I get to Warren Street tube station and to Healing HQ on autopilot. Take a right out of the Tube, a left down Beaumont Place and a right down Huntley Street. It's a short distance, freighted with memories. Today I half walk, half run the gauntlet, and sleepwalk through the automatic doors. Each time I arrive I can't believe it's me heading through those doors. Today is no different. Ten months have passed and I still can't believe that it's me who's got cancer either – or maybe not got it, any more. I wonder if that disbelief ever goes away, for any cancer sufferer.

I walk past the Macmillan volunteer at the main reception desk and the waiting patients, no grimacing at wigs and bald women now, all of us in it together. Up the spiral stairs I go, up to my world of head and neck cancer and the medical elite who devote themselves to it. It is a busy Head and Neck clinic today. There are only two seats free. A man moves his bag for me and I sit down next to him. Wednesday clinic is like Grand Central Station: rammed. I look out for Richard, but don't look at anyone else. I used to, during treatment, guessing at who were the patients and who were the relatives or friends. Often, it is obvious: half a sunken face or a metal mesh in the middle of a neck is a bit of a giveaway. Usually, I look at them and I think, I'm sorry for you. Not today. Today I don't want to be in the cancer club and, selfishly and appallingly, I don't want an inkling of anyone's suffering. The empathy that comes with cancer can be lacerating. I want to switch mine off. Richard arrives, and together we spot one of the Macmillan nurses standing by the reception desk. I will her to keep away from me. 'Hello Genevieve,' she says. Reluctantly, I return the greeting. I've just reminded Richard – as if he needed reminding – that if there is more than one member of staff in the consulting room when I am called in, then the news is bad. A Macmillan nurse in the room is the human equivalent of a box of tissues.

'Genevieve Fox.' A doctor I have never seen before calls my name. My mind computes his stranger status. If I need surgery, then surely Dr Dish would be seeing me today. If it is more chemotherapy I need, it would be Blondie. Richard and I get up and follow the doctor. To my horror, the Macmillan nurse walks alongside us. Get away from me, I hiss in my mind. I don't smile at her. I don't even acknowledge her, which is rude. She makes me feel contaminated. I can't do this, I think, I can't go through more treatment. I want Richard to hold me and keep me in what now seems like a state of blissful hope, benign limbo. Having longed for this time to come, I want time to stand still.

The doctor heads towards one of the consulting rooms. We follow. Just before he enters, the Macmillan nurse peels off and goes into the room before it. Yes! We've shaken her off. The consulting room is empty. Not a single other human being in it. Empty, save for three plastic chairs, a consulting couch, a desk and computer.

The oncologist looks at the screen. He frowns, looks down at his notes, looks back at the screen. I crash. The front of my head is full of wires, fizzing. In this momentary hiatus, my future, our future, the emotional well-being of Reuben and Bassy, and of Richard, too, is a blackout. I can't see it. During the walk to Healing HQ I prayed that I would be given the strength to be brave if the results were bad and I had to go through more treatment. I rehearsed the wording to the boys: 'Just some surgery and then a bit more chemotherapy.' Just.

'The MRI scan was fine,' the doctor says, turning from his screen to me, and quickly back to his screen again. There is no sense of occasion in his voice, no hurrah in it at all. Richard grabs my hand.

'Well done,' he says. I grin. He grins back.

'All the other results are fine. Fine, fine, fine, fine, fine.' Evidently, he is looking at a list of tests but I don't know what they were for and I don't care, either.

'We did a lot of work to try to find the primary,' he continues, 'but we never found it.' He is reading my notes for the first time.

'No, we didn't,' I reply, wondering where this is leading to.

'It only takes one malignant cell to form a cancer.' I picture a cell, see a black nucleus, grind my teeth at the thought of it. Could one still be hiding somewhere?

'Just to clarify,' I say, heaving my heart into my mouth, 'am I now cancer-free?'

'Yes.'

'And the hidden primary, which has never been found, has that been destroyed by the treatment, or could it still be lurking somewhere?'

'It has been destroyed.'

If angels are weightless, then I envy them. Released from fear, I am weightless, too, barely corporeal, and it feels great. I could go anywhere, do anything: I am utterly and completely happy. Not elated, not at this very moment; the elation comes a few minutes later. In this moment I feel peaceful; it is a moment of simplicity, of clarity. I have been given my life back. The ferryman has been cheated. I am back on Planet Earth, back in the club of the living. I feel my feet, and I root into the earth. My body fills out. I am corporeal again.

I am of this earth, but I have also been given wings, the wings I asked for when I had to tell the boys I had cancer and had only arms to protect them, inadequate, not fit for purpose. Today I have wings for them to lean into.

I have opened my arms, and now this gift is given.

I have returned, 'Wing'd-with-Awe, inviolable.'

I am suspended in this state of gratitude and racing-river joy as the registrar explains that I will be seen in clinic once a month for the next year and every three months for an ultrasound scan; every two months the year after; and every three months the year after that. I listen attentively, not like Diagnosis Day, when words washed over me.

We thank the doctor much as one would a GP who has prescribed routine antibiotics, and when we are back in the corridor, Richard puts his arm around me and says well done again. On the way through reception and the waiting patients I make sure I don't smile. I feel guilty, as if I have been let off and they haven't. Is that how an inmate feels when let out of prison, leaving everyone else behind? Or how survivors of a fire feel as they stumble over corpses?

At the foot of the stairs, I skip past a row of pink seats in the main reception, all occupied.

'Save that for outside,' Richard whispers.

And then we are out of the main door and standing on the sidewalk and our arms are around each other. We don't say anything. The relief coursing through us is enough. We have each other back, a shared future, permission to plan again. Richard takes my hand. We walk to the Tube; it is a lifetime since we did this same walk on Diagnosis Day nearly ten months earlier. I say goodbye to Richard and off he goes, back to work, and I go home. It is an unremarkable parting; we slot right back into normality. It is as though we have never been away.

I get home with only ten minutes to spare before the boys are due home from school. Like one of the psychologist's balloons, I am fit to pop. I cannot wait to break the good news. Bassy gets back first, but I want to tell both boys at the same time. I hug him even tighter than I usually do, he squirms and I, for some reason, start yodelling. *Ho-la-la-ee-ay! Ho-la-la-ee-ay!* Bassy shoots me one of his embarrassing mother looks and heads down to the kitchen for a snack. Five more minutes pass, during which I walk up and down the short hall, look out of the living-room window, sit on the sofa, stand up again. Reuben is by now all of three minutes later than he usually is. I call him on his mobile.

'Where are you?'

'I'm walking home.'

'Good. Hurry up!'

'Why? Are you locked out?'

'No. I just need to talk to you.'

That last bit is probably a mistake. They both know I had a hospital appointment this afternoon, though they don't know we were getting the final results.

Reuben is barely through the front door when I summon him, and Bassy, into the living room. 'Sit down,' I say. There is levity in my voice, so I know I am not alarming them, and I've chosen the upstairs living room to break the news. The scene is in every way different to last time: no dead mother on the sofa, no sorrow, no need for obfuscation. The only similarity is that the boys sit either side of me on the sofa.

'We've got good news. You know I was at the hospital today. Well, the treatment was successful. I am cancer-free.'

'Yay!' says Reuben. 'Well done.'

'Well done,' says Bassy.

Their arms are around me. I explain that I will still be going to hospital, regularly, for the next two to three years but that the appointments are never anything to worry about. I don't tell them that if the cancer were to come back, it is most likely to do so in the first two years. They don't need to hear that. I am cancer-free and I want them to be worry-free.

'Can I go down and get something else to eat?' asks Bassy.

Reuben stays with me, hugs me again, tells me he is proud of me. And then he asks:

'When will you be normal?'

I didn't know I ever was, and feel momentarily flattered.

'You mean, when will I be eating again?'

He nods.

'Soon,' I say. 'By your birthday. By Christmas.'

26

RIPPLE EFFECTS

Twenty-four hours after the results I am jiving, spinning, spun out with joy.

Steady, says a voice in my head. You are so quick to be on a high, you haven't even paused to reflect on it all. You're heading for a fall.

Bugger off, I say back. I'll be delirious if I want to.

A week later, I wake up to a text message from Fliff.

How is cancer-free life a week on?

Bloody marvellous, I text back.

You get the green beret, Marine Commando.

I've reached those sunny uplands I dared to dream of ten months earlier. I've got my family back. I do Mum-dancing in the kitchen, with no music. This is the new spectacular: one moment and then another, one minute and then another, hours, days, all so miraculously ordinary; I am back in time, not fighting it. I am a signed-up, functioning player in the continuum of time, not an outsider, stuck on the periphery, jealously watching the well. Fear has skulked off, and real-life anxieties about work and money are lying low.

A month later, the plates shift as a new, post-cancer landscape forms. The emotional aftershocks take me by surprise. There are six of them, and they come after me like the San Andreas Fault. The first, which follows the initial elation after getting the results, is impatience. Then there's gratitude, guilt, compassion, fear and, finally, a sense of failure.

I am wildly impatient for everything to be normal. I want to be able to take control of my eating and to speed up the healing process, end the exhaustion, stop all the internal processing: my mind is a firecracker. Julia and I go to church and there is a sermon about patience, based on Matthew's Gospel. I am incredulous. This is exactly what I need to hear. I want to put my hand up and shout, 'Coo-ee! Over here. Yes, me, thanks for that.' I am emotionally incontinent, and a liability. The old me – or is it the new me? – says: calm down, shut up. Not everything is all about you. Isn't it?

I go and see Dr Suleman and tell him I want to be normal. Too late for that, he might say, if he knew me better. I explain that I want to stop thinking about having had cancer, I want to stop fretting about if and when it will come back, and I want to know how to manage the anxiety caused by still being unable to swallow and eat properly, and more besides. Other people, I tell him, seem to think everything is dandy. When they say: it's so great that you are better, or, it's so great that you are back to normal, I don't know how to respond. I know, I hear myself reply, isn't it fantastic! and that makes me feel alone with my non-normal, wanting-to-be-back-to-normal self. But I can't bang on about how I feel and I also know that friends need to be let off the hook at some stage. I've outstayed my welcome, as it were. But privately the N-word sticks in my sore throat. I don't know how to answer when people ask me how I am. I know the rules. I wrote them, so I say 'great'. They've done their bit. I am releasing them, but tying myself in knots.

Dr Suleman seems to think what I have said is perfectly normal, though of course he does not use that word. Yours is a common response, he says, and he has a solution:

'Have some answers ready that will work for you when people ask you how you are,' he suggests, 'such as: I am doing well, thank you, I am on the road to recovery. Or, the recovery is going well.'

The insertion of the word 'recovery' is the ticket. It is simple, straightforward advice, and it is immeasurably helpful.

It is about this time, some four weeks after getting the results, that the PEG is removed. Halle-bleedin'-lujah. Having two belly buttons may be a bit Victorian freak show, but at least I am on the right track for eating solid food again. I am so grateful.

The trouble is, I am grateful for everything. This is the second aftershock. I walk down our ordinary mishmash of a street in Tufnell Park and I think, wow, such good paving stones, some people won't have paving stones like this. I buy an overpriced takeaway soup that is too spicy for my damaged taste buds and I think, I am so lucky to live in the First World and to be able to buy soup. I choke on a slice of red pepper I have foolishly tried to eat and I think about how fortunate I am to be even trying it. I put some laundry on and I think: this is really fantastic, look at me pulling the dirty clothes out of the basket and putting them in the washing machine, just like that. Somebody tell me: Is this the cancer gremlins, having the last laugh?

Walking on Hampstead Heath is particularly perilous. Grass, leaves, twigs, gnarly nodules on twigs, I compulsively acknowledge them, and then thank each and every one of them. I try to do the same with everything I see. The sky, the sun. It doesn't matter what the sun's doing – even when it is hidden behind a dark cloud, I think, I know you're up there, and my indebted heart comes over all rapturous. I pity

Emerson and those Transcendentalists, and Wordsworth and Coleridge on this side of the pond; I never realised what a lot of energy it took, being moved by nature all the time. Wordsworth and Coleridge had peasants to pity, too. I don't see any of those on Hampstead Heath but I do walk past my 'cancer tree' – it's just a tree halfway up the hill that leads to Kenwood but it's the one I was walking past when I had a premonition of the diagnosis. I photographed it so I could record the moment of knowing. Looking at it now triggers a surge of gratitude. But what has that tree ever done for me? Nothing. Nonetheless I feel grateful to it, and to all trees; feel grateful to be living, just like my cancer tree, and for everything around me. The expression 'fit to burst' was made for me. I open my arms and put my face up to the sky and, ignoring the dog-walkers in both directions on the path, I shout thank you. I want everyone, everything, the whole darn interconnected universe, to know that I am grateful and that I don't take my lucky ticket for granted. Is this normal, post-cancer behaviour?

I ask Dr Suleman. I tell him about the voices in my head and the emotional surges and how I can't think for all the things I have to thank every second of every minute.

'Are you religious?' he asks.

'No,' I say, because that's the simplest answer, plus I want to know if a person would feel like me if they didn't have a sense that there was a spiritual dimension to existence.

'Why?' I ask.

'Because you sound a bit hard on yourself.'

'I just want people to know I am grateful.'

'How could you measure your gratitude?'

'What do you mean?'

'How could you go about showing people how grateful you are? What would be the proof?'

I think for a long time before replying. 'I don't know.'

'That's because there isn't a measure for gratitude. You could go on and on, pushing yourself to be more and more grateful. But you could never be grateful enough because you've got no way of measuring it.'

'Hmmm.'

'So give yourself a break.'

What a relief to be let off the hook. But there's a catch: I am grateful to have survived, and that triggers the third aftershock: guilt. I feel guilty that I got off so lightly, and obsess about all the people who are so much worse off than I am, or did not make it. Survivor's guilt consumes me. The writer Michel Faber recently came to stay and as we sat in the living room talking he broke off, returning from the hall with his overnight bag. He fished out the sheaf of poems he had written about his late wife Eva, and then a pair of red shoes, Eva's shoes. He explained that he carried them with him everywhere he went and that when he was somewhere that he felt she would have liked to be herself, he brought them out. He duly placed them at the feet of the lime-green armchair in which he was sitting, and read us scorching poems about what Eva had to endure, their love, and his universe-altering loss. I watched Reuben's reaction as Faber read, saw his eyes widen. 'They were so sad,' he said the next day after Michel had gone. For my part, I was simply appalled that I made it, and she didn't, this woman I had only met once.

A few days later, I am back on Parliament Hill with the dog and am grappling with the shame of my survivor's guilt, when my thoughts turn to Primo Levi. I catch myself wanting to say to the Italian Jewish chemist, I know how you feel. But Primo Levi was a Holocaust survivor, and all I have had is stage 1b cancer. What am I doing having Holocaust survivors and myself in the same thought? It is obscene. So is my preoccupation with myself when people are dying and being tortured in Syria and child refugees are drowning in the Mediterranean; people are suffering all over the world, properly, unfathomably suffering. My survivor's guilt and concomitant self-loathing are intensified by unprecedented levels of compassion. With this fourth aftershock, it's as if the cancer has wired me up to the suffering of others, suffering which is ordinarily invisible, at least to me. I think that when cancer survivors say they see the world differently, they may, in part, be referring to a heightened capacity for compassion. In my case though it's like an itch you can't scratch: I have the *capacity* for compassion but don't act on it, so it really bothers me, as does the fact that I evidently wasn't compassionate before. Or compassionate enough. What this means in practice is, I'll turn up for a check-up at UCLH, say, and see the sick and the dying, the blindfold I was trying to keep on when I first pitched up here ten months ago now ripped away. But to what end? I can't take away the anguish I now know they must be feeling, and I am left feeling deeply sorrowful, as well as guilty and inadequate all over again.

Meanwhile, there's a new killjoy at the party: what if the cancer comes back? I try hard not to think about this, but functional changes – from impaired eating and diminished taste to the discomfort whenever I yawn – keep my mind focused on the cancer I am hoping I no longer have and the fear of its return. This is the fifth aftershock, and its ripple effects are especially unnerving. When I mention this fact, a friend casually mentions that he has read 'somewhere' that you're more likely to get a second cancer if you've been treated for a first. Hello, what? This is news to me. This time, instead of going on the Internet, I ask Hans the cancer supremo to tell me that this friend is talking nonsense. To which Hans replies, in the plain English I asked for but now wish I hadn't, that yes, a second cancer can develop. 'In essence,' he explains, 'cancer is a genetic disease and cancer cells have relatively large numbers of mutations of their DNA. The chemotherapy and radiation therapy used to kill cancer cells can also cause mutations in the DNA of normal cells. This can explain the observation that the risk of developing a second cancer is slightly increased by the treatment used to get rid of the first cancer. This sounds a bit depressing but remember: the risk of a second cancer remains low compared to the massive benefits of getting rid of an existing cancer. I should also say that 5FU' – one of my two chemotherapy drugs – 'is much safer than other chemotherapy drugs which cause higher levels of mutations.'

Right. That's good then. So, I think, is the fact that were my head and neck cancer to return, it is most likely to recur within the first twenty-four months. When, nine months after the radiotherapy, a routine scan reveals a new lump and a biopsy is taken, I should not be knocked for six, but I am. On the plus side, during the five days we wait for the results, I think, it's OK, I can do this. I thought I wouldn't be able to do more cancer, but I can. Round one has prepared me and got me to the point where I can get my house in order and, if everything goes wrong, do a good handover for Richard. And he will be there for the boys, no better father beneath the visiting moon, no bond stronger. I'm on the other side of my worst fear, my love will endure. I've already had my happy ending: I've discovered the measure of love, and can let go.

The lump turns out to be a false alarm. At ease, then. But, the pressure on me to be even more grateful for what I have right now intensifies. It also prevents me from gaining the psychological distance from the disease I need in order to go back to my old life. Except that there is no going back to my old life. The fear, it turns out, is part of the abnormal new normal of living post-cancer.

'It's like a burglar has got a set of your house keys,' as one cancer survivor put it. 'You never know when they are going to let themselves in.'

The wretched journey metaphor resurfaces next. I have survived Mordor, but have nothing to show for it. Having refused to see cancer as a journey, I nevertheless feel I have fallen short of what is expected of a cancer survivor. The next time I see Dr Suleman I tell him what a failed cancer person I am.

'In what way?'

'I'm supposed to be different.'

'In what way?'

'Better. I'm supposed to be a better person.'

'Who says?'

'Everyone. Everyone says that when you have cancer it's a transformative experience. You see everything differently, and you become good.'

'So how do you see yourself now?'

In that hell between Amsterdam and America, Eco Debbie and her partner went into our garden and planted some chard while I was lying on the sofa. I hate the stuff, and the plant is ugly, but I was too weak to protest. Last week I dug the plants up and put them in the bin.

'Well . . .'

I recently received a text from a homeless charity thanking me for volunteering at a night shelter. I only went twice. The second time, I got locked into a conversation with a former chess champion. On and on he went. I thought: you are egotistical and a bore. Which obviously isn't a very nice thing to think, especially of a homeless person, and yet here I am now, thinking about accepting the invitation. Indeed, I puff up at the very thought.

I decide against sharing these Old Me stories with Dr Suleman, and instead I say: 'Well, you know, room for improvement.'

'Were you good enough? Did you like your old self?'

I've told a few people the night shelter anecdote. The very telling of it lets people know I signed up for a homeless charity, ergo I am a good person. The way to avoid this misunderstanding would have been for me to hold my tongue, to coin a phrase. But holding my tongue is hard for me, proof that in that way, at least, I am back to normal.

'My old self. Hmmm. It was all right, I suppose. Flawed, as I say.' He doesn't know the half of it. 'But yes, I suppose I did like it.'

'Then go back to your old self. Go back to who you were before. I give you permission.'

'Really? No transformation?'

'No transformation.'

I am in my bedroom, sorting through a clothes molehill when a programme about self-love comes on the radio. I latch on to it as to a new scientific discovery, with me the one who has made the discovery. I've got it, I think, sitting on my bed, you need self-love when you are sick, otherwise it is impossible to accept that you need looking after, that you are worth looking after, and that you are entitled to take the love that is being offered to you. It is like being a mother to your self; and what mother would not try to heal her own child with love, after all?

If self-love and maternal love are linked, I've been astoundingly slow on the uptake. On the plus side, my fear of being lost to the boys and of them losing me seems, paradoxically, to have awakened me to the power and reach of a love which, in turn, has revealed its multifarious nature. I thought I knew love's value, but I had not grasped its essence, its immutability and its constancy. In the same way that I've learned the art of motherhood as I go along – as all mothers do – my initiation into chronic disease management and vulnerability appears to have given me an experiential knowledge of love. I know what the form is now. You need to let love in. You don't just give, you take, and the taking both enriches your own giving and increases your capacity to give. Not only am I back in time, I have also taken my place in the continuum of love. It is one side effect my Macmillan team didn't tell me about.

After my half-sister died I inherited the portrait of her by Duncan Grant and two of his watercolours, entitled *Madonna and Child: After Raphael*. I've kept them in a drawer. They are not very good, plus the Catholic veneration of all mothers has continued to grate. It's not only the intellectually fanciful notion of a virgin birth, or the unhelpful idealisation of the mother I have resisted. It's that pesky idea of the bond between mother and child all over again. I chose not to hang a lithograph I acquired by Eileen Cooper, entitled *Offspring*, for the same reason. In it, a kneeling mother stares at what should be her reflection in a puddle; instead, it is that of a child, her son, I presume. They've got quite a connection going.

Since my illness I've put the Eileen Cooper up on my study wall and I am having the Grant sketches framed. I am no longer frightened of, nor wholly resistant to, the veneration of mothers.

There's something else. I look back on how I withheld most of my childhood from the boys and have decided that what is important to any child is not where you, the parent, came from or what you were before they arrived, however flawed, damaged or incomplete. To them, you are whole, and their whole world. What matters is who you are to them, what kind of mother or father you are, how you love, and that they know they are loved. It's all about them, and that's very liberating. The backstory can wait. Or, if it suits you better, can be withheld.

That night, after I've said goodnight to Bassy and closed his door, he calls after me.

'Such love,' he says.

'Much love,' I echo, and my heart races, for all the right reasons.

A few days later we've got friends coming over for a lunch party and Richard and I are cooking up a feast. Reuben asks what the occasion is.

'To mark your mum's survival,' Richard says.

'Hooray,' Reuben replies.

When I explain that we want to say thank you to everyone for being so supportive, Reuben warns me not to 'do an Ebola survivor'. Either he means don't do a God thing, or don't gush. I do the latter, of course I do. Thank you. Sniff. Couldn't do it without you. Blub. Richard says a few words, too. I purr by his side, until he says: 'I was enjoying the Meals on Heels so much I was hoping Genevieve would be ill for a bit longer.'

The other night I shouted at Bassy, ranting about how he had to keep his books and papers in order on his desk, spend more time on his homework. On and on I went.

'Genevieve,' he said, 'what about the study? Why don't you tidy that?'

I am impressed when he addresses me by my name. It's him fighting back, standing up for himself. Given that my study is a tip, I should have met him halfway. Instead, later that afternoon, still fuming, I stomped up to his room and out came my rehabilitated tongue, sharp now:

'I've been ill for the last ten months, I haven't even been working in the study.'

I watched his face shift from defiance to defeat, a sort of crumbling before tears. Not that he would cry, and he certainly wouldn't tell me how he felt. He usually walks away, or shuts the door to hide hurt feelings. A couple of hours later we apologised to each other. I folded into him, guilt-ridden, softened by my love, the underground stream: unseen, constant, mixing with the silt and the chalk, moving forwards, feeding into something bigger than itself: tributaries, rivers, oceans. Indisputably powerful, water the life force, essential, like love.

In the early evening he said, 'I wrote a poem for you.' He must have done so when I was ill – oh, the enormity of using the past tense. I ask if I can read it.

Cancer

It always felt so far away
Never really there.
I heard about it all the time
But this just wasn't fair.
It hit us hard
Like nothing ever felt.
I didn't know what I should do
I wanted to cry for help.
The words she said didn't fit
It really couldn't be true.
My life was spinning in a whirl.
What was happening to you?
Now I fully understand
What they mean by fear.
I was paralysed by what was said
and I couldn't shed a tear.
My perfect world was shattered.
Nothing really mattered.
I didn't want to know what was to come.
I needed to know how this happened to my mum.

A few mornings later, Reuben and I are chatting in the kitchen. He asks me where I stand on milkshakes (fine, it's soups I can no longer bear) and then my PEG comes up in conversation.

'Have you got two belly buttons now?' he says.

'Yes, I am a freak,' I say. He asks to see them so I reveal the double trouble.

'It's all right,' he says, 'just think of them as a battle scar.'

A week later we are both in the kitchen again. Reuben is sitting at the table, surfing on my laptop. I am standing a few metres away. I spot the kumquat someone gave me up on a shelf and which I've been meaning to show the boys. They've never seen one.

'Look at this,' I say.

'What is it?' Reuben is too far away to see it properly.

I run over to him and chuck it down his shirt.

'What are you doing?' he shouts. 'What is it?'

The kumquat comes out the other end and is now perching just by the button of his blue jeans, and he's staring at it. The fruit is tiny and orange, a bit smaller than a Malteser. We both stare at it.

'I thought it was the lump. I thought it was a bit of your tumour.'

I laugh my head off.

ACKNOWLEDGEMENTS

I would like to thank my incisive, inspirational agent, Zoe Ross, for falling off her chair and for her alchemical guidance. Many thanks to my editors at Square Peg, Susannah Otter and Rowan Yapp, to assistant editor Harriet Dobson, and to my editor at Vintage, Alex Russell. Many thanks also to designer Julia Connolly at Vintage for her wonderful cover and to my publicist Mia Quibell-Smith.

For their help and support in the writing of this book, heartfelt thanks to Fliff Carr, Steve Carr, Emma Cook, Gabrielle Le Jeune Cooke, Victoria Finlay, Sally Garner, Marina Kemp, Sarah Lidsey, Clare Longrigg, Sebastian Fox McClure, Reuben Fox McClure, Howard Moody, Blake Morrison, Julia Parry, Vivian Slee, Lu Spinney, Professor Hans Stauss, Bev Thomas, Joanna Kate Thompson and Elif Yesil.

Mighty thanks also to Simone Sultana for the portrait photography and to all my friends for their sparkle and steadfastness.

Thanks, river deep, to Richard McClure, for the wonder of him, and for making this book possible.

AFTERWORD

Some time after I confided my free-fall dream to my friend Howard Moody, he was commissioned to compose a piece by The Southern Cathedrals Festival 2015 as part of the 800th anniversary commemorations of the Magna Carta. 'In The Hand of God' was the result. The anthem was performed at Salisbury Cathedral and broadcast live on BBC Radio 3. Richard, the boys and I were there for the performance. Apart from the Magna Carta, the choice of biblical texts was, according to Howard's programme notes, 'particularly inspired by a friend's account of a dream she had a couple of months before being diagnosed with cancer. In it, she fell through the sky, terrified and certain she would die. Just before she was about to hit earth, a huge hand stretched out and caught her. She knew then that the hand had been there all along, and that she was safe. *In manu Dei sunt*.' In the hand of God.

NOTE

Some names have been changed for privacy.

Sources for quotations include the following:

'The Waste Land', 'Little Gidding' and 'East Coker', from *The Collected Poems and Plays of T. S. Eliot*. © T. S. Eliot. (Faber and Faber Ltd., 1969)

'I Will Survive' performed by Gloria Gaynor, written by Dino Fekaris & Freddie Perren. © Polydor Records, 1978.

'Parts of Speech VI: Her Wisdom', from *The Collected Poems*. © Elizabeth Jennings. (Carcanet Press Ltd., 2012)